MARIJUANA
MEDICINE

MARIJUANA MEDICINE

A WORLD TOUR OF THE HEALING AND VISIONARY POWERS OF CANNABIS

Christian Rätsch

TRANSLATED BY JOHN BAKER

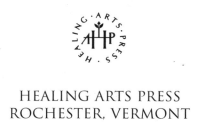

HEALING ARTS PRESS
ROCHESTER, VERMONT

Healing Arts Press
One Park Street
Rochester, Vermont 05767
www.InnerTraditions.com

Healing Arts Press is a division of Inner Traditions International

Note to the reader: This book is intended as an informational guide. The remedies, approaches, and techniques described herein are meant to supplement, and not to be a substitute for, professional medical care or treatment. They should not be used to treat a serious ailment without prior consultation with a qualified health care professional.

Library of Congress Cataloging-in-Publication Data

Rätsch, Christian, 1957–
    [Haus-und heilmittel. English]
    Marijuana medicine : a world tour of the healing and visionary powers of cannabis / Christian Rätsch ; translated by John Baker.
        p. cm.
    Includes bibliographical references and index.
    ISBN 978-089281-933-1
    1. Marijuana—Therapeutic use. 2. Traditional medicine. 3. Medical anthropology. I. Title.

RM666.C266 R3813 2000
615'.7827—dc21

                                                    00-050572

Printed in India

10 9 8 7

Text layout by Kristin Camp
This book was typeset in Goudy with Gill Sans as the display typeface

Do not forget:
The higher we soar,
the smaller we appear to those
who can not fly.

       FRIEDRICH NIETZSCHE
       DAWN (V, 574)

Wake up to find out that you are
 the eyes of the world!

       JERRY GARCIA
       ROBERT HUNTER
       EYES OF THE WORLD

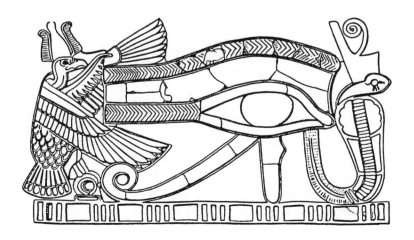

Contents

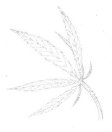

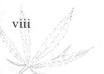

FOREWORD

Dr. Lester Grinspoon

High-ranking U.S. government officials have referred to the concept of medical marijuana as a hoax, a subterfuge designed by proponents of a more liberal policy toward this drug in the hope that its long-standing, harsh prohibition will be rescinded. Ignorant of the role cannabis played in Western medicine from the mid-nineteenth into the early twentieth century, government officials and their many supporters view the notion that cannabis has medicinal properties as a new intrusion into allopathic medicine. The parochialism of this view is highlighted by Christian Rätsch's ethnohistorical study, *Marijuana Medicine*, which documents the ancient uses of this substance as a medicine, as well as the multiplicity of cultures that have incorporated it in their treatment of a large variety of human ailments and discomforts. This palliative use has been so widespread and reports of its toxicity so rare that its dismissal by the Western medicical establishment seems deviant. One might ask why the government of the United States, the leading oppositional force to the idea of medical marijuana, clings so tenaciously to this insular and harmful policy. The answer, of course, is the fear that as people gain more experience with cannabis as a medicine, they will discover for themselves that its toxicity has been greatly exaggerated and its usefulness undervalued—all of this from a substance that has been used for purposes of which the government disapproves. An additional fear lies in the possibility that, having made these discoveries, U.S. citizens will be less supportive of the prohibition of marijuana and the enormous cost of this policy, which includes the annual arrest of almost seven hundred thousand people.

With the publication of its report in March 1999, the National Academy of Sciences Institute of Medicine grudgingly acknowledged that although cannabis has some medical utility, smoking it is too dangerous; patients will have to await the development of pharmaceutical products that would eliminate this hazard. While the report greatly exaggerated the danger of smoking, it failed to provide a discussion of vaporization, a technique that allows patients to inhale the cannabinoids free of the particulate matter present in smoke. Another reason the report suggested patients wait for the "pharmaceuticalization" of marijuana is to allow for the development of cannabinoid analogs that are free of any psychoactive effects. This suggestion is based on the assumption that the psychoactive effects of the substance are unhealthy much as the prohibitionists assume its "high" to be deleterious. This assumption is not supported by anything approaching the mountain of anecdotal evidence supporting marijuana's usefulness as a medicine. While there are some who are not comfortable with its psychoactive effects, those patients are relatively rare; the vast majority find that smoking cannabis not only relieves particular symptoms, but also results in "feeling better." Helping patients feel better, particularly those with chronic diseases, is an important goal of the humane practice of medicine. And there is a growing understanding in the medical field that patients who feel better, respond better physically.

While the Western medical establishment does support governmental resistance to sanctioning the medical availability of cannabis, this has not always been so. Physicians in the United States were enthusiastic about the medicinal uses of cannabis from the middle of the nineteenth century until 1937 and the passage of the first piece of draconian legislation aimed at marijuana—the Marijuana Tax Act. Next, under pressure from the Federal Bureau of Narcotics, the predecessor organization to the present Drug Enforcement Administration (DEA), the *Journal of the American Medical Association* published a vehemently anti-marijuana editorial in 1945 that signaled a sea change in the attitude of doctors toward this drug. Physicians subsequently became both victims and agents of the marijuana disinformation campaign launched by Harry Anslinger, the first Chief of the Federal Bureau of Narcotics. Even today, many physicians suffer from this legacy and fear of the DEA—many so much so that they are afraid to prescribe Marinol (dronabinol), synthetic THC.

Today, the medical establishment takes the position that there is no scientific evidence to demonstrate that cannabis has medicinal usefulness, based on the fact that there is a paucity of double-blind controlled studies addressing this. This scarcity is likely to persist for some time; because the costs of such studies are generally underwritten by pharmaceutical firms who stand to gain if they can demonstrate the therapeutic usefulness of a patented drug and win Food and Drug Administration (FDA) approval for it, and because marijuana is a naturally occurring herb that cannot be patented, these firms will simply not invest the more than $200 million necessary to perform such studies. Consequently, our knowledge of the medical utility of marijuana will continue to rest on anecdotal evidence. Fortunately, a great deal of such evidence has accumulated here in the West and, as Christian Rätsch has demonstrated in this book, all around the world.

Cannabis would not be the first medicine to be admitted to the pharmacopoeia on the strength of anecdotal evidence; such support is the source of much of our knowledge of synthetic medicines as well as plant derivatives. Controlled experiments were not needed to recognize the therapeutic potential of chloral hydrate, barbiturates, aspirin, curare, insulin, or penicillin. It is unlikely that marijuana should or ever will be developed as an officially recognized medicine via the risk-benefit analysis that constitutes the FDA approval process. Over the last three decades, the extensive, multimillion-dollar, government-supported effort of the National Institute of Drug Abuse to establish the existence of a sufficient level of toxicity in marijuana to support its prohibition has instead provided a record of safety that is more compelling than that of most approved medicines. The current FDA protocol is not necessary to establish a risk-benefit estimate for a drug with such a history; to impose this protocol on marijuana is akin to imposing it on aspirin, which was accepted as a medicine more than six decadess before the advent of the double-blind controlled study. Years of experience have shown us that aspirin has many uses and limited toxicity, yet today it could not be marshalled through the FDA approval process. Marijuana too is unpatentable, so the only funding source for the approval process would be the government, which is, to put it mildly, unlikely to be helpful.

Combining the lack of incentive to win FDA approval with today's anti-smoking climate and, most important, the widespread use of cannabis for purposes disapproved by the U.S. government will result in the existence of two distribution systems for medical cannabis in the future. One will be the system of conventional pharmacy-filled prescriptions of FDA-approved, marijuana-derived medicines—isolated or synthetic cannabinoids and cannabinoid analogs. The other will be the currently illegal channels for the acquisition of marijuana. The only difference between the two—an enormous one—will be the continued illegality of whole smoked or ingested marijuana. In any case, increasing medical use by either distribution pathway will inevitably lead to increased familiarity with marijuana and its derivatives. As people learn that its harmfulness has been greatly exaggerated and its usefulness underestimated, the pressure will increase for drastic change in the way we, as a society, deal with this drug.

October 11, 2000

FOREWORD

Dr. William A. Emboden

Most contemporary scholars can be divided into one of two camps: the first is composed of scientists who study amino acids so that they may better understand organisms; the second consists of those synthetic researchers who incorporate the results of their research into a logical system of generalizations. Dr. Christian Rätsch belongs to neither of these groups. Rather, he may be counted among that rare species who work with a scientific background, an immense anthropological knowledge, and an even greater store of personal experiences. Because he proceeds scientifically as well as shamanistically, defying all the rules of normal logic and reasoning, he is able to work veritable wonders. He is a scion of that tree to which belong such shamanic personalities as Bacon, da Vinci, Spinoza, and, at least in his later years, Aldous Huxley.

In this remarkable volume about hemp, Rätsch does not simply present us with yet another compendium on taxonomy, biochemistry, social history, psychopharmacology, and legal history. Instead, we find here for the first time an original interpretation of the role that this plant has played. This work is not unlike the exotic biography of a mystic who has been living for millennia. This sacred plant reveals itself to us in a story so fascinating that the flawless scholarship of the author practically forces us to believe the unbelievable. Reading this book, we are rewarded with stories of ancient rituals, sacred writings, and divine substances, of shamans and their power, of priests and pharaohs, of an eccentric abbess, a Rastafarian, and, ultimately, a mysterious journey into the self.

Christian Rätsch speaks of the knowledge of centuries past with the ease with which we might visit some old friends. He leads us on an amazing journey that takes us into many countries of the world and through more than five thousand years of human history. We have reason to believe that hemp was the milk of the gods at the cradle of civilization—nourishment, medicine, and prophetic plant; a plant which provided fibers for fabric and paper, magical wands for shamanic healing, and resin to close wounds. It could permanently banish worry, soothe the spasms of asthma, and serve as a sedative. Can similar properties be found in any other plant? I am certain that this is not the case.

The great folk healer Abbess Hildegard von Bingen praised hemp in the same way that the *curanderas* (healing women) in the Americas desired it. Was this plant the soma of the ancient Vedic tradition or the haoma of Iran? Was the staff of Asclepius, the symbol of modern medicine, originally the trunk of a hemp plant with a snake wrapped around it, as it appeared among the ancient Chinese texts? What of the rod of Aaron, mentioned in the Bible? Was this too a hemp stem that served as a shamanic staff? These and other questions are pursued in this book. Because of its engaging descriptions, it is one of the most fascinating and informative books that has appeared in recent decades.

If you love history, are interested in the world's cultures, are fascinated by magic and its analogs in medicine, or are a scientist searching for a context in which all of your knowledge of chemistry and pharmacology will make sense, then you can do no better than to carefully consider this extraordinary work. It is rare that an author can so lovingly bring together such various subject areas with such enthusiasm and competence. I can think of no other author who is so well qualified and is so capable of realizing such an interdisciplinary endeavor. More than just a shaman, and certainly a prophet, Christian Rätsch has done us a valuable service by producing a book of this format.

We can only hope that some day this book will appear in a special edition, printed on the finest Japanese hemp paper, sewn with hemp thread, and bound in a cover of hemp. May the winds that once carried the hemp sails of ships throughout the world now contribute to the dissemination of this book.

May 5, 2000

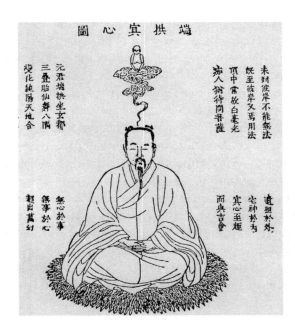

A Taoist alchemist meditates, allowing his spirit to ascend into other spheres. He sits upon a bed of what are clearly hemp leaves. Hemp has always been a part of Chinese culture; shamans, alchemists, physicians, and folk healers have long used it as a medicine and as an elixir of life. (from *Secret of the Golden Flower*, ca. third century C.E.)

PREFACE

When this book was first published in Germany in 1992, the public discussion on the "right to inebriation" was just beginning. This was the result of a sensational judgment rendered by Wolfgang Neskovic, a judge in Lübeck, Germany. At the same time, the discussion about the medicinal value of hemp was at a low point. Obviously, the politics of demonization—disguised as the "War on Drugs"— practiced and exported by the United States was having an effect. No one seemed to remember that hemp is one of the oldest and best known of humankind's healing plants.

In the following year, 1993, a groundbreaking book by Jack Herer and Matthias Bröckers, Die Wiederentdeckung der Nutzpflanze Hanf (The Rediscovery of the Useful Plant Hemp, the German version of *The Emperor Wears No Clothes*) led to a hemp renaissance. Suddenly, the plant was being discussed in public not as a "dangerous drug plant," but as an ecological "savior of the planet." The hemp leaf, once a symbol of those enemies of the state known as the hippies, became an emblem of the environmental movement.

Along with the rediscovery of the plant, the medical and therapeutic potential of hemp was discovered anew. Suddenly, conservative publishers dared to issue books on cannabis. As a result, the plant was judged in a different light. Pharmacological and medical research was taken up once more. Today there is even a scientific society in Germany, the Arbeitsgemeinschaft Cannabis als Medizin e.V. (the ACM, Working Group Cannabis as Medicine).

Carried along on these currents, the "dopers" were once again in the spotlight. They had new arguments for the legalization of their favorite agent of pleasure, namely its ecological uses and its therapeutic potential. Almost overnight, hemp came to be seen as both a cure-all and an ecological wonder. While hemp is indeed a wonderful medicine, it is certainly not a cure-all. And it will not save the world—the world does not even need to be saved, only people want to be saved.

Hemp has also become economically interesting. Not because of the ecologically motivated wearers of hemp clothes, but because of the illegal trade in its psychoactive products. In Switzerland alone, one billion Swiss francs worth of hashish is sold every year (*Berner Zeitung*, June 27, 1997). If hashish was legal and subjected to taxation, this would help fill some of the holes in the national budget. But governments would rather go broke than place their trust in the spirits of the time by removing the legal ban from cannabis. Apparently, their fear that their subjects might be expanding their consciousness is just too great.

The first edition of this book went through a number of printings. Nevertheless, it was time to thoroughly revise the work, expanding it and bringing it up to date. I am very happy that the new edition was published in Switzerland, for Switzerland is an example for the world as far as drug politics and health are concerned. I concur with Günter Amendt, who opined that the Swiss practice a "culture of tolerance." When we are speaking of a medicine, tolerance is the first order of the day.

Christian Rätsch
Hamburg, September, 2000

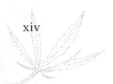

TRANSLATOR'S NOTE

(1) SCHEDULE I
> *(A) The drug or other substance has a high potential for abuse.*
> *(B) The drug or other substance has no currently accepted medical use in treatment in the United States.*
> *(C) There is a lack of accepted safety for use of the drug or other substance under medical supervision.*

21 USC 812

The Comprehensive Drug Abuse Prevention and Control Act of 1970 (P.L. 91-513), which established the current U.S. practice of scheduling drugs, mandated the inclusion of "marihuana" and "tetrahydrocannabinols" in Schedule I, together with such so-called hallucinogenic substances as mescaline, peyote, ibogaine, dimethyltryptamine, bufotenine, psilocybin, and a wide variety of opiates, including heroin. This law effectively ruled that cannabis and its derivatives have no medicinal value and, moreover, are more hazardous than such drugs as amphetamine, methamphetamine, phencyclidine (PCP), cocaine, and phenobarbital, all of which are currently scheduled in less restrictive categories.

The arbitrary assignment of cannabis to Schedule I illustrates the political nature of many of our drug laws. To justify this action, the cannabis opponents often cite a lack of empirical evidence supporting the claims of the advocates of medical marijuana, then blatantly disregard the abundant archaeological and anthropological evidence—the focus of this book—which attests to both the antiquity and the extent of constructive cannabis use. In another expression of this bias, administrative hurdles set up by various agencies within the U.S. government continue to thwart most efforts to conduct legitimate medical research on cannabis. For example, in September 1999 the Food and Drug Administration (FDA) approved an application for a rigorous study designed to test the medical efficacy of marijuana on migraine headaches (Russo 1999:18). To date, however, the National Institute for Drug Abuse (NIDA) has refused to grant the researcher's request to purchase the marijuana necessary for the project (MAPS 2000:5). Moreover, the government has generally refused to fund such research, so that private donations are required. Such actions do not reflect sound scientific thinking, they reflect political maneuvering.

As coincidence would have it, a friend of mine was diagnosed with cancer while I was working on this translation. As part of her presurgical treatment, she had to undergo a month of near-daily radiation therapy along with continuous infusions of a chemotherapy drug. To help her deal with the side effects of her treatment, which included nausea and lack of appetite, her physicians provided her with a prescription for Marinol (pharmaceutical Δ-^{9}-tetrahydrocannabinol). At first, the prescription was a triplicate, a special form of prescription in which one copy is retained by the physician, one copy is retained by the pharmacy, and one copy is sent to the Department of Justice. When it came time for her to reorder her medicine, her pharmacy informed her that Marinol could now be ordered on a normal prescrip-

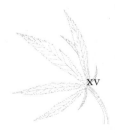

tion form, indicating that requirements for prescribing the drug had been relaxed. What new research appeared to justify this step? I am not aware of any. Rather, it appears to have been a bureaucratic response to the medical-marijuana initiatives that have been approved by the voters of several states. These initiatives ask that individuals be able to grow and possess cannabis if a physician has approved its use for a medical condition. Relaxing the restrictions on Marinol *does* make it easier to obtain for persons who could benefit from its use. But it also undermines the claims of the most vociferous marijuana opponents. By the way, sixty 10 mg Marinol capsules (a twenty-day supply) have a retail price around $825.00. Thus, although my friend did benefit from the medication and obtained relief from her symptoms, the major beneficiary would appear to be the pharmaceutical company that manufactures the capsules.

In 1992, a German judge, Wolfgang Neskovic, stunned his colleagues by suspending the trial of a woman accused of passing a small amount of hashish to her husband in prison. Neskovic cited a German law that allows a judge to suspend a trial to request clarification of a law from a higher court. The brief Neskovic prepared for the higher court summarized the available scientific data concerning hemp, including its toxicity and dangers vis-à-vis other legal drugs, such as alcohol and nicotine, that the state allows, regulates, and taxes (and which, he noted, pharmacologists consider to be significantly more toxic than cannabis). Neskovic argued that in the absence of scientific data to the contrary, hemp should be legal as well. In April 1994, the German High Court ruled that Germany's citizens do have a right to possess and consume small amounts of the plant and its products, and called for the sixteen German states to establish uniform guidelines to regulate such "personal use." Not surprisingly, many conservative politicians were dismayed by the decision, and suggested that possession of amounts as little as two grams of hashish is indicative of intent to distribute. These attempts have been countered by more liberal lawmakers, some of whom have suggested that quantities as high as four kilograms should not be punishable. To date, no uniform agreement has been worked out. But the High Court's decision effectively confirmed that Germany's citizens do indeed have a "right to inebriation" *(Recht auf Rausch)*, opening the door for them to use marijuana for purposes of self-medication. It was against the background of these events that this book was originally written.

Some notes on the translation

The English language, for whatever reasons, is notably poor in terms for describing altered states of consciousness and the agents that can induce them. This is one of the reasons why such street terms as "high," "stoned," "wasted," "hammered," "toasted," "baked," "buzzed," and countless others are often used when discussing such states. While the German language too has its share of such terms, it is also much richer in terms that can be found in a standard dictionary. One of these is *Rausch*, mentioned above in connection with the *Recht auf* ("right to") *Rausch* recognized by the German High Court. The conventional English translation of this term is "intoxication," a term that only very inadequately renders the German meaning. One of the problems with "intoxication" is its root, "toxic." This implies an effect that is physically damaging to the organism, that is, that the substance in question is a "poison." While this may be the case with nicotine, and is certainly the case with alcohol, such effects have not yet been demonstrated with respect to cannabis. In fact, there is not a single known case of death resulting from a cannabis overdose (although there are, of course, instances of people doing stupid things while under its influence, a statement that can also be applied to many other substances, moods, and activities). Thus, I have consciously avoided using the word "intoxication" for *Rausch*, and have instead used the term "inebriation." I am not entirely satisfied with this term either, but it is a step in the right direction.

Another aspect of *Rausch*, and one that is rather foreign to English speakers, is that it can imply an almost sacred event in which one's normal self is transcended, leading to a new level of insight and experience. The ancient Germanic tribes used a variety of plants, skillfully mixed in alcohol, which helped to extract their active ingredients, to *be-rausch* themselves, that is, induce nonordinary (ecstatic) states. And today, many contemporary German speakers use the word *Rausch* to refer to the elation they experience while skiing, dancing, driving, or having sex. This elation has also been described as a "rush," and indeed, the term "goldrush" in German is *Goldrausch*. Here again, "intoxication" is not a suitable word to describe these sensations (although we might use the word "drunk").

Another word that appears quite often in the original version of this work is *Genussmittel*, literally "enjoyment agent." I have translated this term as "agent of pleasure." Many things can be *Genussmittel*, including alcohol and tobacco. The key point is that these agents are consumed for the sheer pleasure of their taste, the effects they induce, and/or the context in which they are used. The idea of an "agent of pleasure" may be unusual to English speakers, but it is certainly a more precise rendering of *Genussmittel* than the more commonly used term: "luxury goods."

In German, medicines and remedies are often referred to as *Heilmittel*, literally "healing agents." While the English term "medicine" does indeed communicate an important aspect of these substances, it tends to ignore another. For the German word *Heil* implies more than just healing. Depending upon the context, it can also mean "well-being," "wholeness," and "salvation." It thus also refers to an extraordinary state of "wellness," of being free of imperfections, worries, and need. Such states never last, of course, but it is important that we experience them from time to time. They help us to transcend our everyday life, to become, even if only for a moment, something more than merely the sum of all the culturally defined roles that we inhabit. A *Heilmittel* can be more than a medicine for the body; it can soothe the mind and restore the spirit. The original title of this work, *Hanf als Heilmittel* (Hemp as *Heilmittel*), expresses this aspect of hemp as well, an aspect that is not easily carried into English. The reader will gain a much greater appreciation of the cannabis plant if she or he keeps this additional meaning in mind. For a true *Heilmittel* is not simply something to take when we need it, but also something that, when used properly, can help us to avoid needing it.

Finally, I would like to make a few comments on the terms "hemp" and "marijuana." In the United States, it has become common to use the term "marijuana" to refer to the leaves and, sometimes, the flowers of *Cannabis* plants when they are used for inebriating purposes. As this book explains, the word "marijuana" comes from Mexican Spanish and is a well-known term in Mexico. Prior to *Cannabis* prohibition in the United States, the plant was commonly referred to as "hemp," regardless of whether one was referring to its fiber or its drug products. As the push for criminalizing the plant progressed, the term "marijuana" came to be applied to the plant as a way of associating it with "foreign" elements and therewith disassociating it from "American" culture. "Marijuana," in other words, was originally a pejorative term, and any connotations that it invoked, including images of criminality, perversion, and insanity, were more than coincidental.

In this book, I have chosen to use *hemp* as a translation for the German word *Hanf*. First and foremost, I do this because it is the correct translation of the term. Beyond this, however, lies another reason: namely, that by using "hemp" instead of "marijuana" it may be possible to introduce a more objective tenor into discussions of *Cannabis*. Because of the recent spate of medical marijuana initiatives throughout the United States, it was thought better to use the word *marijuana* in the title of this book. Yet it is important to remember that hemp is much more than just the marijuana it yields. It is one of humankind's oldest cultigens, a plant that has clothed, housed, nourished, and healed people around the globe for millennia. Perhaps this book will help us remember this fact.

Thanks to her own indomitable willpower, the support of her family and many friends, and the skill and knowledge of her physicians (and with a little help from a tetrahydrocannabinol), my friend was able to beat her cancer. I would like to dedicate this translation to her: *Lebe lang und sei gesund!*

John Baker
October 2000

LITERATURE CITED

Multidisciplinary Association for Psychedelic Studies (MAPS). 2000. Medical Marijuana News, *MAPS Bulletin* 10(1):5.
Russo, Ethan. 1999. Cannabis in Migraine Treatment Project Close to FDA Approval. *MAPS Bulletin* 9(3):18.

ACKNOWLEDGMENTS

As a twentieth-century author, one often does little more than rediscover and compile that which is already known. Nevertheless, it is possible to add something new and fill in a gap in our knowledge here and there. But even for this, we must depend upon the information of others. I have made a serious effort to list the sources available to me in the appropriate bibliographies.

I obtained some information during various field studies and expeditions. Here, Dennis Alegre (Philippines), Rosemarie K. Kern (Dakota), S. Orito (Japan), Count Ossie Urchs (here and there), and Mateo Viejo (Naha'/Mexico) were especially helpful.

Other information was provided by friends and colleagues. Many leads, offprints, newspaper clippings, books, photocopies, addresses, and so forth came from Dr. John Baker, Dr. Andrea Blätter, Dr. Peter Baumann, Prof. Dr. Adolf Dittrich, Dr. Marlene Dobkin de Rios, Dr. William Emboden, Dr. Peter Hess, Dr. Albert Hofmann, Prof. Dr. Harmut Laatsch, Terence McKenna, Dr. Maya Maurer, Dr. Ralph Metzner, Helmut Oberlack, Prof. Dr. Christian Scharfetter, PD Dr. Wolf-Dieter Storl, Herman de Vries, and Dr. Andrew Weil. Many thanks to all of you!

Special thanks are due to Dr. Claudia Müller-Ebeling, the European College for the Study of Consciousness (ECBS), the Albert Hofmann Foundation, Botanical Dimensions, and the Akademie der Neuen Berserker (Academy of the New Berserkers).

Because of the nature of the subject of this book, some data was provided under the seal of silence. I wish to especially thank all of the nameless marijuana users throughout the world who reported on their medical experiences. Without them, I would have never become aware of the universal significance of marijuana as a medicine! Thanks too to Judge Wolfgang Neskovic, whose efforts gave me the courage to write this book. Finally, I would like to thank my friends and German and Swiss publishers, Werner Pieper, Roger Liggenstorfer, and Urs Hunzicker for their honesty, engagement, and enthusiasm.

In the revision of this book, many thanks are due especially to pharmacist Patricia Ochsner, Mike Barten (HanfBlatt), Don Agustín Rivas Vazques, Percy Konqobe, Peter Huber (High Society/Dope Media), Prof. Dr. Rudolf Brenneisen, Jonathan Ott, Rob Montgomery, Dr. Bill Lyons, Margret Madejsky and Olaf Rippe, Jack Herer and Matthias Bröckers, Tamara Graf, Heinz Knieriemen, Ivan Valenčič, Christian Beck, Jace Callaway, Ph.D., Rainer Pliess, Günter Amendt, Kurt Lussi, Dr. Franjo Grotenhermen (ACM), Surendra Bahadur Shahi, Anupama Grell, Hans-Georg Behr, Ralph Cosack (for the Hamburg Hemp Days), Jürgen Neumeyer, Dr. Ulrike Hagenbach, Dr. Michael Schlichting, Dave Pate, Konrad Witt, Achim Zubke, and all of the anonymous respondents to the questionnaire.

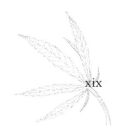

INTRODUCTION

Rising above prejudices and ideological paradigms is the very basis of the scientific approach. Scientists must always keep their eyes open, be receptive to things that are new, and have the courage to cast aside old convictions. If they believe that hemp is a horrible narcotic that causes its users to become addicted and asocial, then they will hardly be able to arrive at a more profound understanding of the role of this unusual plant.

If you travel through the world with open eyes, you cannot avoid noticing the incredible diversity in the ways in which hemp products are used for medicinal purposes. If you study the history of medicine with care, you cannot help but realize that there are few other medicinal plants that are so widely distributed and consistently used in medical systems and doctrines around the globe.

For more than six thousand years, hemp has been used as a medicine wherever it has found the company of humans. *Marijuana Medicine* documents the history of this use, providing an overview of the ethnomedical evidence. This book is not a political treatise, but a cross-cultural survey. The facts speak for themselves.

The Buffalo of Plants

Among plants, the cultural significance of hemp is similar to that of the buffalo in Native American life. The cultures of the Great Plains and prairies were based entirely on the buffalo (*Bison bison*). It provided the Indians with everything that they needed to live. Every part of the buffalo was used. Flesh, fat, and blood were eaten; the bones and sinews were made into tools, ornaments, and other useful objects; the skin and fur were made into clothes and shelter; the horns and skulls were venerated as ritual objects or worn as shamanic dance masks; the entrails were made into kitchen tools (the bladder, for example, was used to fetch water); the testicles were used as an aphrodisiac; the hooves and teeth were made into musical instruments. Every part of the buffalo had a purpose. This multifaceted and thorough use of an animal is unique in the cultural history of our species. The buffalo was nourishment, a source of raw materials, and the spiritual center of Plains Indian religion (Dary 1990; McHugh 1979).

Like the buffalo, hemp is a plant with many uses. Its seeds provide food for both humans and animals and yield an oil with a multitude of applications. The female flowers produce the prized inebriating resin and are used as both a medicine and an aphrodisiac. The roots are used medicinally. Pastes and beverages are derived from the leaves, while the stem provides strong, durable fibers for making ropes, nets, paper, and clothes. The fibers are also used as amulets, and ritually manufactured hemp cord is used for magical protection. Shamanic ritual objects, such as magical wands, are carved from the stems.

In addition to all this, hemp is a plant with few needs. It does not leach nutrients from the soil, and is actually beneficial to other plants growing in its vicinity

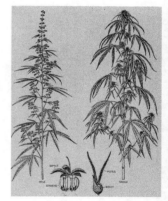

Botanical illustration of the dioecious cannabis plant (*Cannabis sativa*). The flowering male plant is on the left, on the right is the female plant in bloom. (illustration, nineteenth century)

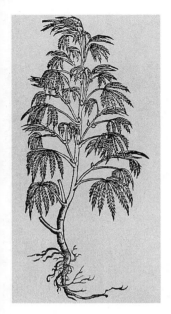

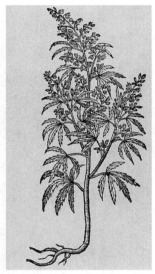

The sexual dimorphism of cannabis was recognized early, but wrongly interpreted. In these illustrations from an early English herbal, the female plant was incorrectly identified as "male"; the male plant was misinterpreted as "female." (facsimile from Gerard, 1633)

(Herer 1990*). The multiple functions of hemp as food, provider of raw materials, medicine, agent of pleasure, and spiritual inebriant have been documented in many early cultures. The ancient Chinese, Indian, and Germanic peoples, for example, all utilized hemp (Bennett et al. 1995*). Today, despite its prohibition, hemp is used in a variety of ways (Behr 1995*; Haag 1995*). In some areas, it is primarily an inebriant, in others it is used mainly for its fibers. It is used for medicinal purposes throughout most of the world. In recent years, hemp has been increasingly cultivated; people view it as a useful plant whose cultivation offers many ecological advantages (Conrad 1993*; Herer and Bröckers 1993*; Hesch et al. 1996*; Nova-Institut 1995; Robinson 1996*; Sagunski et al. 1996*; Waskow 1995*).

Botany and Taxonomy

The botanical and taxonomic history of hemp is as bewildering as the legal situation surrounding its cultivation and use. While the Arabic physicians, the "Fathers of Botany," and the founders of modern binomial taxonomy all recognized a number of types of cannabis, until very recently modern botany held the view that there was only one species—*Cannabis sativa* L.—albeit with local variations (Small 1976). A distinction is often made between fiber, or "useful" hemp, and Indian hemp. It is frequently claimed that only Indian hemp has inebriating effects, a view that carries legal consequences. In many places, it is legal to cultivate the noninebriating fiber hemp, that is, hemp which is free of or has only a very slight THC content, whereas growing the "narcotic" Indian hemp is prohibited and subject to prosecution (Emboden 1974b*, 1981a*, and 1996*).

In the course of botanical history, the following names have been published for species and varieties of hemp:

> *Cannabis sativa* Linnaeus 1737
> *Cannabis lupulus* Scopoli 1772
> *Cannabis indica* Lamarck 1783
> *Cannabis foetens* Gilibert 1792
> *Cannabis erratica* Sievers ex Pallas 1796
> *Cannabis macrosperma* Stokes 1812
> *Cannabis generalis* Krause 1905
> *Cannabis americana* Houghton et Hamilton 1908
> *Cannabis gigantea* Crevost 1917
> *Cannabis ruderalis* Janischewsky 1924
> *Cannabis pedemontana* Camp 1936
> *Cannabis* x *intersita* Sojak 1960

According to the more recent research and field studies by leading botanical authorities Richard E. Schultes and William Emboden, only three valid taxonomic categories exist (Emboden 1974a*, 1981a*; Schultes et al. 1975:34*; cf. Stearn 1975); in other words, there are three species:

---

*Those bibliographic references marked with an asterisk may be found in the Bibliography at the end of this book.

Cannabis sativa Linnaeus 1737—fiber hemp

Synonyms: *Cannabis americana* Houghton
Cannabis chinensis Delile
Cannabis culta Mansfield
Cannabis erratica Sievers
Cannabis generalis Kraus
Cannabis gigantea Crevost
Cannabis intersita Sojak
Cannabis lupulus Scopoli
Cannabis macrosperma Stokes
Cannabis pedemontana Camp
Cannabis sativa monoica Holuby
Cannabis sativa culta Sereb. ex Sereb. et Sizov

Fiber hemp plants grow to be very tall (to 4 meters); have a thick, fibrous stem; few branches; and open foliage. The quantity of psychoactive substances is typically low, sometimes approaching zero.

According to Clarke (1997, 201f.*), this species can be divided into the following subspecies and varieties (however, it is certainly not a good idea to propose an *indica* subspecies as well as variety, as this will only add to the taxonomic confusion):

Cannabis sativa var. *sativa* (the most commonly cultivated hemp)
Cannabis sativa var. *spontanea* (has smaller seeds, grows wild)
Cannabis sativa indica (very rich in cannabinoids)
Cannabis sativa var. *indica* (very small fruits, smaller than 3.8 mm)
Cannabis sativa var. *kafiristanica* (short fruits)

Another proposal (cf. Clarke 1997:203*) distinguishes between four phenotypes (specifically, chemotypes), a distinction that I do not find justified, as the differences in the cannabinoid content within a population can be considerable (Hemphill et al. 1978; Latta and Eaton 1975). Nonetheless, Clarke distinguishes two chemotypes for Africa (Boucher et al. 1977).

Cannabis indica Lamarck 1783—Indian hemp

Synonyms: *Cannabis foetens* Gilibert
Cannabis macrosperma Stokes
Cannabis orientalis Lamarck
Cannabis sativa α-*kif* DC.
Cannabis sativa var. *indica* Lam.
Cannabis sativa indica (Lam.) E. Small et Cronq.

Indian hemp is small, growing to 1.2 m, and very bushy, the stem is low in fiber and branches heavily, and the foliage is dense. The content of psychoactive substances is very high (cf. Edes 1893*).

The wild or feral Indian hemp is sometimes referred to as *Cannabis indica* Lam. var. *spontanea* Vavilov (Schmidt 1992: 641*)

A fool sees not the same tree that a wise man sees.
WILLIAM BLAKE
THE MARRIAGE OF HEAVEN AND HELL
(1790)

Cannabis ruderalis Janischewsky 1924—ruderal hemp

Synonyms: *Cannabis intersita* Sojak
Cannabis sativa L. *spontanea* Serebr. ex Serebr. et Sizov
Cannabis sativa L. var. *ruderalis* (Jan.)
Cannabis sativa L. var. *spontanea* Mansfield
Cannabis spontanea Mansfield

Ruderal hemp plants are very small (60 cm), with a thin, slightly fibrous stem almost devoid of branches. The foliage is open, and the leaves are relatively large. The amount of psychoactive substances is neither low nor high (cf. Beutler and Der Marderosian 1978).

Schultes et al. (1975, 34*) have also recognized the cross *Cannabis* x *intersita* Sojak 1960 between *Cannabis sativa* and *Cannabis ruderalis*.

All hemp species are dioecious, that is, they produce distinct male and female plants. The male plants are generally smaller and exhibit less branching than the females. There are also hermaphrodites. From a cultural perspective, the female plant is much more important. It produces stronger fibers and a higher quantity of psychoactive substances than the male; it also produces the nutritious seeds.

All hemp species and varieties are very variable and can be crossed (cf. Anderson 1980; Meijer 1994; Small et al. 1975; Van der Werf 1994). As a rule, the amount of active substances can be raised significantly through selective breeding (Starks 1981*; Wolke 1995*).[1]

Cannabis was originally assigned to the Urticaceae (nettle) family. However, more recent botanical findings indicate that it belongs to the Cannabaceae (hemp-like) family (Cannabinaceae, also: Cannabiaceae, and Cannabidaceae), a subdivision of the Moraceae (mulberry) family. Cannabis's closest relative is hops, *Humulus lupulus* L., which also belongs to the Cannabaceae family. No other relatives have been described to date (Schultes et al. 1975*).

Cannabis is thought to have originated in Central Asia. From there, it spread throughout the world as a result of human activity. It is possible that the three species may have been developed by humans through selective breeding (Abel 1980*, Merlin 1972*). Schultes et al. (1975*) have distinguished three phases in the history of the plant: the wild form, the cultivated form, and the feral form. In those areas where uncultivated plants are found, such as in Afghanistan, Nepal, northern China, and the Caspian Sea region, it cannot be determined whether these plants are true wild forms or feral descendants of once-cultivated plants. Today, laboratories and nurseries throughout the world are breeding cannabis plants that are either free of psychoactive substances (as in Japan) or are extremely high

Hemp agrimony (*Eupatorium cannabinum* L.) was formerly thought to be a wild relative of cannabis. This plant, however, has no cannabis-like effects. (woodcut from *Tabernaemontanus*)

---

1. There is a voluminous literature describing methods to cultivate all species, types, and crosses of cannabis: Anonymous 1981; Behrens 1996; Bócsa and Karus 1997; Clarke 1997*; Coffman and Gentner 1979; Frank and Rosenthal 1980; Hai 1981*; Marquart 1919; Mountain Girl 1995*; Rosenthal 1990*; Sagunski et al. 1996*; Starks 1981*; Stevens 1980; Waskow 1995*. Special hydroponic methods are used for indoor growing (de Jardin 1997; Storm 1994). A very amusing description of illegal cultivation is contained in a novel by T. Coraghessan Boyle (1990*).

in resin and seedless (as in Holland and California). The seedless, THC-rich strains are usually referred to as *sinsemilla,* the esteemed "Queen of Cannabis" (Mountain Girl 1995*).

As a result of cannabis's chaotic taxonomic history, it is often not possible to precisely state the species used in each of the different medical systems discussed in this book. Where there is unequivocal evidence for a botanical specification it will be noted. Otherwise, the determination of the species actually used must remain a task for future research.

Chemistry and Pharmacology

The production of resin in cannabis plants is very complex, but has been quite well resolved (Lehmann 1995). The plants produce varying amounts of resin with differing concentrations of active substances. The female inflorescences, commonly referred to as buds, exude especially high concentrations of this resin, but it is also distributed unevenly in the stem and leaves: all other parts, that is, but the seeds and roots.

The chemical composition of the resin is now very well understood. The pure resin, known as hashish, contains four primary components: the cannabinoid Δ^1-tetrahydrocannabinol (THC) with three variants. Two of these variants, cannabidiol (CBD) and cannabinol (CBN), result as an artifact only when the resin is stored.[2] These substances are responsible for the psychoactive effects (Murphy and Bartke 1992).[3] The structures of some sixty additional cannabinoids with mild or no psychoactive effects have also been determined (Brenneisen 1996; Clarke 1981*; Hollister 1986*; Mechoulam 1970*; Schmidt 1992*). The resin also contains a number of essential oils (caryophyllene, humulene, farnesene, selinene, phellandrene, limonene), various sugars, flavonoids, alkaloids (choline, trigonelline, piperidine, betaine, proline, neurine, hordenine, cannabisativine), and chlorophyll, none of which are involved in the psychoactive effects of the drug (Binder 1981*; Brenneisen 1996; Hai 1981, 13*).

The structure, pharmacological significance, and structure-activity relationships of THC have been determined by Raphael Mechoulam and his team. They have also ascertained the synthesis path of THC (Mechoulam 1973*; cf. Compton et al. 1993).

THC content can vary greatly in different hemp plants, varieties, and breeds. Some plants have no THC, while in others it can constitute as much as 25 percent of the resin (Hemphill et al. 1978; Latta and Eaton 1975; Starks 1981*). In addition, different methods of preparation and administration can have considerable influence on the concentrations of active substances (Segelman et al. 1975*). Storage does not seem to have much of an impact; studies of old material have shown that even when stored for long periods, THC oxidizes into the much less active CBN at a very slow rate (Harvey 1990).

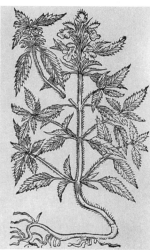

In early modern times, a number of plants were referred to as "wild hemp." These plants are neither botanically nor pharmacologically comparable to cannabis. (woodcut from Gerard, 1633)

---

2. THC and its metabolites have been detected in Egyptian mummies (Balabanova et al. 1992*).

3. Only *trans*-THC is psychoactive, not the isomer *cis*-THC (Smith and Kempfert 1977).

tetrahydrocannabinol (THC)

The dosage of THC needed to produce psychoactive effects is 4 to 8 milligrams. "With reference to the psychotropic dose, the toxicity of THC is very low. When administered orally, the acute lethal dose for rats is 600 mg/kg, and is thus some 6,000 times greater than the [psychotropic] dose effective in humans" (Laatsch 1989:42*). It should be noted, however, that not one human death is known to have occurred as a result of hemp overdose (Schmidt 1992:650f.*). According to a court decision and other legal opinions in Germany, there is "no lethal dose for hashish." Current scientific research indicates that cannabis products are the most harmless inebriants known (Neskovic, cited in Rippchen 1992:16*).

At a dosage of 4 to 8 milligrams (corresponding to about one joint with 0.5 grams hashish or 1 gram marijuana), THC produces an "approximately three-hour-long inebriation characterized by a feeling of detachment that enables a meditative absorption or a surrender to sensory stimuli. The state is generally free of optical and acoustical hallucinations, which can appear at doses four to five times as high. The intensity of sensations when listening to music, looking at pictures, eating and drinking, and during sexual activity are subjectively enhanced" (Binder 1981:120*).

In the blood, THC is converted into the active metabolite 11-hydroxy-Δ^9-THC. This substance is absorbed by fatty tissue after some thirty minutes and is subsequently released back into the blood, metabolized, and excreted. The substance is completely eliminated after just a few days. With chronic use, 11-hydroxy-Δ^9-THC is stored in the fatty tissue and the liver and can be detected for a longer period of time, for example, in urine tests (cf. Rippchen 1996*).

The Most Important Active Substances in Hemp

In addition to essential oil and other substances, the predominant components of hemp resin are the cannabinoids, more than sixty of which are now known structurally and pharmacologically (Grotenhermen and Karus 1998:13ff.*).

The main active ingredient is **delta-9-tetrahydrocannabinol** (Δ^9-THC, corresponding to Δ^1-THC; abbreviated as THC). THC has euphoric, stimulant, muscle-relaxing, antiepileptic, antiemetic, appetite-stimulating, bronchodilating, hypotensive, antidepressant, and analgesic effects.

Cannabidiol (CBD) has no psychoactive properties, but does have sedative and analgesic effects.

Cannabinol (CBN) is mildly psychoactive; its primary effect is to lower intraocular pressure. It also has antiepileptic effects.

Cannabigerol (CBG) is non-psychoactive, but does have sedative and antibiotic effects. It also lowers intraocular pressure.

Cannabichromene (CBC) has sedative effects and promotes the analgesic effects of THC.

Although the internal structures are different, the external structures of THC and anandamide, the body's own neurotransmitter (from the Sanskrit *ananda*, "bliss"), are so similar that both THC and anandamide bind to the same receptors in the nervous system, including receptors in the brain (Devane et al. 1988;

Pertwee 1995).[4] Anandamide appears to be the neurotransmitter responsible for pleasurable and euphoric sensations (Devane et al. 1992; Devane and Axelrod 1994; Grotenhermen 1996*; Kruszka and Gross 1994; Mestel 1993*). Recently, it has been detected in cocoa beans (*Theobroma cacao*) and red wine (Grotenhermen 1996*). Neurological disorders may result if the body does not produce enough anandamide. This suggests that some illnesses caused by a lack of the endogenous neurotransmitter anandamide (such as multiple sclerosis) may be amenable to treatment with THC (Mechoulam et al. 1994).

The "autonomous analgesic efficaciousness of THC" (Geschwinde 1990:33*) is considered its most important medicinal effect. THC also causes a decrease in intraocular pressure and thus has a prominent role to play in the treatment of glaucoma (Roffman 1982*).

Synthetic THC, dronabinol, is better known by its trade name, Marinol. A dose of 20 to 45 milligrams of Marinol produces a "high" some 1 to $1\frac{1}{2}$ hours in duration. (Compare this to the 3-hour high that results from only 4 to 8 milligrams of THC.) Many American patients who have used Marinol have complained that the medicine is ineffective compared to smoked or ingested marijuana or that it has a different, somehow unpleasant effect (Jack Herer, oral communication).

Hemp seeds contain an oil rich in lignan, proteins, and the enzyme edestinase (St. Angelo et al. 1970). The growth hormone zeatin has been found in immature seeds (Rybicka and Engelbrecht 1974). The seeds also contain the alkaloids cannabamine A-D, piperidine, trigonelline, and L-(+)-isoleucine-betaine (Bercht et al. 1973) as well as the rare vitamin K and mineral substances. Recent studies have found gamma-linoleic acid as well as "omega-3"-stearidonic acid (Callaway, Tennilä, and Pate 1997).

> "Obtained from hemp seeds, hemp oil—not to be confused with hash oil—possesses an unusually high amount of mono- and polyunsaturated fatty acids (app. 90 percent), which are of great significance in human nutrition. The essential fatty acid, linoleic acid (50 to 70 percent), and the omega-3-fatty acid, alpha-linolenic acid (15 to 25 percent), merit special mention. Ten to 20 grams of hemp oil are sufficient to meet a person's daily requirements of these two fatty acids."
>
> Franjo Grotenhermen and
> Michael Karus
> *Cannabis als Heilmittel* (1998:21*)

Hempseed oil, obtained by cold pressing the seeds, is very rich in unsaturated fatty acids. It may also contain THC, which can be detected in the urine of those who consume it (Callaway, Weeks et al. 1997).

Cannabis pollen has been shown to contain Δ^9-THC as well as THCA, an alkaloid-like substance, flavone, and phenolic substances (Paris et al. 1975).

---

4. Scientists at the Medical College of Virginia have been able to demonstrate receptors in the nervous system (SAD-Report in the Hamburger Abendblatt, No. 192, p. 5, 1991); cf. Compton et al. 1993, Devane et al. 1988, Matsuda et al. 1990, Mechoulam et al. 1994.

The leaves of *Cannabis sativa* contain choline, trigonelline, muscarine, an unidentified betaine, the cannabamines A-D and, surprisingly, the phenethylamine hordenine, an alkaloid found in many cacti (El-Feraly and Turner 1975). In addition, water-soluble glycoproteins, serine-O-galactoside, and hydroxyproline have been found in leaves from Thai and African populations (Hillestad and Wold 1977; Hillestad et al. 1997).

The roots of *Cannabis sativa* have yielded friedelin, epifriedelinol, N-(*p*-hydroxy-β-phenethyl)-*p*-hydroxy-*trans*-cinnamamide, choline, and neurine as well as the steroids stigmast-5-en-3β-ol-7-on (or 7-keto-β-sitosterol), campest-5-en-3β-ol-7-on, and stigmast-5,22-dien-3β-ol-7-on (Slatkin et al. 1975).

The characteristically scented essential oil, which lends, so to speak, hemp its bouquet, contains among other things eugenol, guaiacol, sesquiterpene, caryophyllene, humulene, farnesene, selinene, phellandrene, and limonene.

The essential oil also contains caryophyllene oxide, a sesquiterpene. This odoriferous substance has been used to train police dogs to detect drugs (Martin et al. 1961; Nigam et al. 1965). Caryophyllene oxide is also present in the essential oils of other plants, such as mugwort (*Artemisia vulgaris* L.) and spice clove (*Syzygium aromaticum* [L.] MERR. et PERRY).[5] Hemp's essential oil is usually free of or contains only trace amounts of THC.

To date, THC has been found only in the three species or varieties of hemp. Hops (*Humulus lupulus* L., *Humulus* spp.) has not yet been found to contain THC or other cannabinoids (Wohlfahrt 1993). It has been claimed that hops can produce THC when grafted to cannabis (Crombie and Crombie 1975). It has also been hypothesized that burning olibanum, the true frankincense (the resin of *Boswellia sacra* FLÜCKIGER, syn. *Boswellia carteri* BIRDW.), will yield THC through pyrochemical reactions (Martinetz et al. 1989:138). Unfortunately, this hypothesis, which is often cited as fact, has not yet been confirmed (Kessler 1991). Nevertheless, olibanum smoke is psychoactive and has inebriating effects (Rätsch 1996e* and 1998:93*).

Until now, we know of few natural substances that produce pharmacological effects similar to those of THC. One such substance is thujone, a close chemical relative of camphor and pinene, whose pharmacological effects are very close (Castillo et al. 1975); it is a component of the essential oils of many plants. High concentrations have been found in wormwood (*Artemisia absinthium* L.), tansy (*Tanacetum vulgare* L.), and in certain arborvitaes (*Thuja occidentalis* L., *Thuja orientalis* L., *Thuja plicata* D. DON). Thujone is also present in the essential oils of yarrow (*Achillea millefolium* L.), garden sage (*Salvia officinalis* L.), muscat sage (*Salvia sclarea* L.), savin juniper (*Juniperus sabina* L.), Atlas cedar (*Cedrus atlantica* [ENDL.] MANETTI), and mugwort (*Artemisia vulgaris* L.) (Albert-Puleo 1978). Not surprisingly, many plants that contain thujone have been used as ersatz marijuana. The chemical is also the main active substance in absinthe liqueur, also known as Green Fairy, the legendary artists' drug of the nineteenth century (Conrad 1988).

The official, state-sanctioned and -supported psychiatry is dominated by the

---

5. This suggests that persons could be suspected of using hashish simply because police dogs are reacting to the presence of these aromatic substances in spices carried in their belongings.

strangest notions and preconceptions about the long-term effects of frequent or chronic cannabis use; for example, it is hypothesized that hemp is a "gateway drug" and that it contributes to the so-called amotivational syndrome (Cutrufello 1980*; Täschner 1981a and b*). These "psychiatric symptoms" are pure inventions and have no empirical basis (cf. Baumann 1989*; Hess 1996*). A politically independent, sociological study of the long-term effects of chronic hemp use yielded an interesting finding: "The chances that a person will think and work creatively and productively while under the influence of hemp increase with increasing experience with hemp" (Arbeitsgruppe Hanf und Fuss 1994:103*). Many studies of long-term use have demonstrated that cannabis products are the most harmless psychoactive inebriants that humans have thus far discovered (cf. Blätter 1992*; Grinspoon 1971*; Hess 1996*; Michka and Verlomme 1993*; Schneider 1984* and 1995*; Tart 1971*).

In Europe recently, there have been discussions concerning the influence of hemp and THC upon driving behavior. In a truly bizarre turn of events, newly enacted laws regard the effects of hemp on motor reflexes as more dangerous than those of alcohol—even though a number of studies have shown that drivers who are high drive considerably slower and with greater care than either sober or drunk drivers (Böllinger 1997:169-184*; Karrer 1995; Robbe 1994 and 1996).

There is also an ongoing discussion as to whether hashish, marijuana, or THC are addictive (so-called dope addiction) or can lead to dependency (Cutrufello 1980*; Stringaris 1939; Tossmann 1987*; Woggon 1974*). The most commonly held position is that psychological dependency[6] can result (cf. Böllinger 1997*; Grotenhermen and Huppertz 1997:99f.*; Grotenherman and Karus 1998:39f.*). One even finds occasional mention of "withdrawal symptoms." This problem appears to be greater in the United States than in other countries; in America, there is an organization analogous to Alcoholics Anonymous: "Marijuana Anonymous" (Kingston 1998).

The Literature and the State of Research

The extant historical sources, which derive from different periods and cultures, have been discussed quite well in the literature on the history of medicine and are widely available. The literature resulting from ethnomedical or ethnobotanical research is quite variable with regard to its value and content. With only a few exceptions, there is no ethnomedical literature specifically dealing with the subject of cannabis as medicine. The subject is usually mentioned only in passing or (depending upon the personal biases of the particular author) neglected entirely. Many ethnologists are afraid of investigating the use of illegal drugs in other cultures, perhaps fearing that they might come under suspicion of being secret sympathizers or even users

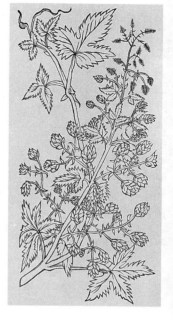

The hop plant (*Humulus lupulus*) is the closest botanical relative of hemp. The two genera are the sole representatives of the family Cannabaceae. The effects of hops, however, tend to be the opposite of those of hemp: hops sedates, soothes, induces sleep, and has anaphrodisiac effects. On the other hand, both hops and hemp are similar in that only the female flowers are usable. (woodcut from Brunfels, *Kräuterbuch*, 1532)

---

6. For example, *Hagers Handbuch der pharmazeutischen Praxis* states: "Cannabis consumption leads to psychological dependency. The tendency to physical dependency is present only slightly or not at all, for after cessation only mild or no withdrawal symptoms appear. The World Health Organization has classified the characteristic features of this dependency as a unique type, the so-called cannabis type" (Schmidt 1992:651*).

themselves. Only a very few ethnologists possess primary data on the medical use of hemp. Many are afraid of experimenting with native drugs and are content to simply reproduce hearsay ("It is said . . . I was told . . . I have heard . . ."). For these reasons, there is considerable variation in the quality of the ethnomedical literature, but I have made an effort to distill a useable extract from that which is available. In addition, I have always endeavored to conduct self-experiments, primarily to verify the evidence I have obtained so that I may better understand and appreciate the native point of view. Much of the data collected through my own studies in many countries of the world (North, Central, and South America; Nepal; India; Southeast Asia; and Japan) have made their way into this book.

As with the ethnobotanical and ethnomedical literature, the conventional medical literature does not present a consistent picture. Some articles simply reproduce the official prejudices that Western governments would have us believe. The literature based on actual experiments with human subjects is very limited. While there are indeed thousands of articles, only a handful are based upon true empirical material. Andrew Weil pointed out this scandalous state of affairs in his revolutionary book *The Natural Mind* (1972* and 1986*). In 1968, Weil was the first physician to carry out a proper scientific experiment with hemp (Weil et al. 1968*). Since then, only a very few studies have appeared: Hess (1973*), Tart (1971*), and Zinberg (1984*). More common are compilations of surveys conducted by medical sociologists, sociologists, and psychologists, such as Grupp (1971*), Schneider (1984*), and Shik et al. (1968*).

On the other hand, the chemical and pharmacological literature on cannabis is very comprehensive. This is probably due to the fact that such research is not as hampered by social or political taboos.

At the end of each chapter, I have included a bibliography of the specific literature cited therein. In addition, there is a bibliography on various aspects of hemp at the end of the book; it also includes publications from bitter opponents of hemp use (for example, Nahas 1979*, Täschner 1981b*). When viewed in the light of modern scientific research, these works can only be regarded as curiosities; even though they are modern, they ignore the scientific evidence available. Legal and political considerations are not treated in this work, but I understand that they may be of interest to the reader; I have included a number of publications on these topics (see for example Burian and Eisenbach-Stangl 1982*; Hellman 1975*; Homann 1972*; Kaplan 1971*; Liggenstorfer 1991*; Rippchen 1992* and 1994*; Scherer and Vogt 1989*). Several "classics" are also included, such as Baudelaire (1972*), Jünger (1980*), Ludlow (1981*), and Moreau de Tours (1973*).

REFERENCES

Albert-Puleo, Michael. 1978. Mythobotany, Pharmacology, and Chemistry of Thujone-Containing Plants and Derivatives. *Economic Botany* 32:65–74.

Anderson, Loran C. 1980. Leaf Variation among Cannabis Species from a Controlled Garden. *Botanical Museum Leaflets* 28(1):61–9.

Anonymous. 1981. *Das Handbuch für den Selbstanbau.* Linden, Germany: Volksverlag.

Behrens, Katja. 1996. *Leitfaden zum Hanfanbau in Haus, Hof und Garten*. Frankfurt am Main: Eichborn.

Bercht, C. A. Ludwig, Robert J. J. Ch. Lousberg, Frans J. E. M. Küppers, and Cornelis A. Salemink. 1973. L-(+)-Isoleucine Betaine in Cannabis Seeds. *Phytochemistry* 12:2457–59.

Beutler, John A., and Ara H. Der Marderosian. 1978. Chemotaxonomy of Cannabis I. Crossbreeding between *Cannabis sativa* and *C. ruderalis*, with Analysis of Cannabinoid Content. *Economic Botany* 32(4):387–94.

Bósca, Iván, and Michael Karus. 1997. *Der Hanfanbau: Botanik, Sorten, Anbau und Ernte*. Heidelberg, Germany: C. F. Müller (Umwelt Aktuell).

Boucher, Françoise, Michel Paris, and Louis Cosson. 1977. Mise en évidence de deux types chimiques chez le *Cannabis sativa* originaire d'Afrique du sud. *Phytochemistry* 16:1445–48.

Brenneisen, Rudolf. 1996. *Cannabis sativa* - Aktuelle Pharmakologie und Klinik. *Jahrbuch des Europäischen Collegiums für Bewußtseinstudien*, 1995:191–8.

Blake, Anthony G. E. 1990. *Intelligenz Jetzt!* Südergellersen, Germany: Verlag Bruno Martin.

Callaway, J. C., T. Tennilä, and D. W. Pate. 1997. Occurrence of *"omega*-3" Stearidonic Acid (*cis*-6,6,12,15-octadecatetraenoic Acid) in Hemp (*Cannabis sativa* L.) Seed. *Journal of the International Hemp Association* 3(2):61–3.

Callaway, J. C., R. A. Weeks, L. P. Raymon, H. C. Walls, and W. L. Hearn. 1997. A Positive THC Urinalysis from Hemp (*Cannabis*) Seed Oil. *Journal of Analytical Toxicology* 21:319–20.

Castillo, J. D., M. Anderson, and G. M. Rubboton. 1975. Marijuana, Absinthe and the Central Nervous System. *Nature* 253:365–6.

Coffman, C. B., and W. A. Gentner. 1979. Greenhouse Propagation of *Cannabis sativa* L. by Vegetative Cuttings. *Economic Botany* 33(2):124–7.

Compton, David R., Kenner C. Rice, Brian R. De Costa, Raj K. Razdan, Lawrence S. Melvin, M. Ross Johnson, and Billy R. Martin. 1993. Cannabinoid Structure-Activity Relationships: Correlation of Receptor Binding and in Vivo Activities. *Journal of Pharmacology and Experimental Therapeutics* 265:218–26.

Conrad, Barnaby. 1988. *Absinthe: History in a Bottle*. San Francisco: Chronicle Books.

Crombie, Leslie, and W. Mary L. Crombie. 1975. Cannabinoid Formation in *Cannabis sativa* Grafted Inter-Racially, and with Two Humulus Species. *Phytochemistry* 14:409–12.

Dary, David A. 1990. *The Buffalo Book*. Athens, Ohio: Swallow Press/Ohio University Press.

Devane, William A., and Julius Axelrod. 1994. Enzymatic Synthesis of Anandamide, an Endogenous Ligand for the Cannabinoid Receptor, by Brain Membranes. *Proceedings of the National Academy of Science* 91:6698–701.

Devane, William A., Francis A. Dysarz III, M. Ross Johnson, Lawrence S. Melvin, and Allyn C. Howlett. 1988. Determination and Characterization of a Cannabinoid Receptor in Rat Brain. *Molecular Pharmacology* 34:605–13.

Devane, William A., Lumir Hanus, Aviva Breuer, Roger G. Pertwee, Lesley A. Stevenson, Graeme Griffin, Dan Gibson, Asher Mandelbaum, Alexander Etinger, and Raphael Mechoulam. 1992. Isolation and Structure of a Brain Constituent That Binds to the Cannabinoid Receptor. *Science* 258:1946–49.

El-Feraly, Farouk S., and Carlton E. Turner. 1975. Alkaloids of *Cannabis sativa* Leaves. *Phytochemistry* 14:2304.

Frank, Mel, and Ed Rosenthal. 1980. *Das Handbuch für die Marihuana-Zucht in Haus und Garten*. Linden, Germany: Volksverlag.

Harvey, D. J. 1990. Stability of Cannabinoids in Dried Samples of Cannabis Dating from Around 1896–1905. *Journal of Ethnopharmacology* 28:117–28.

Hemphill, John K., Jocelyn C. Turner, and Paul G. Mahlberg. 1978. Studies on Growth and Cannabinoid Composition of Callus Derived from Different Strains of *Cannabis sativa*. *Lloydia* 41(5):453–62.

It makes Homo sapiens *hungry, horny, sleepy, and happy*—or afraid. It soothes pain, inhibits movement, lowers the body temperature, and leads to a loss of the sense of time. It influences the memory and distorts thinking and perceptual processes. Why?

"Concerning the question as to why people get high from marihuana, for decades there were as many theories as there were researchers interested in the 421 substances in those serrated marihuana leaves.

JACK HERER AND
MATTHIAS BRÖCKERS
*DIE WIEDERENTDECKUNG
DER NUTZPFLANZE HANF*
(1993:415*)

Hillestad, Agnes, and Jens K. Wold. 1977. Water-Soluble Glycoproteins from *Cannabis sativa* (South Africa). *Phytochemistry*, 16:1947–51.

Hillestad, Agnes, Jens K. Wold, and Thor Engen. 1977. Water-Soluble Glycoproteins from *Cannabis sativa* (Thailand). *Phytochemistry* 16:1953–56.

Janischewsky. 1924. Cannabis ruderalis. *Proceedings Saratov* 2(2):14–5.

de Jardin, Raphael. 1997. *Hanfanbau mit Hydrokultur*. Solothurn, Switzerland: Nachtschatten Verlag.

Karrer, Barbara. 1995. *Cannabis im Straßenverkehr*. Aachen, Germany: Verlag Shaker.

Kessler, Michael, 1991. *Zur Frage nach psychotropen Stoffen im Rauch von brennendem Gummiharz der Boswellia sacra*. Basel, Switzerland: Inaugural-Dissertation.

Kingston, Stephen. 1998. Insane in the Brain. *Sky Magazine* No. 139 (March):48–52.

Kruszka, Kelly K., and Richard W. Gross. 1994. The ATP- and CoA-independent Synthesis of Arachido-noylethanolamide: A Novel Mechanism Underlying the Synthesis of the Endogenous Ligand of the Cannabinoid Receptor. *Journal of Biological Chemistry* 269(20):14345–48.

Latta, R. P., and B. J. Eaton. 1975. Seasonal Fluctuations in Cannabinoid Content of Kansas Marijuana. *Economic Botany* 29:153–63.

Lehmann, Thomas. 1995. *Chemische Profilierung von* Cannabis sativa *L*. Master's dissertation, Universität Bern, Switzerland.

McHugh, Tom. 1979. *The Time of the Buffalo*. Lincoln, Nebraska: University of Nebraska Press.

Marquart, Benno. 1919. *Der Hanfbau, seine Verbreitung, seine Bedeutung und sein Betrieb*. Berlin: Paul Parey.

Martin, L., D. Smith, and C. G. Farmilo. 1961. Essential Oil from Fresh *Cannabis sativa* and Its Use in Identification. *Nature* 191(4790):774–6.

Martinetz, Dieter, Karlheinz Lohs, and Jörg Janzen. 1989. *Weihrauch und Myrrhe*, Stuttgart, Germany: WVG.

Matsuda, Lisa A., Stephen J. Lolait, Michael J. Brownstein, Alice C. Young, and Tom I. Bonner. 1990. Structure of a Cannabinoid Receptor and Functional Expression of the Cloned cDNA. *Nature* 346:561–4.

Mechoulam, Raphael, Zvi Vogel, and Jacob Barg. 1994. CNS Cannabinoid Receptors: Role and Therapeutic Implications for CNS Disorders. *CNS Drugs* 2(4):255–60.

de Meijer, Etienne. 1994. Diversity in Cannabis. Thesis Wageningen (Distributed by the International Hemp Association [IHA], Postbus 75007, 1070 AA Amsterdam, the Netherlands).

Murphy, Laura, and Andrzej Bartke, eds. 1992. *Marijuana/Cannabinoids: Neurobiology and Neurophysiology*. Boca Raton: CRC Press.

Nigam, M. C., K. L. Handa, I. C. Nigam, and Leo Levi. 1965. Essential Oils and Their Constituents XXIX. The Essential Oil of Marihuana: Composition of Genuine Indian *Cannabis sativa* L. *Canadian Journal of Chemistry* 43:3372–76.

Nova-Institut, ed. 1995. *Biorohstoff Hanf: Reader zum Symposium*. Cologne: Nova-Institut.

Paris, M., F. Boucher, and L. Cosson. 1975. The Constituents of *Cannabis sativa* Pollen. *Economic Botany* 29:245–53.

Pertwee, Roger, ed. 1995. *Cannabinoid Receptors*. New York: Harcourt Brace Jovanovich.

Robbe, H. W. J. 1994. *Influence of Marijuana on Driving*. Maastricht, Netherlands: Institute for Human Psychopharmacology, University of Limburg.

———. 1996. Influence of Marijuana on Driving. *Jahrbuch des Europäischen Collegiums für Bewußtseinstudien*. 1995:179–89, Berlin: VWB.

Rybicka, Hanna, and Lisabeth Engelbrecht. 1974. Zeatin in Cannabis Fruit. *Phytochemistry* 13:282–3.

Slatkin, David J., Joseph E. Knapp, and Paul L. Schiff Jr. 1975. Steroids of *Cannabis sativa* Root. *Phytochemistry* 14:580–1.

Small, Ernest. 1975. The Case of the Curious 'Cannabis.' *Economic Botany* 29:254.

———. 1976. The Species Problem in Cannabis. *Science and Semantics*. 2 vols. Toronto: Corpus.

Small, Ernest, H. D. Beckstead, and Allan Chan. 1975. The Evolution of Cannabinoid Phenotypes in Cannabis. *Economic Botany* 29:219–32.

Smith, R. Martin, and Kenneth D. Kempfert. 1977. Δ^1-3,4-*cis*-Tetrahydrocannabinol in *Cannabis sativa*. *Phytochemistry* 16:1088–9.

St. Angelo, Allen J., Robert L. Ory, and Hans J. Hansen. 1970. Properties of a Purified Proteinase from Hempseed. *Phytochemistry* 9:1933–38.

Stearn, William T. 1974. Typification of *Cannabis sativa* L. *Botanical Museum Leaflets* 23(9):325–36.

———. 1975. Typification of *Cannabis sativa* L. In *Cannabis and Culture*, edited by V. Rubin. The Hague, Netherlands: Mouton, 13–20.

Stevens, Murphy. 1980. *Marihuana-Anbau in der Wohnung*. Linden, Germany: Volksverlag.

Storm, Daniel. 1994. *Marijuana Hydroponics: High-Tech Water Culture*. Berkeley, Calif.: Ronin.

Stringaris, M. G. 1939. *Die Haschischsucht*. Berlin: Springer.

Taura, Futoshi, Satoshi Morimoto, and Yukihiro Shoyama.

———. 1995. Cannabinerolic Acid, a Cannabinoid from *Cannabis sativa*. *Phytochemistry* 39(2):457–8.

Van der Werf, Hayo. 1994. *Crop Physiology of Fibre Hemp* (Cannabis sativa L.). Proefschrift Wageningen, the Netherlands. ISBN 90-9007171-7.

Wohlfahrt, Rainer. 1993. Humulus. In *Hagers Handbuch der pharmazeutischen Praxis*. 5th ed. Berlin: Springer, 5:447–58.

de Zeeuw, Rokus A. and Jaap Wijsbeek. 1972. Cannabinoids with a Propyl Side Chain in Cannabis: Occurrence and Chromatographic Behavior. *Science* 175:778–9.

The secret lies in the use of hashish.

FITZ HUGH LUDLOW
DER HASCHISCH ESSER
(1981:15*)

Bum Shankar!

IN THE BEGINNING WERE THE SHAMANS

The shaman connects the past to the future,
thereby creating the present.
AMÉLIE SCHENK

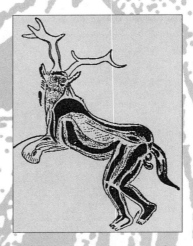

Archaeologists have interpreted the famous cave painting of the "magician" with antlers from Les Trois Frères in the French Pyrenees as the artistic product of a psychedelic trance. Prehistoric finds near Hohen Viecheln, Wismar, have confirmed that Stone Age shamans did indeed wear stag masks. The stag skull mask that is now on display in the Museum in Schwerin comes from the sixth millennium B.C.E., as does the oldest hemp found, and suggests the existence of a Neolithic "stag-hemp-shaman" complex. The alchemist Agrippa of Nettesheim (1486–1535) wrote: "The stag heals the insane and the mad." (*Die magische Werke* II, 37)

Shamanism is not a religion, but a technique of consciousness that is associated with special individuals. It functions especially in polytheistic religions that venerate nature, such as animism, Taoism, Shintoism, Hinduism, and Buddhism (Lamaism) (Scharfetter 1985; Gottwald and Rätsch 1998).

Because the shamans have been called by gods, spirits, demons, or ancestors and have a singular ability to fall into trance and ecstasy, they are persons who always occupy exceptional positions in their culture and society (Eliade 1975*; Halifax 1983). Shamans can fulfill the social functions of physicians, priests, oracles, diviners, magicians, witches, midwives, herbalists, scientists, actors in mystery plays, rhapsodists, and keepers of oral traditions (Lommel 1980).

Shamans are both male and female. All shamans share a worldview in which travel to different worlds or other realities is possible. These normally invisible realities are called by various names, such as heaven, paradise, underworld, hell, spirit world, realm of shadows, blue zone, invisible world, and true reality. Gods, spirits, ancestors, demons, beasts, monsters, and the souls of animals and plants live in these worlds. Shamans communicate with these invisible beings. From them, they learn the secrets of the universe, receive detailed knowledge about the use of medicinal plants, and obtain the power to heal or to cause harm.

In the shamanic universe, illnesses are usually thought to result from a loss of the soul, of different parts of the soul, or of consciousness. The soul of a sick person is sometimes—and for various reasons, including witchcraft, violation of taboos, and misdeeds—carried into the invisible world by negative beings. There, beasts and monsters torment, torture, and imprison the soul. When an illness of this type occurs, the shaman must travel to the otherworld and free the soul that has been taken. Oftentimes, the shaman travels in the form of an animal, such as an eagle, tiger, or jaguar, more infrequently as a snail or a glowworm.

In order to travel to the invisible world, the shaman must enter into a trance and leave the normal world behind. To induce the necessary trance, most shamans use various psychoactive drugs (Furst 1990; Harner 1973; Rosenbohm 1991). The drug, however, does not make a person into a shaman. Instead, the shaman uses the drug as a catalyst that allows him to express and exploit his own abilities. Most shamans use drums or rattles as their "mounts," creating a monotonous rhythm that becomes the bridge into the other reality. Often, shamans wear animal costumes, masks, and cloaks as external signs of their internal reality.

Shamanism is very ancient. There is evidence indicating that it was practiced by the people of the Paleolithic, the Old Stone Age. Numerous cave paintings depict humans in animal costumes, perhaps portraits of Stone Age shamans (Biedermann 1984:69–89). In recent years, many European cave paintings have been interpreted as depictions of shamans, shamanic states of consciousness, and shamanic myths (Clottes and Lewis-Williams 1997; Devereux 1997). But shamanism is not merely some bizarre manifestation of the past; it is alive today, especially in Southeast Asia (Heinze 1991). Its practice has a compelling fascination and attraction here at the dawn of the new millennium (Zinser 1991).

Since ancient times, hemp has been a shamanic drug (Eliade 1975:376ff.*; see esp. Furst 1990:212f.; Knoll-Greiling 1950; Sebode and Pfeiffer 1988:16). Shamans

The shaman moves back and forth between the two realities of his own accord and with solemn purpose. No matter which reality it is, the shaman thinks and acts in the appropriate manner and has as his goal the mastery of both his nonordinary and his everyday activities. Only he who successfully masters his actions in both domains is a master shaman.
MICHAEL J. HARNER
(1994:76F.*)

are generally credited with the discovery of pharmacologically active plants, including the discovery of hemp and its multiple uses (Merlin 1972*). Hemp was used in central and eastern Asia as early as the Neolithic age. The word *shaman* comes from this region. In the Tungusic language, *shaman* refers to the healing and prophesizing artist of consciousness (Sebode and Pfeiffer 1988:7). The earliest literary and ethnohistorical evidence for hemp is found in shamanic texts from ancient China (Li 1974). These texts contain numerous prehistoric descriptions of shamans such as this one:

> The drama of the entrance into the transcendental spiritual and divine realms of heaven with the nonphysical part of his own person led the *saman* that had been initiated in this way into a state of deepest bliss or profound emotion. Overcoming human limits and ordinary standards, *samans* struggled to find adequate expression for indescribable impressions after returning from their visionary journeys. In addition to sculptures and cave paintings, numerous petroglyphs, engravings, and scratches in rocks were made, usually at high-altitude cultic sites. In their simplicity, these often speak an impressively clear language. A Bronze Age petroglyph from the mountainous regions of Southeast Kazakstan, for example, depicts the true origin and home of an earthling: man in the placenta of the stars. (Adrian 1994:76)

The oldest archaeological evidence for the cultural use of hemp also points to a shamanic usage. Hemp seeds, which could be identified as *Cannabis sativa*, were recovered in the Neolithic band ceramic (LBK) layers of Eisenberg in Thüringen, Germany (Renfrew 1973:163; Willerding 1970:358). The layers were dated to around 5500 B.C.E. Hemp seeds have also been found in the excavations of other, somewhat more recent Neolithic layers, such as those in Thainigen, Switzerland; Voslau, Austria; and Frumusica, Romania (Renfrew 1973:163). These finds date from a period of peaceful, horticultural, pre-Indo-European cultures that especially venerated the goddess (Gimbutas 1989) and who very likely practiced shamanism (Probst 1991:239). The band ceramics that lent their name to this Stone Age cultural epoch were decorated with graphics representing the archetypical motifs and patterns of hallucinatory or psychedelic themes (Stahl 1989). All together, there is a great deal of evidence indicating that psychoactive substances were used throughout Europe during Neolithic times (Sherrat 1991).

In Bavaria, prehistoric finds of clay pipe bowls with wooden stems, found during excavations of the barrows of Bad Abbach-Heidfeld, indicate that cannabis products were being smoked more than thirty-five hundred years ago, possibly together with the sleeping poppy or opium *(Papaver somniferum)* (Probst 1996:174).

In Nepal, the tradition-rich Hindu kingdom in the middle of the Himalayas, shamanism is still very important. Most of the cultural groups in Nepal have a mixed religion. Elements from Bön, Tibetan Lamaism *(vajrayana)*, and various schools of Hinduism have fused into a harmonious whole. There are shamans in almost every village; they are frequently known as *jakri*, a word meaning "magician." The jakri live in a polytheistic cosmos in which Buddha is as much at home as the ancient Bön demons and the Vedic and Hindu gods. The shamans venerate Shiva,

"We shamans come from the time before religion. Religions are for those who cannot see."
INDRA B. GURUNG
(AUGUST 1998)

16   Bum Shankar!

whose origins may be traced back to the Vedic Rudra. They consider him to be the original, primordial shaman who has a perfect command of the shamanic arts and who passes the secrets of these arts on to certain chosen persons (Rätsch 1997*).

One Nepalese name for Shiva is *Vijaya*, "the Victor" (Storl 1988:83, 201). The Vedic texts give the same name to hemp. Shiva is also known as Bhangeri Baba, "the Lord of Hemp" (Storl 1988:198). According to shamanic tradition, Shiva discovered hemp and sowed it in the Himalayas so that it would always be there for humans. Shiva also gave people different recipes for its use: "In Nepal, ascetics, shamans, and magicians have consumed small amounts of this substance since ancient times in order to induce trance states" (Gruber 1991:144).

The most common method of ingestion in Nepal is to smoke various hemp products (Knecht 1971). The leaves, the female flowers (*ganja*), or the sticky, aromatic resin (*charas*) are stuffed into a smoking tube, a chilam,[1] either alone or mixed with thornapple leaves (*Datura metel*), henbane (*Hyoscyamus niger*), or tobacco (*Nicotiana rustica*). The chilam, a symbol and attribute of Shiva, is held to the forehead and dedicated to the god of hemp with the words "Bum Shankar" (Hail to the Benefactor).

At this point, it should be noted that not everyone who smokes marijuana is a shaman. Only those who have the gift of and have been called to shamanism are able to smoke hemp and enter into a shamanic trance. Yet as, for example, Fitz Hugh Ludlow (1981*) has so impressively described, hemp users can have experiences with shamanic elements and the contents of shamanic mythologies.

But it is the shamans who are able to use cannabis with the greatest effect. By smoking hemp, the shaman devoted to Shiva can—thanks to his gifts—produce an especially efficacious sacred medicine:

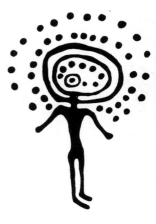

This Neolithic petroglyph from near the Tamgali River depicts a shaman expanding his consciousness. In China, the ritual and medicinal use of hemp was already widespread in the Neolithic. (from Adrian, 1994)

> Smoking is an unbecoming, a dissolution, a process of death. In this small, spinning pyre, the husks of delusion that entwine us burn to ash. The rotting corpses of our transgressions, the cadavers of old karma roast therein and are transformed to snow-white ash. . . . The bolt to the door of the "transcendent" is shattered; the demonic horde of Shiva, the ethereal images of natural forces and the shapes of souls, dance before the eyes of the initiate. The dead appear and the gods! In an even deeper samadhi, all manifestations, all appearances cease, and it simply *is*. In total absorption, Shiva sits on Kailash, the holy mountain, the mountain of snow, the mountain of ash. . . . After the chilam has been smoked all the way to the end and the meditation is over, the shaman takes the ashes and rubs them onto his forehead or he places them on his tongue as *prasad*, for the sacred, white powder is regarded as the best medicine. (Storl 1988:204, 205)

Hemp is also ingested in a drink called *bhang* (Müller-Ebeling and Rätsch 1986:20*). The shamans of the Himalayas drink bhang so that they may enter into the trance or ecstasy required for their healing rituals. They offer bhang to the

---

1. Also spelled *chillum*, pronounced "tschillum."

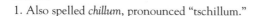

phallus-shaped sacred stones and lingams that are shrines to Shiva. The offering invokes the god's healing power, for no one loves hemp and the state it induces as much as Shiva himself. The inebriated god sends out healing power, which is channeled through the shaman and transferred to the patient. Although it is usually only the shaman who smokes ganja or drinks bhang during the shamanic healing sessions, hemp preparations may also be used medicinally. The patient may be prescribed hemp drinks for various ailments including depression, lack of appetite, inconstancy, or altitude sickness, a common occurrence in the Himalayas (cf. Morningstar 1985*).

These shamanic uses of hemp, which are still found in Nepal today, have their roots in human prehistory. They cast a clear light upon the early shamanic use of this "plant of the gods" as both a means to achieve ecstasy and as a medicine. A number of hemp recipes have been passed down that were or are still used in shamanic practice.

Bhang (Nepal)

Required ingredients:

> Hemp flowers
> Buffalo milk
> Sugar or honey
> Spices (for example, cardamom, cinnamon, cloves, curcuma, nutmeg, pepper)

Optional ingredients:

> Nux vomica seeds (Strychnos nux-vomica)
> Opium
> Thornapple seeds (Datura metel)
> Ground nut meats (for example, almonds, coconut, pistachios)
> Ghee (clarified butter)

Finely chop the hemp flowers and mix with the spices (and the optional ingredients). Dissolve the sugar or honey in the milk. Stir in the hemp/spice mixture.
Use about 2 g of dried hemp flowers or leaves per person.

Tantric Smoking Mix

> Hemp flowers (ganja)
> Fresh or dried cobra venom

This mix can be created in two ways. In the first, crystallized cobra venom—the cobra is a sacred animal and a symbol of Shiva—is mixed with chopped hemp flowers and smoked in a chilam. In the second method, fresh cobra venom is sprinkled over large, dried marijuana flowers (ganja). After it has soaked into or dried on the flowers, chop up the impregnated buds and smoke in a chilam.*

*Very advanced aghoris, adherents of an extreme school of yoga, actually allow themselves to be bitten on the tongue by a live cobra so that they may go on a psychedelic trip (cf. Svoboda 1993 and 1994).

REFERENCES

Adrian, Franciscus. 1994. *Die Schule des I Ging: Hintergrundwissen*. Munich: Diederichs.

Biedermann, Hans. 1984. *Höhlenkunst der Eiszeit*. Cologne: DuMont.

Clottes, Jean, and David Lewis-Williams. 1997. *Schamanen: Trance und Magie in der Höhlenkunst der Steinzeit*. Sigmaringen, Germany: Thorbecke Verlag.

Devereux, Paul. 1997. *The Long Trip: A Prehistory of Psychedelia*. New York: Penguin.

Furst, Peter T. 1990. Schamanische Ekstase und botanische Halluzinogene: Phantasie und Realität. In *Der Gesang des Schamanen*, edited by G. Guntern. Brig, Switzerland: ISO-Stiftung, 211–43.

Gimbutas, Marija. 1989. *The Language of the Goddess*. New York: Harper & Row.

Gottwald, Franz-Theo, and Christian Rätsch, eds. 1998. *Schamanische Wissenschaften: Ökologie, Naturwissenschaft und Kunst*. Munich: Diederichs.

Gruber, Ulrich. 1991. *Nepal*. Munich: Prestel.

Halifax, Joan. 1983. *Schamanen*. Frankfurt am Main: Insel.

Harner, Michael J., ed. 1973. *Hallucinogens and Shamanism*. London: Oxford University Press.

Heinze, Ruth-Inge. 1991. *Shamans of the 20th Century*. New York: Irvington.

Keiling, Horst. 1985. *Steinzeitliche Jäger und Sammler in Mecklenburg*. Schwerin, Germany: Museum für Ur- und Frühgeschichte.

Knecht, Sigrid. 1971. Rauchen und Räuchern in Nepal. *Ethnomedizin* 1(2):209–22.

Knoll-Greiling, Ursula. 1950. Die sozial-psychologische Funktion des Schamanen. In *Beiträge zur Gesellungs- und Völkerwissenschaft, Festschrift for Richard Thurnwald*. Berlin: Gebr. Mann 102–24.

Lewin, Roger. 1991. Stone Age Psychedelia. *New Scientist* 8/91:30–4.

Li, Hui-Lin. 1974. The Origin and Use of Cannabis in Eastern Asia: Linguistic-cultural Implications. *Economic Botany* 28:293–301.

Lommel, Andreas. 1980. *Schamanen und Medizinmänner*. 2nd edition. Munich: Callway.

Probst, Ernst. 1991. *Deutschland in der Steinzeit*. Munich: C. Bertelsmann.

———. 1996. *Deutschland in der Bronzezeit*. Munich: C. Bertelsmann.

Renfrew, Jane M. 1973. *Palaeoethnobotany: The Prehistoric Food Plants of the Near East and Europe*. New York: Columbia University Press.

Rosenbohm, Alexandra. 1991. *Halluzinogene Drogen im Schamanismus*. Berlin: Dietrich Reimer.

Scharfetter, C[hristian]. 1985. Der Schamane: Zeuge einer alten Kultur—wieder belebbar? *Schweizer Archiv für Neurologie, Neurochirurgie und Psychiatrie* 136(3):81–95.

Sebode, Christina, and Rolf Pfeiffer. 1988. Schamanismus. *Salix* 1.87:7–33.

Sherratt, Andrew. 1991. Sacred and Profane Substances: The Ritual Use of Narcotics in Later Neolithic Europe. In *Sacred and Profane*, edited by Paul Garwood, et al. Oxford University Committee for Archaeology, monograph no. 32, 50–64.

Stahl, Peter W. 1989. Identification of Hallucinatory Themes in the Late Neolithic Art of Hungary. *Journal of Psychoactive Drugs* 21(1):101–12.

Storl, Wolf-Dieter. 1988. *Feuer und Asche—Dunkel und Licht: Shiva—Urbild des Menschen*. Freiburg i.B.: Bauer.

Svoboda, Robert E. 1993. *Aghora: At the Left Hand of God*. New Delhi: Rupa.

———. 1994. *Aghora II: Kundalini*. New Delhi: Rupa.

Willerding, U. 1970. Vor- und frühgeschichtliche Kulturpflanzenfunde in Mitteleuropa. Neue Ausgrabungen und Forschungen in Niedersachsen 5, a publication of the Hildesheim Museum.

Zinser, Hartmut. 1991. Zur Faszination des Schamanismus. In *Hungrige Geister und rastlose Seelen: Texte zur Schamanismusforschung*, edited by Michael Kuper. Berlin: Dietrich Reimer, 17–26.

Of the herb which comes from the time before time.

—Three ages before the gods themselves—

In one hundred and seven-fold manner, of that which becomes green will I compose.

Yes, one hundred fold is your kind and one thousand fold is your growth;

well endowed with a hundred powers, make this ailing one well for me!

So go happily into my hand, whether with the flower, with the fruit!

Like the mare who wins the prize, the herb accompanies us to victory.

The watery, the milky, the nourishing, the powerful—

all are here together, to make his harm whole . . .

As once from heaven the herbs did come, they spoke:

if we arrive while still alive, the man shall remain unharmed.

THE SONG OF THE PHYSICIAN
RIG VEDA
(FROM POLLOK 1978:179F.*)

Ma

HEMP IN THE CHINESE HERBAL ARTS

*The heavens have created all living things
which the earth receives, and it is life itself
which the earth has received and which is infi-
nite in its transmission to the descendants,
while the individual in which life is found must
face his finitude by passing on life to the generations that follow.*

WOLFGANG G. A. SCHMID
*DER KLASSIKER DES GELBEN KAISERS
ZUR INNEREN MEDIZIN* (1993:33)

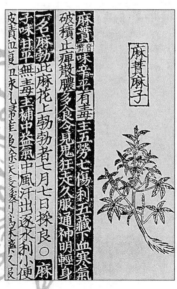

Chinese wood block print of the
hemp plant with descriptive text.
(from the 1234 edition of *Chêng-
lei pên-ts'ao*)

Hemp was present at the dawn of Chinese civilization. It was the first plant to be cultivated by the northern tribes when they became sedentary. Cords, nets, and textiles were manufactured from its fibers (Zheng 1990:16). Hemp stems were used in northern China to produce humankind's first paper (Li 1974b).[1]

The oldest Chinese book extant, the *Shih-Ching* or *Shijing* (following the Pinyin system), the "Book of Songs," was written in northern China sometime between the ninth and sixth century B.C.E. (during the Zhou dynasty), although it is based upon sources two thousand years older (Keng 1974). Frequent mention of cannabis is made in this work, providing us with the first historical mention of the plant. It was listed among the "hundred grains" and associated with shamanism. The text also contains information about growing cannabis (Weber-Schäfer 1967:174):

> Planting hemp, how do you do it?
> You plant it in straight rows.

Hemp was portrayed as a sacred plant in the "New Songs" in the *Ch'u Tz'u* (or *Zhouli*), a collection of cultic lyrics from the third century B.C.E. (Weber-Schäfer 1967:19):

> I pluck the flowers in the sacred hemp field,
> Pluck them for him who is far from me.

It appears that the psychoactive flowers were used for love magic. In the *Zhouli*, hemp stalks were used as oracles in the I Ching (Weber-Schäfer 1967:204). A shamanic or magical use of hemp stalks is described in the *Shu-King*, which is thought to date to 500 B.C.E. There, it is noted that under certain weather conditions, hemp stems can become very woody. When dried, these stems could be carved into magical wands. One illustration in the text depicts a snake curled around a scepter. Magic wands of this type were used in healing. During a typical ritual, a wand would be used by an ill person's relative to hit the patient's bed in order to drive out the spirits that brought the disease (Emboden 1990:217*).

Ancient Chinese shamanism, and probably Paleoasiatic shamanism as well, was seamlessly integrated into Taoism as it emerged (Schmidt 1993; Yu 1988). The ancient New Year's festival took place during the tenth month, concurrent with the harvest festival, which originally took place at the time of the autumnal equinox. Rituals bade farewell to the old and welcomed the new. The leaders of the festival wore white garments (indicating mourning), a leather cap, and a belt of hemp to ensure fertility. They also carried a rod from a hazelnut bush, which was used to drive out spirits (Zheng 1990:93f.). The sparrow is an archaic shamanic bird, a spirit helper, and is called *ma-ch'iao*, hemp bird; it "is said to be the most sensuous of all birds, and this is why the consumption of its flesh is said to strengthen sexual power" (Eberhard 1983:270).

Shen-Nung, or Shennong, is regarded as the (mythical) founder of Chinese herbal lore and pharmacy; his name means "divine countryman." He was born after

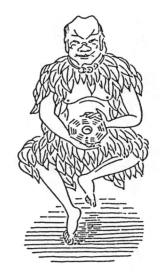

The ancient Chinese culture hero and shaman Fu-hsi, shown here dancing in a garment of leaves, not only gave the I Ching oracle to humans, but also taught them about the medicinal use of hemp. (Chinese woodcut, from Adrian)

The first women to appear as healers in Chinese history were the shamans. They were seers who entered trance while dancing and then uttered incantations in this state. Some of them achieved great fame, especially when they acquired a reputation for being able to predict diseases and death.

PAUL SCHALL
ZAUBERMEDIZIN IM
ALTEN CHINA?

---

1. Chinese hemp was formerly considered a unique species and was named *Cannabis chinensis* DEL. (a synonym today; cf. Keys 1991:137).

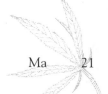

麻醉
麻木
麻痺
麻亂
麻煩

The Chinese word and character for hemp, *ma*, is a component of many composite terms with similar cognitive references:
  narcotic
  anesthetized
  paralysis
  confusion
  troublesome/annoying

his human mother was touched by the head of a heavenly dragon (Zheng 1990:38). Shennong is sometimes portrayed as a human and sometimes as a mixed being with the body of a human and the head of an ox. He is also known as Yandi, or "Red Emperor." It was he who presided over the sacrifice of the herd and brought the blessings of agriculture. He taught early humans how to use the plow and to plant the "five types of grain": hemp, rice, barley, millet, and soy beans (Touw 1981:23*). He tested nourishing, healing, and poisonous plants on himself and produced a pharmacopoeia that is said to be the basis of the *Pen ts'ao Ching* (Weikang 1985:22f.).

The five-finger principle was used to divide and classify plants, foodstuffs, various properties, types of behavior, and similar things. In the Taoist world, painting, medicine, calligraphy, poetry, and t'ai chi ch'uan were officially regarded as the "five excellences." To the alchemistic underground, however, the "five perfections" were something very different: drinking, drugs, women (sex), gambling, and smoking (Olson 1993:66).

In Shennong's pharmacopoeia, which legend says was compiled in the year 2737 B.C.E., but was not written down until the first century, during the Han dynasty, it is said that hemp heals "female weakness, gout, rheumatism, malaria, beriberi, constipation, and absentmindedness" (Emboden 1990:217*). It names the hemp variety *ta-ma* as one of the essential ingredients in an elixir of immortality: "This elixir transforms a mortal into a divine transcendent person. The teachings of the Tao emphasize that one must forget his own consciousness in order to attain the goals of Tao. It is precisely this state which can be attained with Cannabis" (Emboden 1981b:328*). Other ingredients in the early Taoists' "elixirs of immortality" included aconite, foxglove (digitalis), cinnabar, mercury, gold, and arsenic (Cooper 1984:54; Ware 1981). Although different alchemists used different recipes, all mixed in a copious amount of freshly pressed hemp juice for consumption. This psychoactive preparation was to be ingested daily, for then a person could "divide himself into a thousand men and ride through the air." It was also said to improve health (Strickman 1979:172).

The discovery of a pipe bowl in Xianyang, in the Shaanxi province, suggests that the benefits of smoking hemp were already known during the Han dynasty (Weikang 1985:ill.). Necromancers combined hemp with ginseng roots (*Panax ginseng*) so that they could foresee future events (Touw 1981:23*).

The notorious physician Hua-to (ca. 190–265 C.E.), who was also the first surgeon in China, introduced the narcotic anesthetic mixture *ma-yo*. Also known as *ma-po*, it consisted of hemp resin and wine (Emboden 1990:217*), and was also said to have contained monkshood (*Aconitum* sp.) (Thorwald 1985:245), kudzu flowers (*Pueraria lobata* [WILLD.] OHWI; cf. Schneebeli-Graf 1992:21, 25) and wormwood (*Artemisia absinthium* L.). After ingesting a spatulaful, a person was advised to quickly lie down, for a voice would immediately start giving advice (Ware 1981:255). The Chinese, who tended to have a certain aversion to invasive physical operations, wanted nothing to do with the anesthetic: "Hua-to was called to the Chinese Prince Tsao-tsao, who suffered from unbearable headaches. Hua-to recommended that he trephine the skull to open it. But just as the surgeon was beginning the operation, Tsao-tsao was suddenly struck by the suspicious fear that Hua-to intended to murder him on the orders of an adversary. He had the doctor imprisoned and executed. Tradition says that Hua-to left behind many writings on medicine and surgery, but following his wishes, these were destroyed before he died" (Thorwald 1985:246). More than twelve hundred years would pass before another physician would dare to go public with a formula for surgical interventions (Weikang 1985:73).

In 1578, Li-Shih-chen (or Li Shizhen) wrote his famous herbal *Pen-ts'ao*, still considered the fundamental work of Chinese herbalism. In his book, Li Shizhen asserted that hemp can remedy nervous feelings; senility; vaginal discharge, menstrual irregularities; complications during labor; sulfur, lead, or monkshood (*Aconitum napellus*) poisoning; constipation; severe vomiting; skin eruptions, boils, and wounds; tinea; hair loss; dry sensations in the throat; scorpion stings; urine retention; gravel; and hemorrhoids (cf. Emboden 1981b:328*; Lu 1990:168). Li Shizhen also included a recipe for an anesthetic:

> If you collect equal parts of *man-t'o-lo* [white thornapple, *Datura metel* var. *alba*] and hemp in the seventh and eighth month of the year, dry them in the shade, pulverize them, and dissolve them in wine, then this preparation will effect a narcotic anesthesia following ingestion and allow you to carry out minor operations and cauterizations without pain. (cited in Emboden 1981b:328*)

The use of hemp in Chinese medicine can be best understood in the light of the ethical and cosmological systems that underlie it:

> The basic idea that dominates Chinese medicine is that humans and nature are bound closely together. The Chinese physician advocates preventive measures and a natural healing art which utilizes acupuncture, moxibustion, phytotherapy, massage, and other skillful manipulations. Humans, who occupy a place between heaven and earth, must bring themselves into harmony with the outer world. For this reason, medicine is intimately linked to cosmology. It tends to expand the practitioner's field of activity and unite it with the universe. (Wong 1990:49)

In is upon this principle that we can understand the medicinal significance of hemp as a prophylactic agent, a tonic and aphrodisiac, and as a therapeutic medicine (Chin and Keng 1992:49). It has occupied an unshakable position in traditional Chinese medicine (TCM), even into the present day. Listed in all official pharmacopoeia (Beijing Medical College 1985:222), hemp appears under the names *hou-ma-ren*, *ma-jen*, or *ta-ma* and is numbered among both the "sedative agents" and the "asthma agents" (Palos 1990:232, 234). In addition, it is occasionally listed among the purgative agents whose effects "purify downward," for it is regarded as an efficacious laxative for elderly persons (Beijing Medical College 1985:222; Hsu 1986:95f.). In general:

> Every part of the plant finds a medicinal use: the stem has dehydrating and diuretic effects; the oil soothes the irritations of a dry throat; the male flowers are used for "wind ailments" and menstrual disturbances. The resin of the female flowers is slightly toxic and affects the nervous system (hashish). It is used for nervous disorders. Li Shizhen notes that immoderate use can lead to "hallucinations and an unsteady gait." (Reid 1988:89)

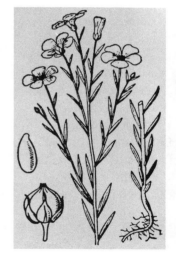

In traditional Chinese medicine, linseed or flax (*Linum usitatissimum* L.), known as *ya-ma-jen*, could be used in place of hemp. (Chinese illustration in an ancient herbal)

Hemp is described in traditional Chinese medicine as having a sweet and neutral character; it has an affinity to the spleen, stomach, and colon. It has laxative effects, stimulates the circulation, functions as an emollient (softening the skin), soothes irritations of the mucous membranes, relieves coughing, and is antiseptic and antidotal. It is usually prescribed for constipation resulting from lack of fluids, especially among older patients, and constipation after childbirth and for urinary retention, menstrual irregularities, vomiting, migraines, rheumatism, cancer, ulcers, infections of the middle ear, and burns. A normal dosage consists of 9 to 30 grams of seeds, powdered, mixed with other drugs, and stirred into fluids or food (from Bensky and Gamble 1986:173f.; Paulus and Ding 1987:247; Reid 1988:89). Linseed can be used in place of hemp: "According to Chinese pharmacology, Semen Cannabis [hemp seed] has the same traditional description of effects as Semen Lini" (Paulus and Ding 1987:248). Sesame seeds are also listed as a hemp substitute (Hsu 1986:96).

As an agent of pleasure, hemp has long been combined with opium. The *Pen-ts'ao kang mu shih-i* notes that "the satisfaction that can be achieved with this is many times greater than with normal tobacco" (Unschuld 1973:145).

Maren Wan (Large Pills with Hemp Fruits)
(from Lee 1996:80)

150 g steamed rhubarb boots (Radix et Rhizoma Rhei)
75 g unripe oranges (Fructus Aurantii Immaturus)
75 g magnolia bark (Cortex Magnoliae Officinalis)
75 g peony roots (Radix Paeoniae Rubra)
56¼ g hemp fruits (Fructus Cannabis)
46⅞ g bitter almonds (Semen Armeniacae Amarum)

Mix the chopped ingredients with enough honey to make the mixture rollable, and form it into pills the size of the seeds of the Empress tree (*Paulownia tomentosa*). Take 50 of these pills with warm water on an empty stomach. This will heal ailments of the lower abdomen.

Laxative

Grind equal parts cannabis seeds and dang gui (*Radix angelicae sinensis*) in a mortar. The dosage is given as 20 grams of this powder. The mixture can also be brewed as a tea.

For Redness, Pains, and Ulcer Formation in the Oral Cavity as a Result of Stomach Heat

Grind equal parts cannabis seeds, jin yin hua (Flos lonicerae japonicae) and gan cao (Radix glycyrrhizae ralensis) and ingest in a dosage of 15 to 30 grams.

I have decided to study agriculture and to go to the market with vegetables.
I have put away my books on the art of war and literature.
The garden is bursting with colorful flowers which gleam in the sun.
On both sides grow dark willow trees, whose branches rock in the wind.
It has rained enough; millet and hemp are thriving well.
The medicinal plants come in small places in the courtyard in late spring.
Before the door lies a great boulder on which one can sit nicely.
Old men say that it is a star which fell from the sky.
                    LI K'AI-HSIEN
                    (MING DYNASTY)

REFERENCES

Beijing Medical College. 1985. *Dictionary of Traditional Chinese Medicine*, Hemel Hempstead, England: Allen and Unwin.
Bensky, Dan, and Andrew Gamble. 1986. *Chinese Herbal Medicine—Materia Medica*. Seattle: Eastland Press.

Chin, Wee Yeow, and Hsuan Keng. 1992. *An Illustrated Dictionary of Chinese Medicinal Herbs*. Sebastopol, Calif.: CRCS Publications.

Cooper, J. C. 1984. *Chinese Alchemy*. Wellingborough, England: The Aquarian Press.

Eberhard, Wolfram. 1983. *Lexikon chinesischer Symbole*. Cologne: Diederichs.

Hsu, Hong-Yen. 1986. *Oriental Materia Medica*. Long Beach, Calif.: Oriental Healing Arts Institute of U.S.A.

Hsu, Hong-Yen, and William G. Peacher, eds. 1982. *Chinese Herb Medicine and Therapy*. Los Angeles: Oriental Healing Arts Institute of U.S.A.

Keng, Hsuan. 1974. Economic Plants of Ancient North China As Mentioned in *Shih Ching* (Book of Poetry). *Economic Botany* 28:391–410.

Keys, J. D. 1991. *Chinese Herbs: Their Botany, Chemistry and Pharmacodynamics*. Rutland, Vt.: Charles E. Tuttle Co.

Lee, Je-Ma. 1996. *Longevity and Life Preservation in Oriental Medicine*. Seoul: Kyung Hee University Press.

Li, Hui-Lin. 1974a. The Origin and Use of Cannabis in Eastern Asia: Linguistic-Cultural Implications. *Economic Botany* 28:293–301.

———. 1974b. An Archaeological and Historical Account of Cannabis in China. *Economic Botany* 28:437–48.

———. 1975. The Origin and Use of Cannabis in Eastern Asia: Their Linguistic-cultural Implications. In *Cannabis and Culture*, edited by V. Rubin. The Hague: Mouton, 51–62. (This source is almost identical to Li 1974a.)

———. 1978. Hallucinogenic Plants in Chinese Herbals. *Journal of Psychedelic Drugs* 10(1):17–26.

Lu, Henry C. 1990. *Chinese Foods for Longevity*. New York: Sterling Publishing Co.

Olson, Stuart Alve. 1993. *The Jade Emperor's Mind Seal Classic*. St. Paul, Minn.: Dragon Door Publications.

Palos, Stephan. 1990. *Chinesische Heilkunst*. Düsseldorf, Germany: Econ.

Paulus, Ernst, and Ding Yu-he. 1987. *Handbuch der traditionellen chinesischen Heilpflanzen*. Heidelberg, Germany: Haug.

Reid, Daniel P. 1988. *Chinesische Naturheilkunde*. Vienna: Orac.

Schall, Paul. 1965. *Zaubermedizin im Alten China?* Stuttgart, Germany: J. Fink Verlag.

Schneebeli-Graf, Ruth. 1992. *Nutz- und Heilpflanzen Chinas*. Frankfurt am Main: Umschau.

Schmidt, Wolfgang G. A. 1993. *Der Klassiker des Gelben Kaisers zur Inneren Medizin: Das Grundbuch chinesischen Heilwissens*. Freiburg, Germany: Herder.

Strickman, Michel. 1979. On the Alchemy of T'ao Hung-ching. In *Facets in Taoism*, edited by Holmes Welch and Anna Seidel. New Haven, Conn.: Yale University Press, pages 123–92.

Thorwald, Jürgen. 1985. *Macht und Geheimnis der frühen Ärzte*. Munich: Droemer-Knaur.

Unschuld, Paul Ulrich. 1973. *Pen-Ts'ao: 2000 Jahre traditionelle pharmazeutische Literatur Chinas*. Munich: Heinz Moos Verlag.

Ware, James R. 1981. *Alchemy, Medicine and Religion in the China of* A.D. *320: The Nei P'ien of Ko Hung*. New York: Dover.

Weber-Schäfer, Peter. 1967. *Altchinesische Hymnen*. Cologne, Germany: Hegner. This book contains the *Book of Songs* and the *Songs of Ch'u*.

Weikang, Fu. 1985. *Traditional Chinese Medicine and Pharmacology*. Beijing: Foreign Languages Press.

Wong, Ming. 1990. Die altchinesische Medizin. In *Illustrierte Geschichte der Medizin*, edited by R. Toellner. Salzburg, Austria: Andreas und Andreas.

Yu, Chaishin. 1988. Korean Taoism and Shamanism. In *Shamanism: The Spirit World of Korea*, edited by C. Yu and R. Guisso. Berkeley, Calif.: Asian Humanity Press.

Zheng, Chantal. 1990. *Mythen des alten China*. Munich: Diederichs.

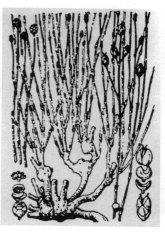

Chinese ephedra (*Ephedra sinica* STAPF) is called *ma-huang* in Chinese, a name which contains the word *ma*, "marijuana." Ephedra has potent stimulating effects and is an excellent medicine for asthma and hay fever. Ephedra leaves are sometimes mixed with hemp for smoking. (Chinese illustration in an ancient herbal)

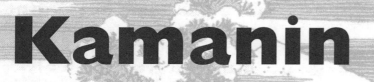

Kamanin

HEMP IN JAPANESE MEDICINE

What is Buddha?
Three pounds of hemp!
JAPANESE KOAN

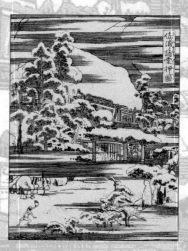

The Japanese ritual hall of Urasa, in which hemp was a required offering. In Japan, the scattering of hemp flowers was once a widespread fertility magic that symbolized "the real sowing on the fields still slumbering under snow." (woodcut, Japan, nineteenth century)

As in China and Korea, shamanism stands at the beginning of Japanese medical history. The Ainu, the indigenous people of Japan (only a few of their descendants exist today, repressed and brutally culturally assimilated, on the northern island of Hokkaido), developed a religion that venerated nature, at the heart of which was a bear ritual. Ainu medicine was usually practiced by female, occasionally by male, shamans (Ohnuki-Tierney 1980). Much like the Siberian peoples, Ainu shamans are known to have used a variety of psychoactive plants, such as wild rosemary (*Ledum palustre* L.) (Mitsuhashi 1976; Ohnuki-Tierney 1980:134). Unfortunately, we do not know whether they knew of cannabis, and if they did, whether it was used for medicinal, ritual, or recreational purposes.

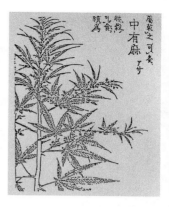

Wood print of cannabis in the Japanese edition of a medicinal herbal originally from China. (from Okamoto Otori, *Mao-Shih-ming-wu-t'zu-kao*, ca. 1785)

During the Neolithic period, a number of Asian peoples migrated from Korea to Japan, bringing with them the shamanism that was practiced in eastern Asia. In doing so, they laid the foundations of what would ultimately become Shintoism (Chang Chu-kun 1988). Shamans have been a permanent fixture in Japanese society ever since that time, and they can still be found there today (Eder 1958).

Korean physicians introduced Chinese medicine to Japan around 400 C.E. It was incorporated into the Shinto culture and made Japanese. The traditional Shinto god Okuni-nushi no Mikoto (Exalted Master of the Great Land) was proclaimed the protector of medicine and expert on herbs. During the centuries that followed, "Japanese medicine" was increasingly influenced and shaped by Korean physicians whose work was based primarily on the Chinese system. It was also enriched by Ayurvedic concepts, which trickled in with Buddhist missionaries (Briot 1990).

A Chinese monk named Chu Ts'ung arrived in Japan in 562 C.E. In his baggage were 164 books on medicine, among them classic works on acupuncture and the *Pen ts'ao ching*, the basic pharmacopoeia of the Chinese, which included knowledge of the medicinal efficacy of marijuana (Briot 1990: 652), and thus hemp officially entered into Japanese medicine. All subsequent Japanese pharmacopoeias have their roots in the *Pen ts'ao ching*. Evidence of the first pharmacy comes from the year 757 (Rosner 1989:19).

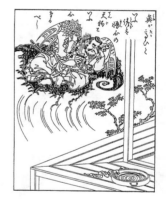

The Japanese Tengu, a shamanic "fly agaric goblin," had an enchanted leaf, a magical fan, which he used to perform his tricks and magic. In some traditional illustrations, Tengu's magical leaf of has obvious similarities to a hemp leaf. Depicted here is Flying Tengu, who produces wind with his leaf fan. (illustration by Ishikama, Toyonobu, Edo period)

Around 808 C.E., the Japanese Emperor Heizei commanded all his governors to collect home medical recipes and traditions from the cloisters and old families in their provinces. These traditional recipes were published by Hizumo Hirosada and Abe Manao in the hundred-volume *Daido-rui ju-ko* (Recipe collection from the Daido era). Unfortunately, most of this invaluable work of folk medicine, in which hemp was certainly mentioned, has been lost (Briot 1990:656).

The oldest, fundamental Japanese work on the use of herbs that has been preserved, the *Honzowamyo* (The names of plants), by Sukahito Fukae, is from 918 C.E., the Heian Period. It is essentially a Japanese adaptation of the large, much older Chinese pharmacopoeias (Hodge 1974:128).

In 1607, a Chinese edition of the *Pen-ts'ao kang-mu* by Li Shih-chen (1518–1596) came into the possession of the personal physician of the Shogun. This work had a great influence on the medical and pharmacological assessment of the plants that flourish in Japan (Rosner 1989:67).

The Japanese physician Hanaoka Seishu carried out the first breast amputation in Japan in 1805. He induced a general anesthesia, using a preparation based on the

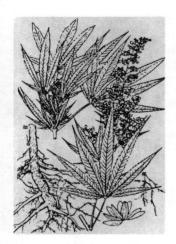

Japanese depiction of *kamanin* (*Cannabis sativa*) in a medical book. (from Kimura)

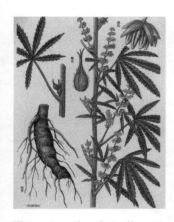

Illustration of medicinally useful hemp (*Cannabis sativa*) in a Japanese book on healing plants. (from Mitsuhashi 1988:23)

Mafusan, the famous recipe of Hua-to (Namba 1980:201). It utilized eight parts *Datura tatula* (= *Datura stramonium* var. *tatula* TORR) and two parts each of *Aconitum japonicum*, *Angelica anomala*, *Angelica acutiloba*, *Cnidium officinale*, and *Arisaema japonicum*; the combined ingredients were chopped and boiled in water. The anesthesia began to work some one to two hours after ingestion and lasted for five to six hours (Briot 1990:669). Hanaoka's recipe differed from the Chinese original in that it omitted hemp. Why Hanaoka left out hemp is unknown.

After officially adopting Western medicine toward the end of the nineteenth century, the Meiji government wanted to do away with the traditional system of medicine (*Kampo*, or the Chinese method) that had developed over the centuries. Chinese medicines were viewed with particular suspicion, and were gradually suppressed (Briot 1990:677). Yet, as in other countries, twentieth-century pharmacologists began to reinvestigate such traditional healing plants as ma-huang (*Ephedra sinica*), ling-chih (*Ganoderma lucidum*), and ginkgo (*Ginkgo biloba*) (Rosner 1989:1).

In the *Shino-Honzo-Sutra* (Teachings about Herbs), a pharmacopoeia that was adopted from China at a very early date, hemp is referred to as *masho*. The following is noted about its effects:

> This hemp heals five ailments and seven types of injuries. But if you take too much, you will go crazy. (cited in Namba 1980:201)

In traditional Japanese medicine (*Kampo*), the dried fruits of hemp (Cannabidis Semen), known variously as mashinin, kaminin, or taimanin, were most frequently used (Tsumura 1991:113).

> Mashinin is a medicine for the spleen, stomach, and intestines. It moistens the intestines and makes the passage smooth, so that it is used to treat constipation. Its effects are like those of sesame, but sesame is useful for nourishing the blood and for the kidneys, while mashinin is useful for moistening and smoothing the intestines. For this reason, mashinin is used to treat constipation caused by a lack of fluids resulting from stomach fever, and sesame is utilized to treat constipation due to kidney ailments and anemia. (Namba 1980:202)

As for the range of applications:

> Mashinin is utilized as a laxative for the elderly, children, pregnant and nursing mothers, and for those who are still weak after a serious illness. It is also used as a remedy for coughs or to moisten. Today, it is primarily used as food, as in the mixture of seven hot spices; as bird food; as a raw material for the oil industry; and so forth. (Namba 1980:202)

In centuries past, hemp's psychoactive resin was also used as a sedative and analgesic, and to induce a medicinal hypnosis (Kimura and Kimura 1978:22).

Kampo medicine has little significance in modern Japan, with its strong Western orientation (Ohnuki-Tierney 1992; Tsumura 1991). Only a few traditional herb shops remain. Kampo is occasionally encountered in such traditional cities as Kyoto and Nara, and in rural areas. Only seeds that are free of cannabinol (namanin) are allowed to be sold. Otherwise, the possession of cannabis products is strictly prohibited. Anyone possessing, cultivating, or trafficking in marijuana faces a jail sentence of no less than five years. In the Japanese underground, hashish is worth its weight in gold. The police crackdowns are brutal and merciless. This notwithstanding, some rituals cannot be conducted without it:

> When a woman has died during labor, her name is written on a piece of raw hemp cloth, which is then stretched out horizontally between bamboo poles. Passersby spray water on this cloth. The cloth then gradually rots and a hole appears, the deceased has then gone on to eternal rest. (Eder 1958:377)

Fiber hemp has long been cultivated in the Japanese prefectures of Ibaragi, Zochigi, Hiroshima, Nagano, Saga, and Kumanoto. There, the plant grows two to four meters tall and blooms in August or September. It is claimed that Japanese hemp exudes relatively little psychoactive resin:

> Japanese hemp for textiles actually contains no toxic part [cannabinol], but has recently become poisonous as a result of hybridization. Lately, however, it has been possible to separate the Japanese variety through gene technology, so that the cultivation of safe hemp has been revitalized. The fibers, such as those for hemp canvas, are produced from the stem cortex. The inner woody portion of the stem is used to manufacture coal for pocket warmers or coal powder for gunpowder. Hemp oil, which is used for dyes, waterproofing, and so forth, is obtained by pressing the seeds. (Kimura and Kimura 1978:22)

Although it is considered a crime to possess medicinal hemp preparations in Japan and violations are punished severely, hemp is still a part of everyday life, for it is an ingredient of the famous spice mix Kaori Shichimi, which is used to season grilled skewers (yakitori). As with so many Asian spice mixtures, Kaori Shichimi is composed according to medicinal principles. It is said to stimulate digestion (especially because of the hemp) and generally promote good health.

Sha-kanzo-to

(from Tsumura 1991:206f)

  6 g dihuang roots (Rehmanniae Radix)
  6 g ophiopogonis tubers (Ophiopogonis Tuber)
  3 g cinnamon bark (Cinnamomi Cortex)
  3 g Chinese dates (Zizyphi Fructus)
  3 g ginseng root (Ginseng Radix)
  1 g ginger (Zingiberis Rhizoma)
  3 g hemp seeds (Cannabidis Semen)
  3 g licorice root, roasted (Glycyrrhizae Radix)
  2 g extract of horse leather (Asini Gelitinum)

This Kampo medicine is prescribed for debility, heart palpitations, and shortness of breath.

Hemp for the ritual purification of ritual sites:

When all [participants] have left the ceremonial hall, then the mountain chief is to spread hemp hulls there, as is customary. The next morning he should bring consecrated wine as an offering, whereby he is to walk backward toward the god, who does not like it when you approach him looking forward. All of the hemp hulls that were scattered the previous evening will now have been broken into little pieces. The people explain this in the following manner: After the people and the mountain chief all went away, the gods came together and did their own dancing, whereby, of course, they tread upon the hemp hulls.

All of these divine events are like children's games, but one should not attempt to understand them with normal reasoning. Certainly, similar things occur in other places; I have reported on them here so that one may compare them with other events of this type.
BOKUSHI SUZUKI
LEBEN UNTER SCHNEE
(1989:251)

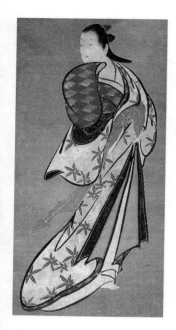

Cannabis once occupied a position in Japanese culture: this Japanese color woodcut from the eighteenth century depicts a woman wearing a kimono adorned with cannabis leaves.

Kaori Shichimi (Fragrant Seven Tastes)

chimpi (dried orange peel)
cannabis seeds
poppy seeds *(Papaver somniferum)*
sesame seeds
aosa (seaweed)
Guinea pepper *(Capsicum annuum var. longum)*
sanshō (Japanese pepper tree—*Zanthoxylum piperitum*)

Mix together equal parts of each ingredient, grind, and sprinkle over food according to taste.

REFERENCES

Briot, Alain. 1990. Die japanische Medizin, in *Illustrierte Geschichte der Medizin*, edited by R. Toellner. Vol. 2. Salzburg, Austria: Andreas und Andreas.

Chan Chu-Kun. 1988. A Correlation of the Ancient Religions of Japan and Korea, in *Shamanism: the Spirit World of Korea*, edited by R. W. I. Guisso and Chai-shin Yu. Berkeley, Calif.: Asian Humanities Press.

Eder, Matthias. 1958. Schamanismus in Japan. *Paideuma* 6(7):367–80.

Hodge, W. H. 1974. Wasabi—Native Condiment Plant of Japan. *Economic Botany* 28:118–29.

Kimura, Koiti, and Takeatsu Kimura. 1978. *Medicinal Plants of Japan* (in Japanese). Osaka: Hoikusha Publishing Co.

Lowell, Percival. *Occult Japan: Shinto, Shamanism and The Way of the Gods*. Boston: Houghton-Mifflin, 1894. Reprint, Rochester, Vermont: Inner Traditions International.

Mitsuhashi, Hiroshi. 1976. Medicinal Plants of the Ainu. *Economic Botany* 30:209–17.

———, ed. 1988. *Illustrated Medicinal Plants of the World* (in Japanese). Tokyo: Hokuryukan.

Namba, Tsuneo. 1980. *Coloured Illustrations of Wakan-Yaku (The Crude Drugs in Japan, China and the Neighbouring Countries)* (in Japanese). 2 vols. Osaka, Japan: Hoikusha Publishing Co. (Contains a genealogy of Japanese herbals.)

Ohnuki-Tierney, Emiko. 1980. Ainu Illness and Healing. *American Ethnologist* 7(l):132–52.

———. 1992. *Illness and Culture in Contemporary Japan: An Anthropological View*. Cambridge, England: Cambridge University Press.

Rosner, Erhard. 1989. *Medizingeschichte Japans*. Leiden, Germany: E. J. Brill.

Suzuki, Bokushi. 1989. *Leben unter dem Schnee: Geschichten und Bilder aus dem alten Japan*. Munich: Diederichs.

Tsumura, Akira. 1991. *Kampo: How the Japanese Updated Traditional Herbal Medicine*. New York: Japan Publications.

Vijaya

HEMP IN AYURVEDIC MEDICINE

Phytotherapy, the science of healing with plants, "was originally 'envisioned' by people with spiritual knowledge. In the course of thousands of years of practical experience, phytotherapy has been refined. Seen from this perspective, Ayurveda is probably the oldest and most highly developed science of phytotherapy in the world that is based on spiritual insight."

VASANT LAD AND DAVID FRAWLEY
DIE AYURWEDA-PFLANZEN-HEILKUNDE
(1987:17)

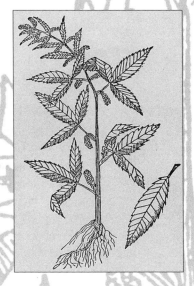

The earliest European illustration of the Indian hemp plant, published under the name *bangue*. (woodcut from Garcia da Orta, sixteenth century)

The Vedas, or Vedic scriptures, constitute the oldest literature of India. *Veda* can be roughly translated as "knowledge"; even today, the Vedic scriptures are regarded as the original knowledge of Indian culture (Mylius 1981). The Rig-Veda, a collection of religious hymns, was written down sometime between 1200 and 100 B.C.E., perhaps even earlier. A number of these hymns sing the praises of a psychedelic superdrug known as soma.

Soma is the name for a plant, for a meadlike inebriating beverage produced from this plant, and for a male god. In the Vedic literature, it is especially the thunder god Indra who is constantly inebriating himself with soma. The plant, which has not yet been botanically identified (Ott 1994), grew on the highest peaks of the Himalayas. From there, the falcon Syená, who can fly as "fast as thought," either stole or abducted it and brought it to Indra in heaven. As an inebriating beverage, soma inspired poetry and possessed the magical power to make offerings effective. ("The falcon brought you from heaven, oh juice that is adorned with all [poetic] thoughts," Rig-Veda IX 86, 24.) The beverage bestowed indispensable mental and physical powers upon the gods; it even became "the element which created the world" (Schneider 1971:vii). According to shamanic tradition, Indra, the original Vedic deity, discovered cannabis and sowed it in the Himalayas so that it would always be available to people, who could then attain joy, courage, and stronger sexual desires by using the plant (Haag 1995:78*). Hashish is also called *indracense*, "incense of Indra." From the post-Vedic period, we know that the soma ritual was conducted using *Cannabis indica* and *Ephedra gerardiana*. It seems likely that "soma" was in fact a generic term that was used in a manner not unlike the ways we currently use the words "drug," "entheogen," "psychedelic," and so forth. The word *soma* has also become a synonym for the "perfect drug."

While soma was attributed with the power to bestow divine vision, it was also a healing agent. Considerably more recent than the Rig-Veda is the Atharva Veda, a collection of medicinal texts and incantations from the seventh century B.C.E. Soma is also mentioned in these texts, as is medicinal hemp, which is referred to as *vijaya,* the "victor." Although the botanical identity of the soma plant remains uncertain, more recent Indian medical literature often equates it with hemp. What we do know with certainty is that hemp was being used as a medicine during Vedic times. The name victor is indicative of its great power in overcoming the demons of illness. Both soma and vijaya are regarded as *rasayana,* elixirs with the greatest healing power (Müller 1954). According to the Atharva Veda, hemp is a sacred plant because "a guardian angel [deva] lives in its leaves" (Touw 1981:25*).

One Puranic myth relates how Dhanvantari, the physician or shaman of the gods, was born during the stirring of the primordial sea, the ocean of space. He appeared holding a milk-white chalice in his hands that was filled with amrita, the elixir of immortality. The moon is considered to be the vessel of amrita. This vessel refills itself every time it is emptied; this is why the moon wanes and waxes. Dhanvantari brought something in addition to the drink of immortality: he brought Ayurveda:

> According to the medical textbook of Śuśruta, he received the Ayurveda, that
> is, "the Veda of the full span of life," from Brahmâ himself. In the Puranic con-

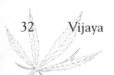

ception, the mere mention of his name is sufficient to destroy the disease. Only a few temples are dedicated to him, but he gave rise to some interesting conceptions because he joined together the two sides of the Indian healing arts: the ability to extend life and the art of defending against illnesses and demons. In the course of time, he became a manifestation of Viśnu. (Gonda 1978:232)

The writings contained in the Vedas form the foundation of the "knowledge" of Ayurveda, the ancient Indian "science of life." Ayurveda literally means "the knowledge of life," and this includes, of course, the knowledge of how to prevent and treat diseases, states of exhaustion, and chronic ailments. Among the most significant fundamental treatises are the *Charaka-Samhita*, the writings of Charaka (ca. 500 B.C.E.), and the *Shushrata-Samhita*, written by Shushrata in the fifth century B.C.E. (Sharma 1985). The most important Ayurvedic textbook from the Indian Middle Ages (800–1500) is the *Sarngadhara-Samhita* (Murthy 1984; Sharma 1981). In these and all other Ayurvedic books, hemp is known as *vijaya* or *bhanga* (Chopra and Chopra 1957). In addition, many sources refer to hemp as *siddhi* (Nadkarni 1976:260). Siddhi is also used to refer to the "wondrous properties and abilities" of yoga and of consummate yogis.

Ayurvedic medicine, which is becoming more widely known in the West, is not a system of folk medicine. It has always been practiced by Ayurvedic physicians and scholars, and has been refined over the centuries. It combines experience with wisdom, the art of living, religion (Hinduism), yoga, and a knowledge of herbs. It is a scientific method that is based upon a rich literature and is taught at universities. In modern India, the physician *(vaidya)* typically receives two educations: one in traditional, classical medicine—Ayurveda—and one in Western medicine. In most Indian hospitals, the two medical systems are utilized alongside one another and are often combined (Scharfetter 1976). Ayurveda has had a significant influence upon the medical systems of the Asian continent. It is, for example, one of the foundations of Tibetan medicine as well as Southeast Asian medicine, and has left its marks on both Chinese and Japanese medicine.

Since early times Ayurveda has defined eight clinical domains. This is especially well documented in the *Shushrata-Samhita* (cf. Scharfetter 1976; Wallnöfer 1990):

1. Salya-Tantra: the doctrine of surgery, specifically, the removal of foreign objects from the human body
2. Salakya-Tantra: the doctrine of general surgery
3. Kaya-Cikitsa: therapeutics; general diseases of the body not associated with organs
4. Bhuta-Vidja: knowledge; beliefs about demons and exorcism
5. Kamara-Bhritya: pediatric diseases and child care
6. Agada-Tantra: toxicology
7. Rasayana-Tantra: the knowledge of rejuvenation
8. Vajikarana-Tantra: the doctrine of the devices of love

Hemp and its products play significant roles, especially in the last two domains of Ayurveda, but is just one of hundreds of plants that have occupied a firm place in the Ayurvedic pharmacopoeia since Shushrata's time. Healing plants are

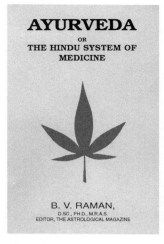

The title page of this book on Ayurvedic medicine clearly shows the central role of hemp as medicine (1994, reprint from 1947).

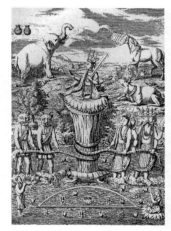

Amrita, the drink of immortality (and a terrible poison), was produced when the milk ocean was stirred. Cannabis is said to have sprouted from a single drop of amrita. (copperplate engraving, nineteenth century)

regarded as divine gifts and are to be honored as such. In Ayurveda, humans enter into an intimate relationship with medicinal plants:

> To properly use a plant or healing plant means to participate in it. When we have become one with a plant, it will vitalize our nervous system and increase our perception. This means that we should consider the plant as something sacred, as a means to take part in all of nature. In this way, every plant, like a mantra, can help us to realize every potential of cosmic life, of which it is a representative. (Lad and Frawley 1987:23)

In this sense, of course, the psychoactive hemp in particular fulfills its role as a cosmic intercessor. It is the plant of the god Shiva, and is thus associated with eroticism, asceticism, and healing (Majupuria and Joshi 1988:167ff.) Tantrics use it as a euphoria-inducing aphrodisiac, ascetics as an aid to concentration, contemplation, and meditation. Shamans use it for their ecstatic trance, and physicians prescribe it for numerous illnesses and ailments (Fisher 1975).

The effects of hemp are characterized as *sattvik nasha,* "tranquil inebriation" (Morningstar 1985:144*). The *Raja Valabha,* a Sanskrit text from the seventeenth century, states: "The gods gave humans hemp out of compassion so that they could attain enlightenment, lose their fear, and maintain their sexual desire" (Morningstar 1985:148*). Contemporary Ayurvedic teachings attribute the following properties to hemp:

> Leaves are bitter, astringent, tonic, aphrodisiac, antidiarrhoeic, intoxicating, stomachic, analgesic, and abortifacient. They are used in convulsions, otalgia [earaches with no organic cause], abdominal disorders, diarrhoea, somatalgia, and heamatorrhoea. Its excessive use causes dyspepsia, cough, impotence, melancholy, dropsy, hyperpraxia, and insanity. The bark is tonic, and is useful in inflammations, haemorrhoids and hydrocele [accumulation of serous fluid]. Seeds are carminative, astringent, aphrodisiac, anti-emetic, and anti-inflammatory. (Sala 1993 I:322)

The Ayurvedic pharmacy utilizes four hemp products:

1. *Charas,* the resin rubbed from the female buds with the hands (contains approximately 40 percent active substances)
2. *Ganja,* the fresh or dried female buds, preferably without seeds (contains approximately 15 to 25 percent active substances)
3. *Bhang,* the upper leaves of the female plant (contains up to 10 percent active substances)
4. *Seeds* (contain no psychoactive substances)

Each of these products may be mixed with many other ingredients and made into powders *(churnas),* brewed in tea mixtures, or combined with ghee (clarified butter). Hemp products are the main ingredients in a wide variety of medicines used to treat diarrhea, cholera, jaundice, tetanus, rheumatism, sleep disorders, pain, coughs, indigestion, impotence, malaria, asthma, neuralgia, migraines, and alcoholism (Fisher 1975:251). The leaves, usually mixed with black pepper and sugar, are prescribed for chronic and acute diarrhea, sleep disorders, tetanus, and menstrual problems. A paste from the fresh leaves is applied externally to treat tumors and furuncles. Freshly pressed juice from the leaves is massaged into the scalp to treat dandruff and lice. Dried hemp powder is applied to oozing wounds and itchy areas of the skin. A paste made from the leaves is applied to treat hemorrhoids, eye ailments, and orchitis (testicular inflammation). Pulverized leaves are used to make a snuff to "cleanse the brain" (Nadkarni 1976 I:258, 262f.)

Great attention has always been paid to the domain of recipes (*vajikarana*) that have general tonic and invigorating as well as aphrodisiac effects (Bose 1981). Every recipe collection, such as the *Rudrayamala Tantra*, from the eighth century, and the *Davasita*, from the twelfth century, includes numerous examples. These recipes usually contain high dosages of hemp, and often include opium, thornapple seeds (*Datura metel*), nux vomica seeds (*Strychnos nux-vomica*), and many spices; less frequently, metals (such as mercury), minerals (such as realgar, oripiment, borax), and animal products (such as musk and toad extract) (Chaturvedi et al. 1981).

Vajikarana
(from the *Rudrayamala Tantra*)

Vilva *(Aegle marmelos)*
Nirgundi *(Vitex negundo)*
Tulasi *(Ocimum sanctum)*
Durva *(Cynodon dactylon)*
Hemp
Milk

Mix equal parts vilva, nirgundi, tulasi, and durva with two parts vijaya (hemp), stir into milk, and drink. The effects are said to be astonishing; it makes humans "equal to the gods and immortal"!

Rasayana
(from the *Davasita*, cf. Vaghji 1985:41)

Mix 1 pound gum resin from the catechu acacia *(Acacia catechu)*
Wheat flour
30 g hydrophilia *(Hydrophilia spinosa)*
30 g *Padellium muracus*
30 g asparagus *(Asparagus ascendens)*
30 g cowitch seeds *(Mucina pruriens)*
30 g broad-leafed orchis *(Orchis* spp.)
30 g cinnamon bark *(Cinnamomum verum)*
30 g broad-leafed Buchanania *(Buchanania lanzan)*
30 g nutmeg *(Myristica fragrans)*
30 g tamala cinnamon *(Cinnamomum* sp.)
30 g cloves *(Caryophyllus aromaticus)*
30 g henbane *(Hyoscyamus niger)*
30 g hemp *(Cannabis indica)*
30 g tulasi or sacred basil *(Basilicum sanctum)*
30 g seeds from Indian bamboo *(Bambusa* spp.)
30 g Layia (?)

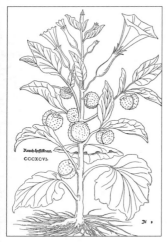

The dried leaves of the thornapple (*Datura metel*) are particularly well suited for use as a tobacco substitute. They are often mixed with and smoked together with cannabis products. The medicinal usefulness of such mixtures is especially pronounced with asthma and bronchitis as well as colds. (woodcut from Fuchs, *Kreutterbuch*, 1543)

The best healing plants are said to have sprung with the sacred soma plant from amrita [ambrosia], the immortal, which trickled down from the fig tree of heaven onto the Himalayas. Because they are under the influence of higher powers they are personified as demons and called upon in cases of illness.

KURT POLLAK
*DIE HEILKUNST DER FRÜHEN
HOCHKULTUREN* (1978:178*)

30 g cardamom *(Elettaria cardamomum)*
30 g paleteri root (?)
30 g China root (perhaps *Panax ginseng*)
30 g pepper *(Piper nigrum)*
30 g poppy seeds *(Papaver somniferum)*
30 g dates *(Phoenix dactylifera)*
30 g ginger *(Zingiber officinarum)*
30 g almonds.
Ghee (clarified butter) to taste
Syrup to taste

Mix gum resin with wheat flour. Add the remaining ingredients. Mix. Knead in ghee and syrup. Bake as you would cookies. In the *Davasita*, it is said that "if a man eats one of these cookies upon rising, he will feel strength, health, and virility in his body."

Jatiphaladi
(from the *Sarngadhara Samhita*, circa the fourteenth century)

One part each:
Jatiphala (nutmeg) *Myristica fragrans*
Lavanga (cloves) *Caryophyllus aromaticus*
Elaici (cardamom) *Elettaria cardamomum*
Tejpatra (tamala cinnamon) *Cinnamomum tamala*
Dalacini (cinnamon) *Cinnamomum verum*
Nagakesara (ironwood tree) *Mesua ferrea*
Karpura (camphor) *Cinnamomum camphora*
Candana (sandalwood) *Santalum album*
Tila (sesame) *Sesamum indicum*
Bamsalocana (bamboo) *Bambusa arundinacea*
Tagara (valerian) *Valeriana wallichi*
Avala (Indian gooseberry) *Phyllanthus emblica*
Talisapatra (East Himalayan silver fir) *Abies webbiana* (syn. *Abies spectabilis*)
Pippali (long pepper) *Piper longum*
Haritaki *Terminalia chebula*
Sthula jiraka (fennel flower) *Nigella sativa*
Citraka (plumbago) *Plumbago zeylanica*
Sunthi (ginger) *Zingiber officinale*
Vidanga *Embelia ribes*
Marica (black pepper) *Piper nigrum*

Mix all the ingredients with 20 parts of bhang and 40 parts of sugar. Daily dose is one tola (approximately 12 grams), corresponding to approximately 3 grams of hemp leaves. To be ingested over an extended period for chronic diarrhea; this powder is also considered an aphrodisiac.

Majun

Mix bhang, charas, ganja, opium, poppy seeds, thornapple seeds and leaves, cloves, olibanum (incense), aniseed, cumin, cardamom, wheat flour, sugar, butter, milk, and flour and add to ghee (clarified butter). This yields a sweet, but slightly bitter, candy that can be eaten for hedonistic, ritual, or medicinal purposes. The effects have been described as "ecstasy, an elation, the sensation of flying, increased appetite, and burning sexual desires" (Thakur 1977:317).

REFERENCES

Bose, A. K. 1981. Aphrodisiacs—A Psychosocial Perspective. *Indian Journal of History of Science* 16(1):100–3.

Chaturvedi, G. N., S. K. Tiwari and N. P. Rai. 1981. Medicinal Use of Opium and Cannabis in Medieval India. *Indian Journal of History of Science* 16(1):31–5.

Chopra, I. C., and R. N. Chopra. 1957. Use of Cannabis Drugs in India. *Bulletin on Narcotics* 9: 4–29.

da Orta, Garcia. 1987. *Colloquies on the Simple and Drugs of India*. 1913. Reprint, Delhi: Sri Satguru Publications.

Fisher, James. 1975. Cannabis in Nepal: An Overview. In *Cannabis and Culture*, edited by V. Rubin. The Hague: Mouton.

Gonda, Jan. 1978. *Die Religionen Indiens: I Veda und älterer Hinduismus*. Stuttgart, Germany: W. Kohlbammer.

Hummel, K. 1959. Aus welcher Pflanze stellten die arischen Inder den Somatrank her? *Mitteilungen der Deutschen Pharmazeutischen Gesellschaft*. 29:57–61.

Kashikar, C.G. 1990. *Identification of Soma*. Research Series No. 7. Pune, India: Tilak Maharashtra Vidyapeeth.

Lad, Vasant, and David Frawley. 1987. *Die Ayurweda Pflanzen-Heilkunde*. Haldenwang, Germany: Edition Shangrila.

Mahdihassa, S. 1963. Identifying Soma as Ephedra. *Pakistan Journal of Forestry* Oct. 1963:370ff.

———. 1991. *Indian Alchemy or Rasayana*. Delhi: Motilal Banarsidass Publ.

Majupuria, T. Ch., and D. P. Joshi. 1988. *Religious and Useful Plants of Nepal and India*. Lalitpur, India: M. Gupta.

Müller, Reinhold F. G. 1954. Soma in der altindischen Heilkunde, in *Asiatica—Festschrift Friedrich Weller*. Leipzig: Otto Harrassowitz.

Murthy, K. R. Srikanta, ed. 1984. *Sarngadhara-Samhita (A Treatise on Ayurveda)*. Varanasi, Delhi: Chaukhamba Orientalia (Jaikrishnadas Ayurveda Series No. 58).

Mylius, Klaus ed. 1981. *Älteste Indische Dichtung und Prosa*. Wiesbaden, Germany: VMA.

Nadkarni, K. M. [and A. K. Nadkarni (revision)]. 1976. *Indian Materia Medica*. Bombay: Popular Prakashan.

Ott, Jonathan. 1994. La historia de la planta del 'soma' después de R. Gordon Wasson, in *Plantas, Chamanismo y Estados de Consciencia*, edited by J. M. Fericgla. Barcelona: Los Libros de la Liebre de Marzo.

Rätsch, Christian. 1995. Mahuang, die Pflanze des Mondes. *Dao* 4/95:68.

Sala, Arya Vaidya, ed. 1993. *Indian Medicinal Plants*. Madras: Orient Longman.

Scharfetter, Christian. 1976. Ayurveda. *Schweizerische medizinische Wochenschrift*. 106:565–72.

Schneider, Ulrich. 1971. *Der Somaraub des Manu: Mythus und Ritual*. Wiesbaden: Otto Harrassowitz.

Sharma, Priyavrat V. 1981. Contributions of Sarngadhara in the Field of Materia Medica and Pharmacy. *Indian Journal of History of Science* 16(1):3–10.

———. 1985. *Caraka-Samhita—Critical Notes*. Varanasi, Delhi: Chaukambha Orientalia (Jaikrishnadas Ayurveda Series No. 36).

Stein, Sir A. 1932. On Ephedra, the Hum Plant and Soma. Bulletin of the School for Oriental Studies. London Institution, 6:501ff.

Thakkur, Ch. G. 1977. *Ayurveda: Die indische Heil- und Lebenskunst*. Freiburg, Germany: Bauer.

Vaghji, Muni. 1985. *Davasita—ein achthundert Jahre altes Buch indischer Heilmethoden und Rezepte*. Augsburg, Germany: Maroverlag.

Wallnöfer, Heinrich. 1990. *Ayurveda: Wissenschaft vom langen Leben*. Stuttgart, Germany: Verlag Stefanie Nagelschmid (edition hannemann).

In India, cannabis was referred to in ancient times as the "giver of delight" and "soother of distress." Today, the antidepressant effects have been most clearly demonstrated for reactive depressions, that is, depressive moods that are reactions to particular events, such as serious physical illnesses. Many people also use cannabis for everyday depression and sadness.

FRANJO GROTENHERMEN
AND RENATE HUPPERTZ
HANF ALS MEDIZIN
(1997:85*)

Bhanga

HEMP IN INDIAN AND NEPALESE FOLK MEDICINE

To the Hindu the hemp plant is holy. A guardian lives in the bhang leaf. . . . To see in a dream the leaves, plant, or water of bhang is lucky. . . . A longing for bhang foretells happiness. . . . It cures dysentery and sunstroke, clears phlegm, quickens digestion, sharpens appetite, makes the tongue of the lisper plain, freshens the intellect, and gives alertness to the body and gaiety to the mind. Such are the useful and needful ends for which in his goodness the Almighty [Shiva] made bhang. . . . the quickening spirit of bhang is the spirit of freedom and knowledge. In the ecstasy of bhang the spark of the Eternal in man turns into light the murkiness of matter. . . . Bhang is the Joy-giver, the Sky-flier, the Heavenly-guide, the Poor Man's Heaven, the Soother of Grief. . . . No god or man is as good as the religious drinker of bhang.

HEMP DRUG COMMISSION REPORT (1884)
(CITED IN ANDREWS AND VINKENOOG 1968:145*)

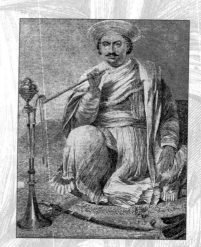

Nena Sahib was a renowned nineteenth-century Indian Brahman who fiercely resisted the British colonial power and urged his people to turn their backs on "all that was English." He is shown here with a water pipe, an Indian necessity for smoking hemp. Brahmans should consume hemp daily for meditation, contemplation, and to study the Vedas. (engraving, nineteenth century)

Hemp grows wild throughout the Himalayas and it is also cultivated on a large scale in some regions, including Manali and Langtang (Atkinson 1989; Malla et al. 1982:61). If you wander through the Himalayas in October, you will see magnificent plants reminiscent of Christmas trees everywhere you turn—even at elevations over three thousand meters. Since Himalayan hemp exudes especially large amounts of resin (*charas*), anyone who wants to harvest some need only rub his hands on the flowers that adorn the sides of the paths and enough for that night and the next will stick to the surface of his hands.

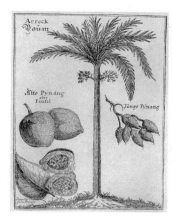

In India, betel nuts, the stimulating fruits of the *Areca catechu* palm were mixed with the leaves and fruits of marijuana and the leaves of the nutmeg tree (*Myristica fragrans*) and consumed to stimulate the appetite and to pleasurably enhance the mood. (copperplate engraving from Georg Meister, *Der Orientalisch-Indianische Kunst- und Lustgärtner,* 1692)

In addition to its traditional use as a universal agent of inebriation at such gatherings as the Holi festival (Patnaik 1993:34), hemp plays an important role throughout India and Nepal in Hindu folk medicine, which has been strongly influenced by Ayurvedic concepts. In folk medicine contexts, hemp preparations are used to combat worms, stimulate the appetite, and treat intestinal ailments, bronchitis, colds, coughs, cramps, delirium, epilepsy, cuts, indigestion, ear ailments, eye disorders, gonorrhea, labor pains, constipation, skin eruptions, paralysis of the tongue, wounds, tetanus, and hemorrhoids. It is also used as a nerve stimulant and as a sleeping pill (Jain 1991:43).

In Nepal, hemp preparations are used for almost every illness (Singh et al. 1979:193). The Bhils in the Jhabua District smoke hemp to treat the pains associated with broken bones. In the Kumaon District of northern India, juice pressed from fresh plants is applied externally to treat hemorrhoids. The fresh juice of the leaves is drunk for stomachaches. It is also given to cattle that exhibit symptoms of upset stomach or stomach pains.

> In India, hemp has long found a multitude of uses, including in veterinary medicine, where the leaves and stems of the plant are used to treat fever and colic in cattle. (Reininger 1941:2792f.*)

Hemp seed is used as bird food in the Himalayan region, just as it is in Germany and other countries (Kaul 1997:108). In the mountainous areas of Nepal, hemp seeds are also pickled for human consumption, while the oil obtained from the seeds is used for frying (Malla et al. 1982:61). Food made from hemp is considered healthy. Hemp is also widely praised as an aphrodisiac (Patnaik 1993:34).

A Nepalese story tells of how hemp came to humans: Shiva was married to Parvati and lived with her in a beautiful house at the foot of the Himalayas. Shiva, however, liked to roam about in the area and amuse himself with other goddesses, and thus was seldom at home. This made Parvati angry. She said to herself: "What am I going to do? My husband is always wandering around while I sit alone in our house." She then saw a hemp plant in bloom. She plucked a few of the magnificent, resinous, fragrant flowers. When Shiva returned home, she gave him the flowers to smoke. Then Shiva smoked ganja for the first time in the history of the world. It made him happy and excited. His third eye opened and he beheld the divine Parvati. Recognizing her as the most beautiful being in the universe, he enthusiastically told her: "Now this is most wonderful. I will stay with you always." And so Shiva and Parvati smoked ganja and drank bhang. And this is why people today still smoke ganja to honor Shiva and drink bhang on his birthday, Shivarattri.

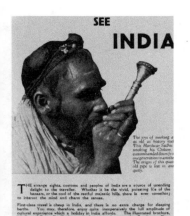

This advertisement uses a chilam-smoking sadhu ("holy man") to call attention to a London travel agency organizing and offering trips to India. Clearly, the ritual and religious use of marijuana has exerted a strong attraction for quite some time. (from *The Illustrated London News*, Oct. 6, 1934, p. 496)

Humankind had been given its aphrodisiac. And this is how the medicine of the gods came into the hands of men.

In Kashmir, gout sufferers are advised to smoke copious amounts of ganja (Vetschera and Pillai 1979:19). In the same region, unripe buds and roasted leaves from the female plant are mixed with honey and swallowed to help induce sleep. Fresh leaves are placed upon the eyelids to treat eye problems (Shah 1982:298). In Kashmir and Ladakh, bhang is made from the larger hemp leaves and various fruits (Kaul 1997:108).

Throughout India, *thandai*, a cold, refreshing beverage containing a small amount of hemp, is generally considered good for one's health, especially when the drink contains asafetida as well (Hasan 1975:240). Many Hindus believe that regular consumption of thandai has aphrodisiac effects and promotes virility (Morningstar 1985:141*). Similar expectations are attached to quids of betel to which hemp has been added (Hartwich 1997:14*).

Hemp is also smoked to treat asthma, especially in combination with thornapple *(Datura metel)*.[1] The smoke is literally swallowed to treat stomachaches. Even hemp ashes, especially those from the smoking tubes, or chilams, of the holy men (sadhus) and yogis, are regarded as a magical medicine. In fact, people do not generally regard the hemp-smoking, long-haired sadhus only as holy men, but consult them for all types of ailments, problems, and diseases (Bokhare 1997).

In India and Pakistan, ganja and charas are used to treat nervous diseases, indigestion, and gonorrhea. Ganja smoke is swallowed to counteract orpiment poisoning and applied rectally to treat inguinal hernias. Charas is used to treat malaria, periodic headaches, migraines, acute mania, imbecility, delirium, whooping cough, cough, asthma, anemia, nervous vomiting, tetanus, cramps, and nervous breakdowns. A tea made from seeds is prescribed for gonorrhea (Dastur 1985:44f.)

---

1. Information about the various devices used for smoking was published in Europe at the beginning of the nineteenth century (Solvyns 1811).

Bhang

50 g marijuana leaves
Black pepper
Cucumber seed
Melon seed
1/2 liter milk
1/2 liter water
Sugar to taste

Carefully wash and finely chop the hemp leaves. Mix with black pepper, cucumber seeds, and melon seeds. Stir in water and milk and sweeten with sugar. This recipe makes approximately one day's dose.

Ten grams of dried leaves can be used in place of the fresh leaves. They should be soaked in water for one hour and rinsed several times before use.

Thandai

Grind equal parts of almonds, pistachio nuts, rose petals, black peppercorns, aniseed, and cloves. Moisten with water to produce a paste, and stir into milk. Add a pinch of asafetida (*Ferula asafoetida* resin) and finely chopped hemp leaves. Sweeten with brown or caramelized sugar to taste.

A psychoactive dose is said to contain about 10 g of fresh or 2 g of dried hemp leaves per person.

REFERENCES

Atkinson, E. T. 1989. *Economic Botany of the Himalayan Regions*. New Delhi, India: Cosmo Publications.

Bokhare, Narendra. 1997. *Religion and Magic in Urban Setting*. Jaipur, India: Illustrated Book Publishers.

Dastur, J. F. 1985. *Medicinal Plants of India and Pakistan*. Bombay: D. B. Taraporevala.

Hasan, Khwaja A. 1971. The Hindu Dietary Practices and Culinary Rituals in a North Indian Village. *Ethnomedizin* 1:43–70.

———. 1975. Social Aspects of the Use of Cannabis in India. In *Cannabis and Culture*, edited by V. Rubin. The Hague: Mouton.

Jain, S. K. 1965. Medicinal Plant Lore of the Tribals of Bastar. *Economic Botany* 19:236–50.

———. 1991. *Dictionary of Indian Folk Medicine and Ethnobotany*. New Delhi, India: Deep Publications.

Jain, S. K., and Namita Dam (nee Goon). 1979. Some Ethnobotanical Notes from Northeastern India. *Economic Botany* 33(1): 52–6.

Jain, S. K., V. Ranjan, E. L. S. Sikarwar, and A. Saklani. 1994. Botanical Distribution of Psychoactive Plants in India. *Ethnobotany* 6:65–75.

Kaul, M. K. 1997. *Medicinal Plants of Kashmir and Ladakh: Temperate and Cold Arid Himalaya*. New Delhi: Indus Publishing Company.

Malla, Samar Bahadur et al., eds. 1982. *Wild Edible Plants of Nepal*. Kathmandu: Ministry of Forests.

Moser-Schmitt, Erika. 1981. Sozioritueller Gebrauch von Cannabis in Indien. In *Rausch und Realität*, edited by G. Völger. Vol. 1. Cologne: Rautenstrauch-Joest-Museum für Völkerkunde.

Patnaik, Naveen. 1993. *The Garden of Life: An Introduction to the Healing Plants of India*. New York: Doubleday.

Shah, N. C. 1982. Herbal Folk Medicines in Northern India. *Journal of Ethnopharmacology* 6:293–301.

Singh, M. P., S. B. Malla, S. B. Rajbhandari, and A. Manandhar. 1979. Medicinal Plants of Nepal—Retrospects and Prospects. *Economic Botany* 33(2):185–98.

Solvyns, Baltazard. 1811. *Les Hindoûs (Tome troisième)*. Paris: Mame Frères.

Vetschera, Traude, and Alfonso Pillai. 1979. The Use of Hemp and Opium in India. *Ethnomedizin* 5, 1/2(1978/79):11–23.

Myan rtsi spras

HEMP IN TIBETAN MEDICINE

Buddhists consume cannabis in order to obtain a mystical experience, the primary goal of which is detachment from worldly things.

NICOLAUS NEUMANN
HASCH UND ANDERE TRIPS
(1970:96*)

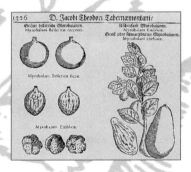

In Tibetan medicine, a number of recipes whose main ingredient is myrobalan (*Terminalia* spp.) have hemp as an additive. Myrobalan is not only a sacred plant, but also a symbol of the Medicine Buddha and of Tibetan medicine in general. (woodcut from Tabernaemontanus)

Tibetan medicine has its roots in the original shamanic religion of Tibet, Bön, and in early Tantric teachings (Baker and Shrestha 1997). Buddhism was introduced into Tibet around the end of the first millennium C.E.; this led to the adoption of Ayurvedic-Buddhist medical concepts as well (Clifford 1984). Tibetan medicine was also strongly influenced by cultural exchanges with the Chinese and the Mongolians (Pálos 1981).[1] Thus, many elements of Taoism, Chinese alchemy, Mongolian herbalism, and the folk botanical knowledge of the high mountain nomads flowed together, so that Lamaistic medicine (that which was taught in the monasteries) developed from these influences but is clearly distinct from Tibetan folk medicine (Devoe 1981). Lamaistic medicine is essentially a comprehensive system of formal medicine that is intensively studied in the Lamaist monasteries.

Of all the worlds, the imaginary was the earliest. Of all origins, the deliberate was the earliest. Of all creations, the reason for arising was the earliest.

TIBETAN MYTH
DAS LIED VOM URSPRUNG DER WELTEN
(1996:16)

> The medical lamas were required to study grammar, mathematics, astronomy, astrology, logic, and, of course, philosophy and Buddhism. Before the examination leading to the diploma, the students would go into the mountains between the 1st and the 13th of July to collect plants. During the examinations, first prize was awarded to the one who could identify 200 plants. The theoretical studies were followed by practical exercises. Ultimately, the government [in Lhasa] would decide to which parts of the country to send the trained physicians. Accounts differ as to the length of the studies. One characteristic was that the texts had to be learned by heart. (Finckh 1991:9)

Because of its gentle treatment methods, Tibetan medicine is now receiving worldwide recognition. Many westerners have had good experiences with Tibetan medicine (Asshauer 1997; Kaufmann 1985), which even offers a hopeful prospect for persons with AIDS (Baratti 1991). Today, Tibetan-Lamaistic medicine is practiced in Tibet, Nepal, Bhutan, China, India, Ladakh, Sikkim, Darjeeling, Mongolia, and even in Switzerland, where Western physicians increasingly advocate an acceptance of traditional Tibetan remedies (Reichle 1997:106f.).

The basis of Lamaistic medicine is the so-called Tibetan medical tree, which, like a tree of life, provides a red thread that runs through the Tibetan medical system (Finckh 1990). The principle text on medicine, the *rGyub bzi* (Four Tantras) is organized along the lines of the medical tree. This work contains the basic treatises on cosmology, anatomy, etiology, diagnosis (use of the pulse and urine analysis), therapy (moxibustion, dietetics, and surgery), the doctrine of medicines, and pharmacology (Finckh 1991). The Four Tantras are illustrated with a series of traditional medicine *thangkas*, rolled pictures with didactic and encyclopedic text (Aris 1992; Byams-pa et al. 1987).

The Lamaistic-Tibetan conception of medicine is based upon the doctrine of the three fluids (the Ayurvedic tridosha) or humors: wind, bile, and mucus. These are the fluids that affect us and determine our health. Diseases result when the

---

1. For example, the five-finger principle, which has had such a dominant effect upon Chinese medicine and alchemy, also plays a prominent role in Tibetan cosmology. The creator god Töndo Chosug is the protector of the five life essences or the five elements (Gruschke 1996:42).

relationships between these fluids are disturbed; the relationships must then be restored to harmony. To achieve this, dietary guidelines and instructions for meditations and rituals (lifestyle) are provided and medicines are prescribed. Tibetan medicines are derived from the plant, mineral, and animal kingdoms. Every individual medicine (raw drug) is a combination of the five elements (fire, water, earth, wind, ether) and thus has a characteristic "taste," that is, a particular mechanism of action. There are six different tastes: sweet, sour, salty, acrid, bitter, and astringent. These tastes are linked to and affect the three bodily fluids. For example, remedies for wind diseases are sweet, sour, salty, or acrid. The effects of the medicines are described by eight qualities: heavy, greasy, cool, coarse, light, bland, hot, and acute. Wind diseases, for example, are treated with medicines that produce heavy and greasy effects. Discussions of the tastes and effects of medicines occupy a large place in the Tibetan medical literature and are always related to the three fluids. Elaborate mixtures of medicines are composed according to these principles (Donden 1990; Finckh 1991).

Hemp has been an enduring component of the Tibetan pharmacopoeias since ancient times (Hübotter 1957; Pálos 1981:25, 35). It is mentioned in the Four Tantras, and the *thangkas* portray two different forms (Aris 1992:64; Byams-pa et al. 1987:190). Both are female. Next to the illustrations of the plants are depictions of vessels with seeds. One of the plants is simply called *myan rtsi spras*, "hemp"[2]; the other bears the additional comment "inferior hemp from Tibet" (Aris 1992:63, 219). Apparently, foreign, that is, imported hemp (which was most likely Indian hemp), was more esteemed from a medicinal perspective. And in fact, hemp that is grown in the warm south does contain a much higher concentration of active substances. Hemp also appears in various Tibetan pharmacopoeias under the synonyms *kha lu mu ta*, *ba lu mu tra*, *su ksnai mu la*, *sug sme la nu la*, *ha ri ta*, *szo yi*, *dzam yam*, *sza yi tri dza yam tri*, *dza ya nitri*, *bi dza ya*, *a ba ra ti*, and *apa ra ti* (Dash 1987:346f.). The medicinal properties of hemp are precisely defined:

> Hemp is bitter in taste, hot in energy, acrid, constipating, light, antiflatulent, soothes kapha [mucus], and aggravates pitta [bile]. It produces feelings of elation, inebriation, and stimulates the digestion. It makes a person talkative. (cited in Dash 1987:347)

The psychoactive effects of hemp products are noted in the medicine *thangka* "Poisons and Their Composition," which corresponds to the eighty-seventh chapter of the medical text *Man-ngag-rgyud, Vaidurya sNgon-po*. It describes "a mixture of fish, butter, radish, egg, plant oil, and hemp seeds. The digestion of such a mixture causes inebriation" (Byams-pa et al. 1987:341).

Hemp is *pittala*; it is used primarily as a medicine to treat diseases and disorders that are caused by pitta, or bile. The bile regulates the activating, warming metabolic functions, and is concentrated in the liver. A pittala medicine stimulates the

---

2. This cannabis "species" has also been construed as *Hibiscus cannabinus* L. (Deccan hemp) or *Hibiscus abelmoschus* L. [syn. *Abelmoschus moschatus* Medik.] (Eibisch) (Aris 1992:219).

functions of the liver and thus the fires of digestion. Because of its antiphlegmatic (mucous inhibiting) effects, hemp is prescribed for internal use to treat nervous disorders as well as diseases of the digestive organs, the respiratory tract, the skin, the lymphatic system, and the genitals. The list of complaints for which hemp is used includes rheumatism, animal bites, scorpion stings, inflammations, leprosy, cramps, diarrhea, cholera, inability to urinate, head cold, coughs, and intestinal worms. It is frequently taken internally for suppurating diseases, especially those of the ear. Suppuration of the ears occurs as a result of excessive fluid production in the head. Hemp dries out this excess fluid and stops the flow of pus (Touw 1981*).

Reports of a Tibetan medicine known as *momea* or *mumio* have come down to us from centuries past. This tonic agent is said to have been composed of bitumen, excrement, human flesh, cranial bones, and hemp (Rätsch n.d.). This recipe is reminiscent of black-magic Bön practices for manufacturing an elixir of immortality (David-Neel 1983). The natural remedy *mumeo*, available today from Russia, is a type of bat guano collected in caves in the mountains of Central Asia.

As a folk medicine home remedy, hemp is either drunk or smoked in order to relax; it is also used as an aphrodisiac (Sharma 1977b*). In Tibetan psychiatric practice, persons suffering from mental illness are often prescribed aphrodisiacs. The assumption is that increasing or promoting sexual activity will have healing effects upon the mind (Clifford 1984; Müller-Ebeling and Rätsch 1986*).

Hemp preparations are occasionally given during childbirth or shortly thereafter in order to strengthen mothers weakened by labor and to protect them from puerperal fever and postpartum depression. Pulverized leaves of young plants are mixed with honey and ingested as a tonic. This combination is said to maintain youthfulness, enhance vitality, increase sexual potency, and maintain or improve the color and the condition of the hair (Touw 1981*). Hemp is also used to increase performance during high-altitude treks and to treat dizziness and altitude sickness—information that has delighted many a foreign trekker.

Hemp seeds and the oil they yield (not to be confused with hashish oil) are an important source of nutrition. In addition, rope and paper are manufactured from the fibers.

Tibetans consider hemp to be a sacred plant, and they often cultivate it in proximity to monasteries and courtyards. In the Lamaistic tradition, it is said that Buddha nourished himself with just one hemp seed a day during the six ascetic years preceding his enlightenment. As a result, hemp seeds are an important food for fasting ascetics. Books in monasteries have been printed on hemp paper since the adoption of Buddhism.

In Tantric Buddhism (*Vajrayana*), psychoactive hemp drinks continue to be used when meditating on the cosmic union of Buddha and his shakti (*yab/yum*) as well as for the actual physical union between temple servants and priests (cf. Grieder 1990:152ff.). Here, the aphrodisiac hemp is regarded as the "food of Kundalini," the female subtle creative energy that transforms sexual energy into a spiritual experience. The drink is consumed 1½ hours prior to meditation or the yab/yum ritual so that the culmination of its effects occurs at the beginning of the spiritual or physical activity. When used in this manner, hemp increases meditative concentration,

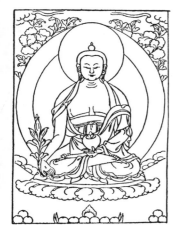

Not only is the Medicine Buddha said to have introduced the art of healing with plants, but one goal of meditation is to merge with him in order to overcome mental and physical ailments. Hemp, of course, is one of the Medicine Buddha's medical treasures. (wood block print, Tibet/ Mongolia, ca. twentieth century)

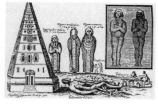

In former times, mummies and the products obtained from them were prized as medicines throughout the world. The name *mumeo*, which was derived from "mummy" (mumia), has survived in the Himalayas into the present day and is occasionally used to refer to a hemp preparation. (engraving from Pierre Pomet, *Der aufrichtige Materialist und Specerey-Händler*, Leipzig 1717, chapter on "Mumia")

improves attentiveness to the ceremony, and stimulates sexuality (Aldrich 1977*; Touw 1981*).

Today, hemp is a component of many important and oft-used Tibetan combination preparations that appeared in ancient medical texts (from Tsarong 1986).[3] The names of the recipes are derived from the principal component of the mixture and the number of ingredients.

---

3. "The overall effect of a plant mixture can be quite different from that of the individual ingredients. Thus, in one recipe, the various plant parts may have no effect when taken alone, but together may have a strong flushing effect. This synergistic effect is the main problem when evaluating a plant medicine . . ." (Asshauer 1997:122). This problem is apparent in, for example, the increasingly popular remedy Padma 28.

A-RU 35—Myrobalan 35

Ingredients:

Plants: *Terminalia chebula, Carthamus tinctorius, Rubia cordifolia, Mucuna prurita, Symplocos crataegoides, Swertia chirata, Cupressa torulosa, Eletteria cardamomum, Terminalia belerica, Emblica officinalis, Caesalpinia bonducella, Eugenia jambolana, Verbascum thapsus, Malva verticillata, Mirabilis himalaica, Acorus calamus, Aconitum spicatum, Tribulus terrestris, Polygonatum cirrhifolium, Pholgacanthus pubinervius, Tinospora cordifolia, Shorea robusta, Cassia tora, Cannabis sativa, Sinapsis alba, Saussurea lappa,* and *A'-'bras* (A'-'bras is a Tibetan plant substance not yet identified)

Animal products: crab shells, musk, donkey's blood

Minerals: bitumen, Gya-tsod salt, saltpeter, cinnabar

Uses: Used to treat kidney inflammation, hip pain, gout, arthritis, lymphatic diseases, suppurative urine

Dose: Take 1–1.5 g mornings or evenings in warm water.

bSAM-'PHEL NOR-BU—Spirit Increasing Jewel

Ingredients:

Plants: *Carthamus tinctorius, Bambusa textilis, Eugenia caryophyllata, Myristica fragrans, Elettaria cardamomum, Amomum subulatum, Santalum album, Pterocarpus santalinus, Aquilaria agallocha, Terminalia chebula, Glycyrrhiza glabra, Verbascum thapsus, Terminalia belerica, Emblica officinalis, Foeniculum vulgare, Nigella sativa, Piper longum, Zingiber sp., Cinnamomum verum, Cinnamomum camphora, Cassia tora, Cannabis sativa, Inula racemosa, Saussurea lappa, Fragaria nilgeernsis*

Animal products: oyster shells, stag horn, crab shells, elephant gallstones, musk

Uses: Use for inflammations of the nerves and blood vessels; to strengthen the brain and spinal cord; and to treat cramps in the extremities; defective functions of the sensory organs; pains in the kidneys, hips, and vertebrae; and contortions of the mouth and eyes

Dose: Ingest 2–3 g twice daily with hot water.

ZHI-BYED 29—Quiet 29

Ingredients:

Plants: *Inula racemosa, Terminalia chebula, Plumbago zeylanica, Myristica fragrans, Piper longum, Cassia tora, Elettaria cardamomum, Asiantum pedatum, Piper nigrum, Amomum subulatum, Zingiber officinale, Rheum palmatum, Tinospora cordifolia, Carthamus tinctoris, Aristolochia moupinensis, Cinnamomum camphora, Cannabis sativa, Hedychium spicatum,* soot, and radish ash

Animal product: calcined cowry shells (*Cypraea* spp.)

Minerals: calcite, sodium carbonate, limestone, bitumen, black salt

Uses: Use for pain (as an analgesic), tumors, digestive disorders, and stomach, abdominal, and liver pains

Dose: Ingest 2–3 g twice daily with hot water.

BYI-THANG 7—Embelia 7

Ingredients:

Plants: *Embelia ribes, Allium sativum, Butea frondosa, Cannabis sativa, Iris ensata, Artemisia nestita*

Animal product: musk

Uses: Use for hemorrhoids and worm infestations

Dose: Ingest 2–3 g in the morning with hot water on an empty stomach, or use rectally as an enema. Apply externally as an ointment for itchy skin.

KLU-bDUD 18—Codonopsis 18

Ingredients:

Plants: *Codonopsis nervosa, Aconitum balfourii, Cassia tora, Corydalis meifolia, Acorus calamus, Tinospora cordifolia, Terminalia chebula, Gymnadenia crassinervis, Terminalia belerica, Cinnamomum camphora, Cannabis sativa, Acacia catechu, Commiphora mukul, Veronica ciliata, Emblica officinalis, Aconitum heterophyllum, Saussurea lappa*

Minerals: bitumen

Uses: Use for disorders of the lymphatic system, inflammations, pains, rheumatism, gout, swollen feet, diseases of the nasal sinus passages, abscesses, itching, leprosy

Dose: Ingest 2–3 g once during the night with hot water.

bSE-RU 25—Rhinoceros 25

Ingredients:

Plants: *Myristica fragrans, Eugenia caryophyllata, Elettaria cardamomum, Bambusa textilis, Amomum subulatum, Crocus sativus, Saussarea lappa, Santalum album, Pterocarpus santalinus, Mesua ferrea, Cassia tora, Cannabis sativa, Foeniculum vulgare, Meconopsis grandis, Veronica ciliata, Geranium* sp.*, Terminalia chebula, Emblica officinalis, Hippophae rhamnoides, Onosma hookeri*

Animal products: rhinoceros horn, stag horn, mountain sheep horn, elephant gallstones

Uses: Use for all diseases of the lungs and respiratory organs, especially to promote expectoration and to expel blood or serum from the lungs

Dose: Ingest 2–3 g daily in the morning or midday with hot water or yak milk.

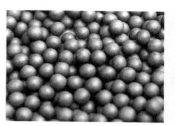

Tibetan medicine primarily uses compound medicines (*composita*) that combine many plants and some minerals, along with other substances into pill form. Hemp is a component of many of these pills.

dNGUL-CHU 18—Mercury 18

Ingredients:

Plants: *Cannabis sativa, Bambusa textilis, Commiphora mukul, Carthamus tinctorius, Terminalia chebula, Eugenia caryophyllata, Ferula jaeschkeana, Myristica fragrans, Acorus calamus, Elettaria cardamomum, Amomum subulatum, Aconitum balfourii, Cinnamomum camphora, Oxytropis chiliophylla, Cassia tora, Acacia catechu*

Animal product: musk

Minerals: purified and detoxified mercury

Use: Use for inflammations and pains in the limbs, vertebrae, and joints; rheuma-tism; and head colds

Dose: Ingest 1 g daily with hot water.

dNGUL-CHU 25—Mercury 25

Ingredients:

Plants: *Cannabis sativa, Bambusa textilis, Commiphora mukul, Carthamus tinctorius, Eugenia caryophyllata, Ferula jaeschkeana, Myristica fragrans, Acorus calamus, Elettaria cardamomum, Amomum subulatum, Cinnamomum camphora, Oxytropis chiliophylla, Verbascum thapsus, Mucuna pruriens, Caesalpinia bonducella, Eugenia jambolana, Gnaplium affine, Saussarea lappa, Cassia tora,* and *A'-'bras*

Animal product: musk

Minerals: purified and detoxified mercury, sulfur, rock salt, bitumen

Uses: Use for epilepsy, leprosy, tumors, edema, swelling of the lymph nodes, inflammations of the throat and epiglotis, swollen feet, gout, rheumatism, and especially for disorders of kidney function

Dose: Ingest 1 g daily with hot water.

sPOD-KHYUNG 15—Garuda of Camphor 15

Ingredients:

Plants: *Cinnamomum camphora, Cassia tora, Cannabis sativa, Terminalia chebula, Terminalia belerica, Emblica officinalis, Veronica ciliata, Tinospora cordifolia, Acacia cate-chu, Saussurea lappa, Commiphora mukul, Acorus calamus, Aconitum balfourii*

Animal product: musk

Mineral: bitumen

Uses: Use for inflammations, pains, hyperacidity (of the stomach), swelling and pains in the joints

Dose: Ingest 1–2 g with hot water before going to bed.

It is noteworthy that most of the ingredients in these recipes are spices (cloves, nutmeg, cinnamon, asafetida, pepper, fennel, ginger, cardamom), food stuffs (bam-boo, garlic, fruits), or aromatic substances (musk, camphor, yellow or red sandal-wood, aloeswood, catechu). Drugs with strong pharmacological effects (such as Aconitum) are seldom mentioned.

Unfortunately, the Tibetan pharmacopoeias almost never provide information about the proportions and amounts to be used. In general, equal amounts of the ingredients are often used when mixing the medicines.

REFERENCES

Ardussi, John A. 1977. Brewing and Drinking the Beer of Enlightenment in Tibetan Buddhism: The Doha Tradition in Tibet. *Journal of the American Oriental Society* 97(2):115–24.

Aris, Anthony, ed. 1992. *Tibetan Medical Paintings*. 2 vols. London: Serindia Publications.

Asshauer, Egbert. 1997. *Tibets sanfte Medizin: Heilkunst vom Dach der Welt*. Freiburg, Germany: Herder.

Baker, Ian A., and Romio Shrestha. 1997. *The Tibetan Art of Healing*. London: Thames and Hudson.

Baratti, Alfredo. 1991. Von Einsicht, Hoffnung und Wohlergehen. *Dao* 2:51–5.

Byams-pa 'Phrin-Las, Wang Lei, and Cai Jingfeng. 1987. *Tibetan Medical Thangka of the Four Medical Tantras*. Lhasa, Tibet: People's Publishing House of Tibet.

Clifford, Terry. 1984. *Tibetan Buddhist Medicine and Psychiatry: The Diamond Healing*. York Beach, Maine: Samuel Weiser.

Dash, Vaidya Bhagwan. 1987. *Illustrated Materia Medica of Indo-Tibetan Medicine*. Delhi: Classic India Publication.

David-Neel, Alexandra. 1983. *Liebeszauber und schwarze Magie*. Basel, Switzerland: Sphinx.

Devoe, Dorsh Marie. 1981. An Introduction to Tibetan Folk Medicine. *curare*, 4:57–63.

Donden, Yeshi. 1990. *Gesundheit durch Harmonie: Einführung in die tibetische Medizin*. Munich: Diederichs.

Finckh, Elisabeth. 1990. *Der tibetische Medizin-Baum*. Uelzen, Germany: Medizinisch Literarische Verlagsgesellschaft.

———. 1991. Tibetische Medizin: Eine Einführung. *Salix* 7(1):5–43.

Germer, Renate. 1991. *Mumien: Zeugen des Pharaonenreiches, Zurich*. Munich: Artemis und Winkler.

Grieder, Peter. 1990. *Tibet: Land zwischen Himmel und Erde*. Olten, Germany: Walter-Verlag.

Gruschke, Andreas. 1996. *Mythen und Legenden der Tibeter*. Munich: Diederichs.

Hajicek-Dobberstein, Scott. 1995. Soma Siddhas and Alchemical Enlightenment: Psychedelic Mushrooms in Buddhist Tradition. *Journal of Ethnopharmacology* 48:99–118.

Hübotter, F. 1957. *Chinesisch-Tibetische Pharmakologie und Rezeptur*. Ulm: Karl Haug Verlag.

Kaufmann, Richard. 1985. *Die Krankheit erspüren: Tibets Heilkunst und der Westen*. Munich: Piper.

Pálos, Stephan. 1981. *Tibetisch-Chinesisches Arzneimittelverzeichnis*. Wiesbaden: Otto Harrassowitz.

Rätsch, Christian. n.d. *Mumio: Neues aus der Dreckapotheke*. Manuscript.

Reichle, Franz, ed. 1997. *Das Wissen vom Heilen: Tibetische Medizin*. Bern, Stuttgart, Germany: Haupt.

Tsarong, T.[sewang] J.[igme] 1986. *Handbook of Traditional Tibetan Drugs*. Kalimpong (Darjeeling): Tibetan Medical Publications.

———. 1991. Tibetan Psychopharmacology. *Integration* 1:43–60.

Kancha

HEMP IN SOUTHEAST ASIAN MEDICINE

Ganja came from India or the Himalayan region to Cambodia, which was Hindu from the first to the fourteenth centuries, and there may be no other people which know how to use the plant in so many ways as the Khmer.

STEFAN HAAG
HANFKULTUR WELTWEIT
(1995:94*)

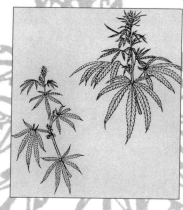

In Thailand, hemp is known as *gan-chaa*. It is numbered among the traditional medicines, but is now illegal. (from Ponglux et al.)

oday, hemp is found throughout Southeast Asia, on both the mainland and the islands. The common names used in this region, *kancha, kanhcha, kân-hcha:, kan xa,* and *cân xa,* all indicate that hemp came to Southeast Asia from India or the Himalayas. It has a long history of use for both medicine and pleasure. Now its use has even spread to indigenous peoples of the Philippines, such as the Igorot (Alegre 1980:38, 60), and to the Papua peoples of New Guinea (Sterly 1979).

The medical systems of Southeast Asia are mixed forms rooted in a variety of traditions. Elements of Chinese medicine, Ayurveda, indigenous healing systems, and rural folk medicine have merged with animistic, shamanic, Buddhist, Islamic, and Western scientific influences. There is even an Ayurvedic group in Thailand. Despite the multitude of influences, the medicinal use of hemp and hemp products in East and Southeast Asia is quite uniform (Perry and Metzger 1980).

The tribal peoples of the Golden Triangle, the area where Thailand, Laos, and Burma come together, also cultivate hemp for its fibers, which they use to manufacture the material for their clothing (Anderson 1993:24, 157). The Hmong smoke or eat hemp for its psychoactive effects (ibid: 159, 183).

In Thailand, the hedonistic use of hemp (known as *gan-chaa*) has been illegal since 1971, and folk medical use is regulated by law. Hemp (leaves, flowers, stalks) may only be prescribed and used in combination with other medicines (Martin 1975:67). The Ayurvedic use of hemp in Thailand is very similar to the Indian practice. Traditionally, hemp has been used as a sedative and to treat painful indigestion, cancer, ulcers, migraines, neuralgia, and rheumatism (Ponglux et al 1987:62). A cough medicine is prepared from dried hemp chopped on a board made from the wood of the nux vomica tree *(Strychnos nux-vomica).* Hemp is mixed with shavings of this wood, which contains strychnine.[1] This medicine is also made in Cambodia (Martin 1975:67).[2]

In Thailand, hemp is combined with white sandalwood *(Santalum album* L.) to make a tea used to relieve dizzy spells and to stimulate the functions of the heart, liver, and lungs. Strong preparations of hemp are ingested for cholera; the water from a water pipe may also be consumed (Martin 1975:71). Because the hemp laws often lead to a shortage of the drug in Thailand, various plants are used as substitutes, including leaves of the kratom tree *(Mitragyna speciosa* KORTH.)[3] and the stems and leaves of a plant in the Compositae family, *pa-yaa-mutti (Grangea maderaspatana* POIR.). Roots of a plant known as *ra:k ya: nang dêng* (probably *Melanorrhoea usitata)* are consumed as a tea or decoction to counteract cannabis inebriation (Martin 1975:69).

---

1. Interestingly, in the nineteenth century *Cannabis indica* was a recommended antidote for strychnine poisoning (Schmidt 1992:650*).

2. It has recently been discovered that in Cambodia, pieces of the wood of the *shlain* tree, whose botanical identity has not yet been determined, are added to ganja to potentiate its effects (Rätsch 1998:219, 615f.*).

3. Kratom is also considered an opium substitute and is used to treat "opium addiction" in Thailand and Malaysia (Beckett et al. 1965:241; Jansen and Prast 1988). The Hmong pulverize the leaves and stems, roast these, and apply the resulting product as a poultice on broken bones (Anderson 1993:136).

The country with the harshest drug laws in the world is Malaysia. There, hemp is completely illegal, and anyone convicted of possessing more than 200 grams is sent to the gallows (Haag 1995:102f.*). As a result, both the hedonistic and the medicinal uses of hemp have declined significantly in recent years. The psychoactive effects are well known to Malay healers, shamans known variously as *bomor, pawang,* or *poyang* (Eliade 1975:329*). A number of hemp preparations are included in their store of traditional medicines. Hemp is a component of a narcotic, aphrodisiac mixture used in Kelantan (Gimlette 1981:220). A Chinese hemp recipe was introduced to Malaysian medicine at the turn of the twentieth century. The medicine, known as *tai foong chee,* consists of seeds from *Hydnocarpus anthelmintica* PIERRE and *Cannabis indica.* It is used to treat leprosy (Gimlette and Thomson 1968; Lu 1991:142).

In Laos, Cambodia, and Vietnam, hemp is legal as a medicine and is available to all. Throughout the region, it is regarded as a means to obviate pain and to relax, especially in cases of migraines and stiffness. These properties are recognized in both folk medicine traditions and in the government pharmacopoeias of these countries (Martin 1975:70).

In Cambodia, hemp is not solely an agent of pleasure. The entire dried plant is freely sold in the markets, for it is an important ingredient in the spicy, stimulating soups *(sngao, sngao moon)* that are offered in numerous Cambodian restaurants and consumed with gusto (cf. Huu 1987). The Khmer consider smoking marijuana (leaves and flowers) a sign of good manners, and it is a mandatory part of social events (Haag 1995:94f.*; Martin 1975:74). Marijuana is primarily regarded as a medicine, no matter whether it is used prophylactically (hedonistic and recreational use) or as part of a therapy. Sick persons, irrespective of the cause of their ailments, often receive small amounts of marijuana mixed into the rest of their medicines. This makes them feel better and also stimulates their appetites. They may also be given a decoction of the entire plant to drink twice daily (before lunch and dinner) or a joint to smoke (Haag 1995:95f.*; Martin 1975:70).

Cigarettes made from hollow stems of the *chkaê sraêng* plant (*Cananga latifolia,* a ylang-ylang plant) stuffed with hemp foliage are smoked daily to cure nasal polyps; they recede and then entirely disappear. A smoking blend of hemp and tobacco is said to inhibit excess bile flow. Malaria sufferers are advised to add 500 g of male and female hemp flowers to a water bath and inhale the vapors twice daily (Haag 1995:97*; Martin 1975:70, 71).

In Cambodia, new mothers often ingest hemp teas, flower decoctions, and tinctures in order to restore their strength and general well being after giving birth. Hemp preparations are also ingested to stimulate the production of milk. Postpartum complications are usually attributed to a violation of food taboos during pregnancy. When these occur, an alcohol or water extract of hemp and other medicinal plants is ingested three times a day until the complaints have subsided.

In Vietnam, hemp use is similar to that described in traditional Chinese medicine, the system that has probably had the most important influence upon the traditional Vietnamese healing arts. The Vietnamese primarily utilize the seeds, dried or roasted, for medicinal purposes. These are prescribed for disturbances of memory,

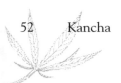

states of confusion, premature aging, labor pains, amenorrhea, and blood poisoning (Martin 1975:72).

Even though hemp is still legal in Laos (Haag 1995:101*) it is used much less frequently than in adjacent countries, because the most important folk remedy in the country is opium. Drinks made from hemp leaves and flowers are administered to treat abdominal pains and stomach swelling. Indigenous magicians use hemp smoke to treat possessed persons. The smoke is also commonly offered to the spirits of possession (Martin 1975:72f.).

Medicine to Treat Cramps (Thailand)

kancha (*Cannabis indica*)
ma ha hing (*Ferula* sp.)
rong thäng (*Garcinia hanburyi*)
kläy tubers (*Dioscorea* sp.)
sa mä thai fruits (*Terminalia chebula*)
sa mä phi phek fruits (*Terminalia belerica*)
sa khàn fruits (*Piper* sp.)
di phli fruits (*Piper retrofractum*)
ka dàt thâng song (an Araceae)
kan phlu (*Eugenia aromaticus*)
khon thi sä leaves (*Vitex trifolia*)
swàt leaves (*Caesalpinia* sp.)
thiam dam (*Abroma augustum*)
thian khaw leaves (*Lawsonia inermis*—Henna)
òp choy stems (*Cinnamomum* sp.)
prik thai fruits (*Piper nigrum*)
matum fruits, unripe (*Aegle marmelos*)
same hearts (*Aegiceras corniculatum*)

Hemp, the main ingredient, is ground and mixed with honey and the other chopped plants.

Hemp Tincture (Thailand)

kancha flowers (*Cannabis indica*)
kòt cù la lampha foliage (*Artemisia vulgaris*—mugwort)
can fruits/flowers (*Myristica* sp.)
peppercorns (*Piper nigrum*, *Piper chaba*, *Piper* sp.)
ginger (*Zingiber officinale*)
òp choy bark (*Cinnamomum* sp.)
sà mun la weng (*Cinnamomum* sp.)
khop chà nang thang song (*Salacca flavescens*)
sannu—arsenic (?)

Chop all the ingredients, mix, and macerate in pure alcohol. Strain. This tincture is used to treat hemorrhoids, laryngeal polyps, and ulcers in the intestinal and genital areas.

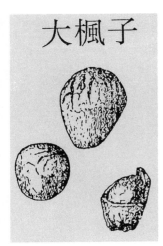

大楓子

Seeds of *Hydnocarpus anthelmintica* PIERRE, known as *dafengzi*, have been used in traditional Chinese medicine since ancient times to kill worms, as an antidote, and to treat leprosy. The plant is found throughout Southeast Asia and is also used in mixtures containing hemp. In Thailand, the plant is called *gra-bao*. (illustration from an ancient Chinese herbal)

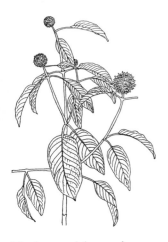

The leaves of the tree known as *gra-tom* or *kratom* (*Mitragyna speciosa*) are used as a folk medicinal substitute for hemp in Thailand and other countries of Southeast Asia. (from Ponglux et al.)

Asthma Smoking Mix (Thailand)

kancha flowers (*Cannabis indica*)
tobacco (*Nicotiana rustica*)

Mix equal parts of hemp and tobacco and smoke in cigarette form as needed to treat asthmatic symptoms. Draw the smoke deeply into the lungs.

Narcotic/Aphrodisiac Mix (Malayan)

ganja (hemp flowers)
chandu (opium)
kechubong (seeds of *Datura metel* var. *fastuosa*)
ikan keli (mucous secretion of a silurid, such as catfish)
merunggai (juice of the horseradish tree, *Moringa oleifera* or *Moringa pterygosperma*)
sago (juice of the pith of the sago palm, *Metroxylon sagu*)

Unfortunately, I have no information about the amounts of each ingredient to use. This mixture is strongly reminiscent of the Oriental Joy Pills (Rätsch 1990b*).

Tai Foong Chee (Chinese/Malaysian Leprosy Medicine)

2 parts chaulmoogra seeds (*Hydnocarpus anthelmintica*)
1 part hemp flowers and leaves (*Cannabis indica*)

Crush and sift the chaulmoogra seeds. Mix these with the hemp flowers and leaves. Use for external, local treatment. (In Chinese medicine, the leprosy remedy consists of *Hydnocarpus* seeds, calomel, and sesame oil.)

Pain and Relaxation Medicine (Cambodia, Thailand, Laos, Vietnam)

Boil sun-dried hemp leaves (usually male and female). Use approximately 5 grams per ¼ liter of water. Other aromatic plants may also be added. This decoction is ingested before going to bed or before dinner to treat migraines and stiffness.

Digestive Drink (Cambodia)

têpiru bark (a myrtle plant)
sâmbä lvêng (*Cinnamomum* sp.)
kânhcha (*Cannabis indica*)

Mix the ingredients and boil in water. Drink one full glass before every meal.

Milk-Producing Drink (Cambodia)

sâmbä lvêng stems (*Cinnamomum* sp.)
kânhcha flowers (*Cannabis indica*)
dâng kwen (*Tetracera loureiri*)
sdok sdao (*Walsura villosa*)
vä kro:c (*Illigera* sp.)

Mix and boil all the ingredients. Drink one glass twice daily.

> ## Medicinal Hemp Tincture (Cambodia)
>
> kâncha flowers *(Cannabis indica)*
> têpiru bark (a myrtle plant)
> khtom bark *(Mitragyna* sp., *M. speciosa* [?])
> sâmbä lvêng stems *(Cinnamomum* sp.)
> sdok sdao bark *(Walsura villosa)*
> matum bark *(Aegle marmelos)*
>
> Cover all the ingredients with pure grain alcohol and allow to macerate for sev-
> eral days. Use to treat stiffness following childbirth.

REFERENCES

Alegre, Dennis G. 1980. *Sagada: A Survey of the Folk Herbal Practices of the Sagada Igorots in Mountain Province and Some Important Implications.* Los Baños/Luzon: College of Agriculture, University of the Philippines (MS).

Anderson, Edward F. 1993. *Plants and People of the Golden Triangle: Ethnobotany of the Hill Tribes of Northern Thailand.* Portland, Oregon: Dioscorides Press.

Beckett, A. H., E. J. Shellard, and A. N. Tackie. 1965. The *Mitragyna* Species of Asia—The Alkaloids of the Leaves of *Mitragyna speciosa* KORT.: Isolation of Mitragynine and Speciofoline. *Planta Medica* 13(2):241–6.

Gimlette, John D. [1929] 1981. *Malay Poisons and Charm Cures.* Reprint, Kuala Lumpur: Oxford in Asia Paperbacks.

Gimlette [John D.] and Thomson. 1968. A Dictionary of Malayan Medicine, 1939. In *The Book of Grass,* edited by G. Andrews and S. Vinkenoog. New York: Grove Press, page 146.

Huu, Tien 1985. *Augen lachen, Lippen blühen: Erotische Lyrik aus Vietnam.* Munich: Simon und Magiera.

———. 1987. *Liebe im Reisfeld: Die erotische Kochkunst Asiens.* Munich: Simon und Magiera.

Jacquat, Christiane. 1990. *Plants from the Markets of Thailand.* Bangkok: Duang Kamol Book House.

Jansen, Karl L. R., and Colin J. Prast. 1988. Ethnopharmacology of Kratom and the *Mitragyna* Alkaloids. *Journal of Ethnopharmacology* 23:115–9.

Lu, Henry C. 1991. *Legendary Chinese Healing Herbs.* New York: Sterling Publishing Co.

McMakin, Patrick D. 1993. *Flowering Plants of Thailand: A Field Guide.* Bangkok: White Lotus.

Macmillan, H. F. 1991. *Tropical Planting and Gardening.* 6th ed. Kuala Lumpur: Malayan Nature Society.

Martin, Marie Alexandrine. 1975. Ethnobotanical Aspects of Cannabis in Southeast Asia. In *Cannabis and Culture,* edited by V. Rubin. The Hague: Mouton, pages 63–75.

Perry, Lily, and Judith Metzger. 1980. *Medicinal Plants of East and Southeast Asia.* Cambridge, Mass.: MIT Press.

Ponglux, Dhavadee et al., eds. 1987. *Medicinal Plants.* Bangkok: Victory Power Point.

Sterly, Joachim. 1979. Cannabis am oberen Chimbu, Papua New Guinea. *Ethnomedizin* 5(1/2):175–8.

Penka

THE HEMP RITUAL OF THE SCYTHIANS

Among other things, hemp was used [as an incense] in order to be able to see into the future and to speak with the dead, but also for sleep disorders and migraines or to come into contact with the higher self.

FRED WOLLNER
DUFTENDER RAUCH FÜR DIE SEELE
(1998:141)

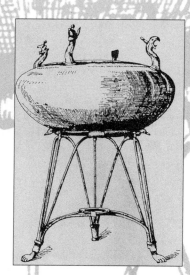

In ancient times, incense was usually burned in bronze tripods. Hemp, frequently used as an ingredient in incense mixtures, was known as "Scythian fire." It was used in this form as a ritual incense in the sacred cult of Asclepius. (illustration, nineteenth century)

Herodotus of Halicarnassus (ca. 500–424 B.C.E.) is considered the founder of ethnography as well as of adventure and educational tourism. The Greek fled from his home because of political turmoil, studied for a long time in Athens, lived on Samos, and between 455 and 444 B.C.E. undertook extended journeys to Egypt, Syria, Cyprus, Asia Minor, northern Greece, Thrace, Macedonia, and high into the Crimean peninsula. He wrote the standard work of antiquity on the geography, history, and ethnography of the eastern Mediterranean region. His *Nine Books of History* still provide us with valuable ethnohistorical material on the cultures of the Egyptians, Babylonians, Libyans, and Hyperboreans, as well as on the Scythians. In ancient times, the name *Scythian* was a collective term used to refer to nomadic horse peoples who lived on the Black Sea, along the Danube, and in southern Russia, and who spoke a variety of Indo-Iranian languages or dialects (Pavlinskaya 1989:19). Many Scythian tribes established extensive trade relationships with the Pontus Greeks. They were regarded as wild warriors and were feared and respected by all. They also stopped the brutal invasion of the Persians into Pontus.

Herodotus dedicated an extensive chapter of his work to the culture of the Scythians. In it, he described Scythian social structure, religion, mythology, and customs, which he repeatedly compared to his own Greek, or Hellenistic culture. He was particularly impressed by a burial ritual or ritual of the dead:

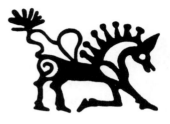

The Scythians were a nomadic people who were closely associated with the horse, as can be seen in many prehistoric petroglyphs found in their territory. Because of their great mobility, they helped to widely disseminate the cannabis throughout Asia. (petroglyph on an "altar rock," West Iran, ca. first millennia B.C.E.)

> After the burial, the Scythians purify themselves in the following manner: When they have washed and applied ointment to their heads, they begin the following cleansing ritual: they lean three poles against one another, and then spread woolen felt blankets over these. After they have stuffed the blankets together as tightly as they can, they toss glowing stones taken from a fire into a basin standing in the middle of the room made of poles and felt blankets.
>
> Now in their land grows hemp, which looks very much like flax but is much thicker and taller. It grows by itself, but is also sown; indeed, the Thracians even use it to make fabrics for themselves that are very similar to the linen ones, and anyone who does not precisely know of these things will have difficulty distinguishing whether they are from flax or hemp. But anyone who has never seen hemp will think it is flax.
>
> After they slip under the felt tent, the Scythians take of the seeds of this hemp and throw these on the red-hot stones. This produces a smoke and a steam, against which no Hellenic sweat bath can compete. This gives the Scythians such delightful satisfaction that they shout with joy. It serves them in the place of a bath, for they do not bathe in water. Only their women use water as part of a mixture of cypress, cedar, and olibanum wood, which they rub on a coarse stone. They smear this over their whole body and face; for it lends them a delightful fragrance, and when they remove the plaster the following day, they have a clean and shining skin. (IV, 73–75)

It seems likely that the hemp seeds were still lodged in the flower buds, for how else could there have been a "smoke and a steam" that would have caused the Scythians such jubilation? According to Jettmar (1981:310) this could be "a description of a cult activity in which the deceased's next-of-kin accompanied the soul of the departed into the other world in a shamanic trance. This was a form of 'family shamanism,' in which there was as yet no distinct specialization." This ritual, in other words, served to promote the well-being of both the soul of the deceased and of the souls of those who remained behind (Eliade 1975:376ff.*) Here, hemp loosened the boundaries of death and allowed humans to take part in the immortality of the soul by utilizing the purifying effects of the drug on the body and spirit to collectively overcome sorrow and prevent depression. This is probably the reason why hemp has been known as "Scythian fire" since late antiquity. It has even been suggested that hemp "is probably the oldest of plants that humans have used for fumigation" (Wollner 1998:140).

Similar rituals were also known among other ancient tribes. The Thracians, for example, knew how to produce a healing inebriation. The Massagets, a nomadic tribe from central Asia, camped together around fires in which certain "fruits" were tossed, causing the participants to spring up enraptured after inhaling the smoke (Jettmar 1972, 1981).

In his *Books of History*, Herodotus provides us with the following story from Assyria:

> Of the River Araxes [Jaxartes/Syr Darja], some say that it is larger than the Istros, others that is smaller. Numerous islands are said to lie within it, about the size of the island of Lesbos, and these are inhabited by people who dig out all kinds of roots in the summer and nourish themselves from these, but in winter they live from the fruits of trees, which they collect and store after they have ripened. They also have other trees which bear very special fruits. When many people have come together, they light a fire, sit around it in a circle, and throw these fruits into the fire. When the smell of the burning fruits enters their noses, they become inebriated like the Greeks from their wine. They throw more and more fruits into the fire, so that they become more and more inebriated and finally jump up to dance and to sing. This is what is said about the way they live. (II, 202)

The "fruits" burned here as an incense sound suspiciously like female hemp flowers, while the manner of their use is strongly reminiscent of the Scythian purification ritual. However, it is not possible to know their identity with certainty.

The Scythians, who have left us a rich and very characteristic art with animal ornamentation and other shamanic themes, had already penetrated deep into central and eastern Asia by the fifth century B.C.E. (Pavlinskaya 1989). A great deal of archaeological evidence of the Scythian culture has been excavated from the Altai Mountains of Mongolia. For example, the barrows of Pazaryk in the High Altai were frozen in the high mountain ice and thus perfectly preserved. Excavations of these barrows, which began in 1929, have provided sensational confirmation of the reports of Herodotus. The Russian archaeologist S. I. Rudenko recovered various bronze incense vessels, above which a frame covered with felt still stood (Clarke 1995). According to Rudenko's report on the excavation,

In addition to the stones already mentioned, both vessels were found to contain a large amount of hemp seeds (*Cannabis sativa* L. of the variety *C. ruderalis* Janisch). Hemp seeds were also in one of the leather bottles described previously, which was attached to one of the poles of the hexapod which stood over the vessel in the form of a Scythian kettle. The stones in the incense vessels had been scorched, a portion of the hemp seeds blackened. In addition, the handles of the kettle that had been used as an incense vessel were wrapped around with birch bast. Clearly, the vessel had been so heated by the glowing stones that it could not have been picked up with the bare hands. . . . Consequently, we have here complete sets of those utensils which were necessary to carry out the purification ritual which Herodotus so precisely recorded in reference to the Pontic Scythians. (cited in Jettmar 1981:311)

In Turkmenistan and Tajikistan, hemp pollen and the remains of other psychoactive substances were discovered in ritual drinking utensils found in many temple complexes that date to around the second millennium B.C.E. and which may have been associated with the Scythian culture (Sarianidi 1994; Sherratt 1995:29).

As well as being known as "Scythian fire," hemp was also known as "Scythian incense," both clear indications of the preeminent position of the plant in Scythian ethnobotany. However, late ancient writers such as the lexicographer and grammarian Hesychius of Alexandria (fifth/sixth century C.E.) were rather critical of "hemp, a Scythian incense, which has the power of stealing the youthful vigor of all who stand near" (cit. in Hartwich 1997:9*).

The ancient Scythians also used hemp for hedonistic purposes (Rocker 1995). Recently, a Scythian shaman was discovered in a frozen, undisturbed grave in the Altai Mountains. She possessed hashish as well as other hemp products (*Stern* 18/94, p. 194ff.).

In the Middle Ages, hemp was still known in some parts of Russia as *penka*, a word that is said to be of Scythian origin (Golowin 1989:160) and that is reminiscent of the ancient Iranian *bhanga*, "inebriating agent." Penka was consumed in familiar company as tea.

Today, the species *Cannabis ruderalis* grows throughout the region once inhabited by the Scythians. It still finds use in both Russian and Mongolian folk medicine, especially to treat depression. Recently, the Mongolian Academy of Sciences sponsored a project aimed at documenting all the shamanic, folk, and Lamaistic knowledge about medicinal plants (oral communication from Mr. Günther, Ulan Bator). This project found that in the Mongolian tradition, *Cannabis sativa* and *Cannabis ruderalis* are used for different medicinal purposes. *Cannabis sativa* is used primarily as a source of oil, whereas *Cannabis ruderalis* is esteemed more for its psychoactive properties. It is very likely that Mongolian shamans in the Altai used *Cannabis ruderalis* in addition to juniper (cf. Jettmar 1981) or savin juniper (*Juniperus sabina*) to induce shamanic trances. Clearly, the Scythians have left a legacy that has continued into our times (cf. Sikojev 1985:325). This includes the use of hemp from the Altai Mountains. A Mongolian medicine named *bagaschun*, said to be a type of cure-all and apparently made from hemp, juniper, and bat guano, comes from the

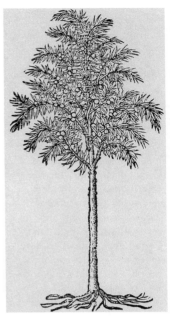

In Eurasia, juniper needles (*Juniperus* spp.) were often mixed with marijuana flowers to make shamanic incenses. Juniper is one of the oldest incenses of humankind, and is utilized by shamans and folk healers wherever it grows. (woodcut from Gerard, 1633)

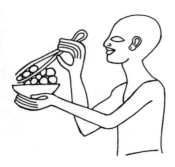

Altai. This preparation is also known as *mumio*, and is esteemed as a tonic in Russian folk medicine.

During Herodotus's lifetime it was a common and widespread practice to fumigate with aromatic plants and resins. In Mesopotamia and Egypt, incense mixtures were rolled into pills. Some of the recipes contained hemp flowers. As a result of the Scythian incense rituals, hemp was also occasionally referred to as "sacred incense." (relief in a grave, Memphis, nineteenth dynasty)

Recipe for Shamanic Incense

Female hemp flowers (*Cannabis* spp.)
Juniper needles (*Juniperus communis* L.)
Wild thyme (*Thymus serpyllum* L.)
Spruce resin (*Picea* spp.)

Mix equal parts of each ingredient together in a bowl. Toss the mixture onto glowing coals. Deep inhalation will induce psychoactive effects.

The tips of branches of the savin juniper (*Juniperus sabina* L.) can be used in place of the juniper needles, garden thyme (*Thymus vulgaris* L.) can be substituted for wild thyme, and fir or pine resin (*Abies* spp., *Pinus* spp.) can be used instead of spruce resin.

A similar shamanic incense with psychoactive effects can be mixed from equal parts of hemp flowers, the tips of juniper branches (*Juniperus communis* L., *Juniperus recurva* Buch.-Ham., *Juniperus* spp.), thyme (*Thymus* spp.), and wild rosemary (*Ledum palustre* L.).

REFERENCES

Clarke, Robert C. 1995. Scythian *Cannabis* Verification Project. *Journal of the International Hemp Association* 2(2):194.

Golowin, Sergius. 1989. *Das Reich des Schamanen*. Munich: Goldmann.

Herodotus. 1984. *Neun Bücher der Geschichte*. Essen, Germany: Phaidon.

Jettmar, Karl 1972. Schamanismus in Nord- und Zentralasien. In *Ergriffenheit und Besessenheit*, edited by J. Zutt. Bern, Switzerland: Francke, pages 105–15.

———. 1981. Skythen und Haschisch. In *Rausch und Realität*, edited by Gisela Völger. Vol. 1. Cologne: Rautenstrauch-Joest-Museum, pages 310–3.

Meuli, K. 1935. Scythia. *Hermes*. 70/1, Berlin.

Pavlinskaya, Larisa 1989. The Scythians and Sakians, Eighth to Third Centuries B.C. In *Nomads of Eurasia*, edited by Vladimir Basilov. Los Angeles: Natural History Museum and Seattle: University of Washington Press, pages 19–39.

Rocker, Tom 1995. Hanfkonsum im Altertum: Die Skythen. *Hanfblatt* 2(11):19.

Rudenko, S. I. 1970. *Frozen Tombs of Siberia: The Pazaryk Burials of Iron Age Horsemen*. Berkeley: University of California Press.

Sarianidi, V. 1994. Temples of Bronze Age Margiana: Traditions of Ritual Architecture. *Antiquity* 68:388–97.

Sherratt, Andrew. 1995. Alcohol and Its Alternatives: Symbol and Substance in Pre-industrial Cultures. In *Consuming Habits*, edited by J. Goodman et al. London: Routledge, pages 11–46.

Sikojev, André. 1985. *Die Narten—Söhne der Sonne: Mythen and Heldensagen der Skythen, Sarmaten und Osseten*. Cologne, Germany: Diederichs.

Wollner, Fred. 1998. *Duftender Rauch für die Seele: Vom praktischen Umgang mit Räucherwerk*. Munich: Goldmann.

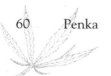

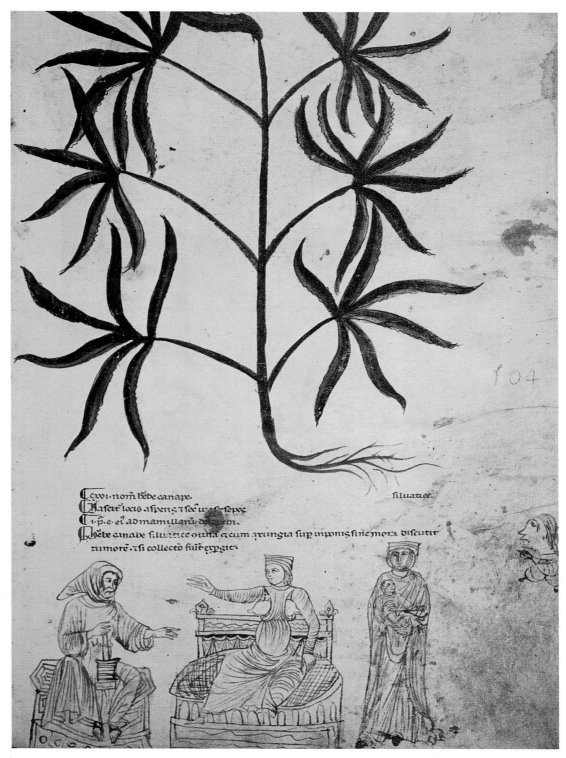

The hemp plant, here referred to as *canape*, as
depicted in the manuscript *Medicina antiqua* (ninth
century), attributed to Pseudo Apuleius. It is listed as
a remedy for nipple pains and frostbite. (*Codex
Vindobonensis* 93, 108r)

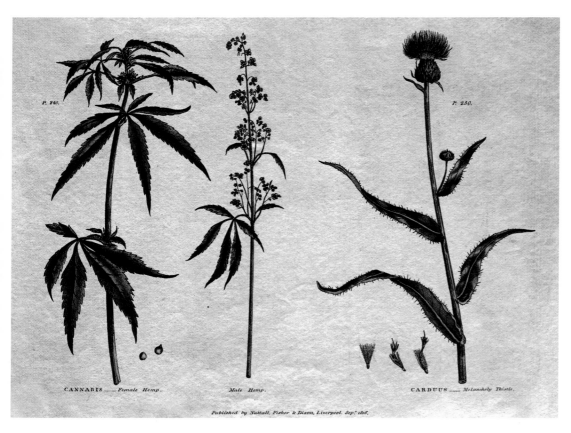

Botanical illustration of dioecious hemp. (hand-colored copperplate engraving, England, 1816)

Botanical representation of *Cannabis sativa*
 A. male plant in flower
 B. female plant in fruit
 1. male flower
 2. anther
 3. anther, viewed from the opposite side
 4. pollen grain
 5. female flower with bract
 6. female flower without bract
 7. ovary in longitudinal section
 8. fruit with bract
 9. fruit without bract
10. seed
11. seed in cross-section
12. seed in longitudinal section
13. seed with seedcoat removed
(from *Köhler's Medizinal-Pflanzen,* 1887)

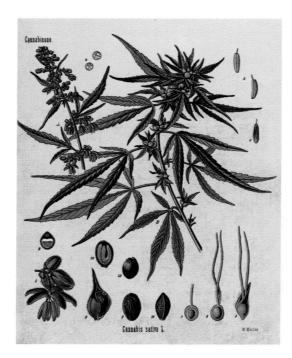

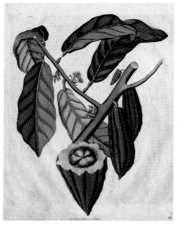

New research has revealed that chocolate, which is produced from the cacao tree *(Theobroma cacao),* contains anandamide, the same substance that binds to the THC receptor sites in the human nervous system and produces pleasant states of consciousness. (hand-colored copperplate engraving, Germany, nineteeth century)

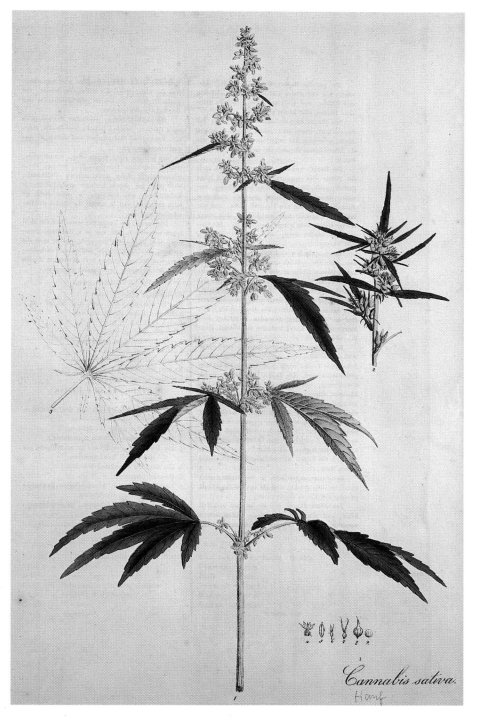

Fiber hemp *(Cannabis sativa)* is one of the traditional cultigens of Central Europe. In the center is a male plant in bloom; a female flower is shown at right. (antique colored copperplate engraving, 1850)

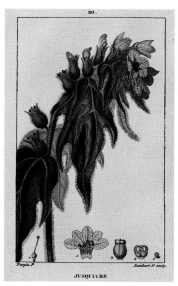

Above: Black henbane *(Hyoscyamus niger)* is a popular tobacco substitute and is smoked together with hemp in many countries of the world. (copperplate engraving from Tabernaemontanus, 1731)

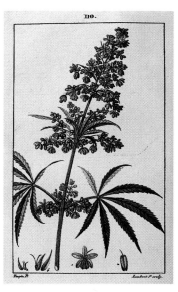

Below: In earlier times, the plant that modern botany now recognizes as the male hemp plant was thought to be the "little female," probably because it contains only a small amount of active substances and is of little value. (copperplate engraving from Tabernaemontanus, 1731)

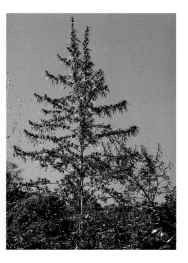

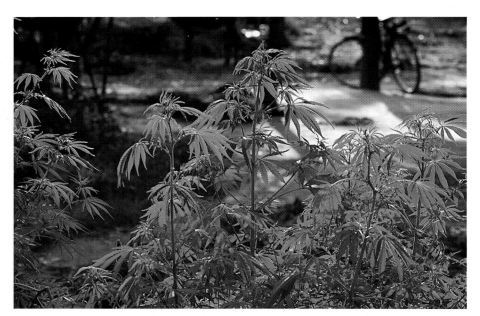

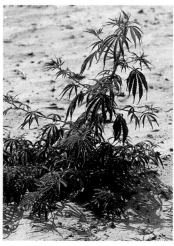

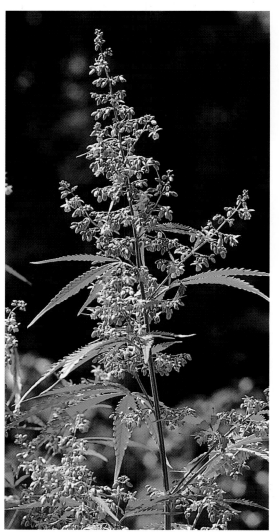

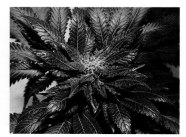

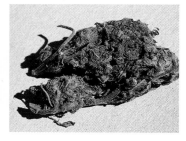

Above left: In the Himalayas in Nepal, *Cannabis indica* is still a true wild plant. Full-grown female specimens often resemble Christmas trees. (photographed near Sikeh, Nepal)

Below left: In Uttar Pradesh, North India, *Cannabis sativa* occurs as a true wild plant, fields of which can be very large.

Above right: Hemp (*Cannabis sativa*) is a very adaptable plant. In North India, wild plants even thrive in sand! (on an island in the Ganges at Septarishi, near the sacred pilgrimage city of Hardwar)

Below middle: The inflorescence of a male cannabis plant.

Small photo above: The female flower of an indoor-grown *Cannabis indica* plant is very rich in THC and covered with tiny drops of resin.

Below: The dried, resinous inflorescences of the female cannabis plant are commonly referred to as marijuana, ganja, or grass.

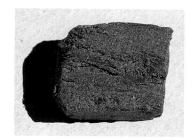

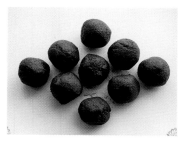

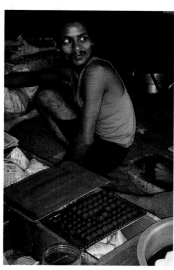

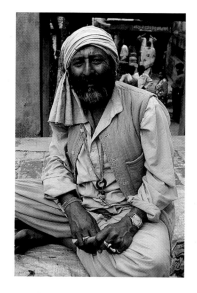

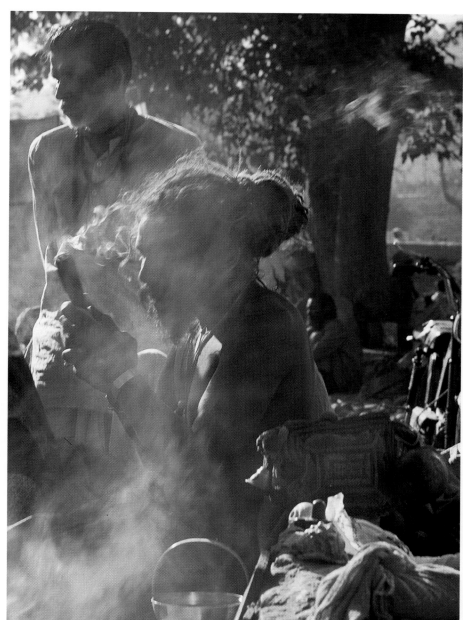

Left, from top to bottom:
The resin rubbed from the female inflorescences is called *charas* in the Himalayas, but is typically sold as hashish in the West. This photo shows a Swiss product.

Balls of bhang, from Varanasi, India.

In Varanasi (Benares), the "City of Light" sacred to Shiva, there are small shops that sell bhang.

North Indian folk healers use magical objects as well as medicinal plants, especially hemp, when treating their patients.

The sadhus, the holy men of India and Nepal, practice a variety of forms of yoga. They also smoke copious amounts of *charas* (hashish). Because of the psychoactive effects of the drug, they are able to control their body and their bodily functions at will. Most sadhus possess a good knowledge of Tantric medicine and yogic alchemy. (photographed in Hardwar during the 1998 Kumbha Mela)

65

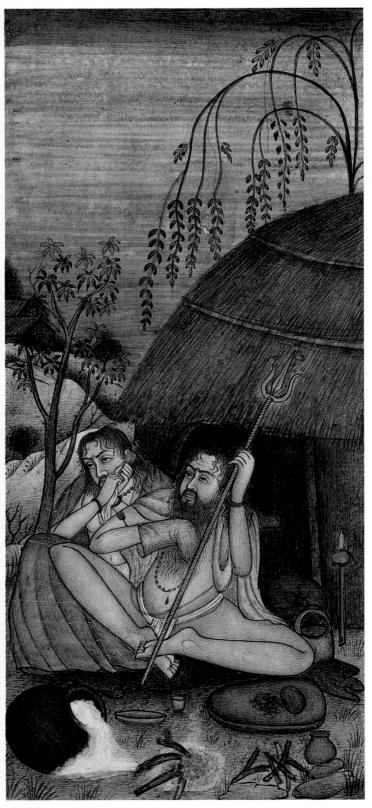

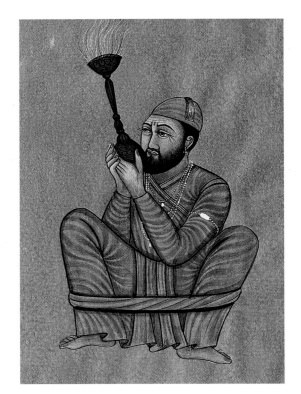

Above: In India's Muslim culture, smoking hashish in a hookah is a regular part of daily life. It is also done for medicinal and spiritual purposes. (miniature, Rajasthan, twentieth century)

Left: Chilam-smoking sadhus or yogis in front of their hermitage. (miniature, Rajasthan, twentieth century)

Facing page: Hindus, especially members of the Brahman caste, smoke hemp products for relaxation, inspiration, religious insight, spiritual development, and improved health. (colored copperplate engraving from F. Baltazard Solvyns, *Les Hindoûs*, Vol. 3, Paris, 1811)

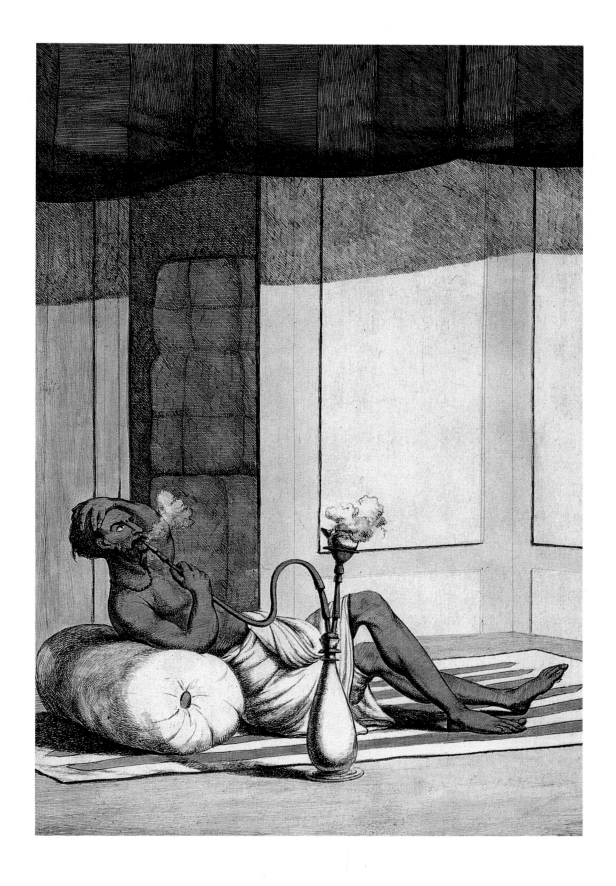

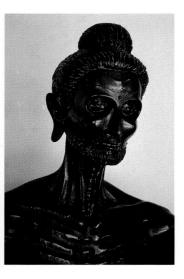

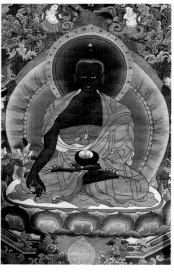

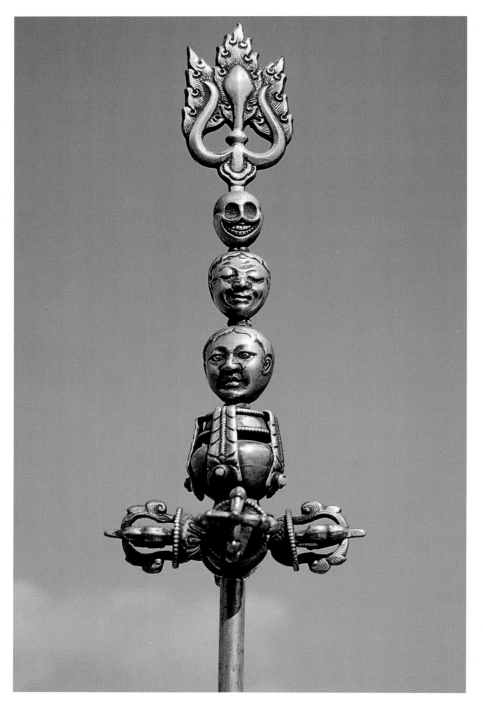

Above: During the period preceding his enlightenment, the fasting Buddha is said to have nourished himself with just one or two hemp seeds per day. (Thai copy of an ancient sculpture from Pakistan)

Below: In the Himalayas, the Medicine Buddha is venerated as the god of healing plants. One of his sacred herbs is hemp. (Newari-Tibetan thangka, twentieth century)

In Tibetan and Tantric medicine, elixirs of life (nectar, amrita, soma) based upon secret recipes are still being manufactured. Many of these recipes include hemp. This Tantric scepter (*kathvanga*), an attribute of Padmasambhava, is one of the magical shamanic weapons related to the spirit dagger (*phurba*). The ritual device depicts the vessel of amrita as well as the three stages of aging. The vessel rests upon a double thunderbolt, symbol of the Tantric path, and is crowned by Shiva's trident. In worldly rituals, the inebriating and vision-producing soma drink is seen as the counterpart of the divine amrita.

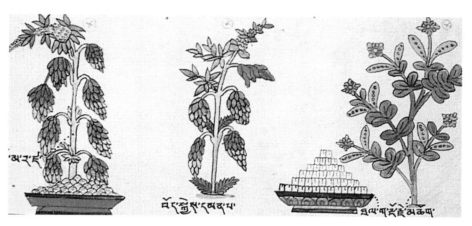

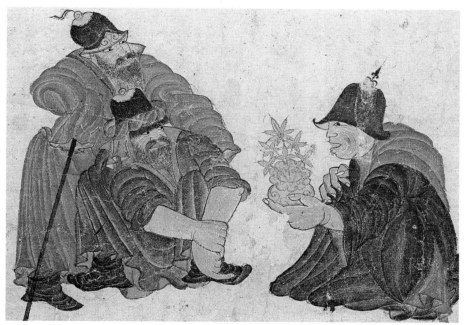

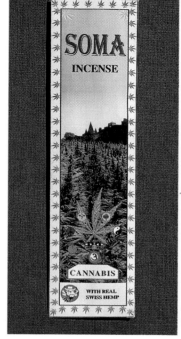

Above: In many cultures, hemp fumigations are used for medicinal purposes. In Switzerland, incense sticks containing hemp are sold under the historically significant name *soma*. Unfortunately, these incense sticks have no effects and do not live up to the promise of their name.

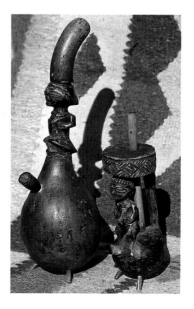

Above: Traditional Tibetan illustration of hemp (two types; left and center) on a medicine thangka (detail).

Below: This Mongolian painting from the Middle Ages (by Master Siyah Qalem) depicts a scene of deference to a shaman. The offering is a golden hemp plant.

Left: Water pipes such as these are used to smoke *dagga* (hemp) in many parts of Africa.

Right: The Japanese spice mixture *Kaori Shichimi* is thought to promote health and digestion. It contains hemp seeds.

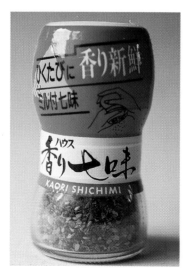

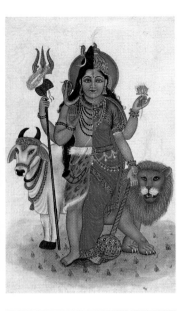

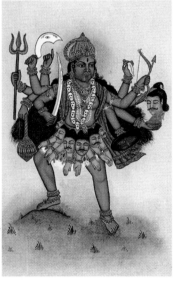

Above: The Hindu god Shiva is shown here as half male, half female. In this form, the god of hemp embodies the unity of the two poles of the universe, a unity that leads to enlightenment. (miniature, Rajasthan, India, twentieth century)

Below: Kali, the "Terrible Goddess," is a manifestation of Parvati, the wife of Shiva. She is said to have been the first to discover the hemp plant, which she served to Shiva as an aphrodisiac. (miniature, Rajasthan, India, twentieth century)

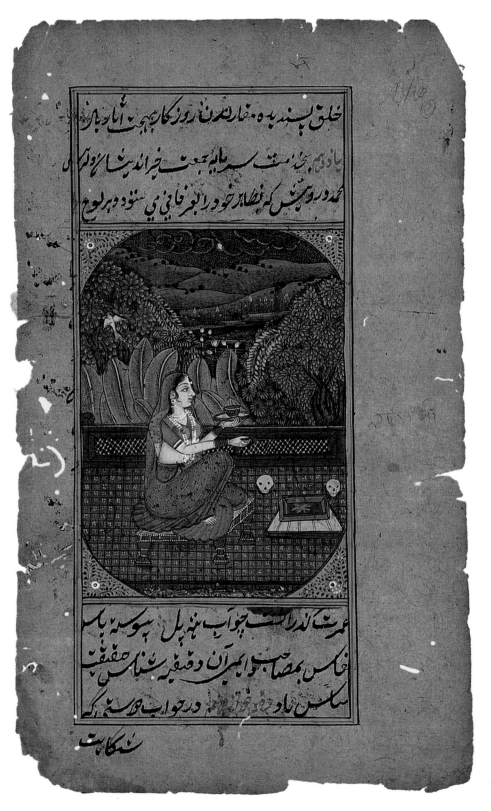

A North Indian healer preparing medicaments. Hemp is a component of numerous recipes. (miniature, Rajasthan, India, ninteenth century)

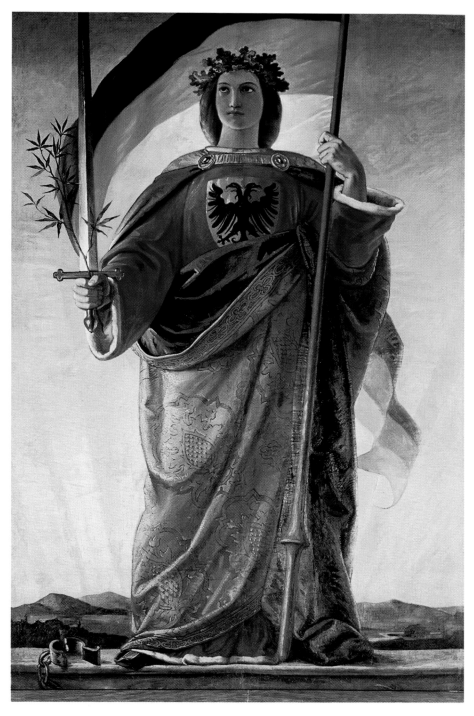

Germania, the personified spirit of the
1848 German Revolution, holds a
hemp branch, a symbol of peace and
liberation, in her right hand.
(*Germania* oil painting by Philipp Veit,
1848)

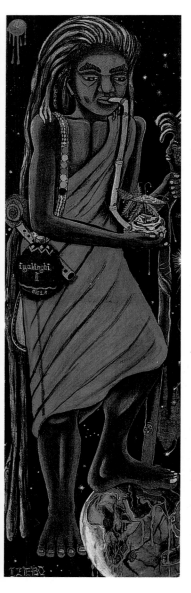

This oil painting by the Jamaican Rastafarian artist Ras Izebo (1978) illustrates the cultural and religious significance of hemp for the Rastafarians.

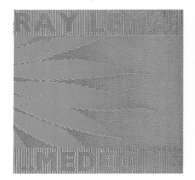

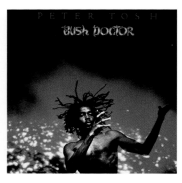

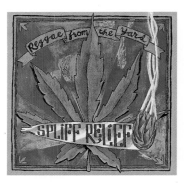

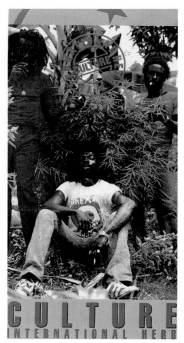

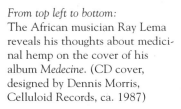

From top left to bottom:
The African musician Ray Lema reveals his thoughts about medicinal hemp on the cover of his album *Medecine*. (CD cover, designed by Dennis Morris, Celluloid Records, ca. 1987)

The reggae star Peter Tosh sings about the medicinal qualities of hemp on his album *Bush Doctor*. (Record/CD cover, EMI Records, 1978/1988)

The reggae anthology *Spliff Relief* used a postcard from California as inspiration for the layout of its cover. (Mesa Records, 1994)

The Jamaican reggae band Culture praises the wondrous effects of the "sacred herb" on their album *International Herb* (CD cover, Shanachie Records, 1990)

This postcard from Amsterdam makes a statement about the beneficial effects of hemp. (ca. 1990)

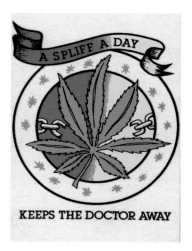

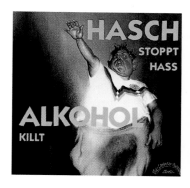

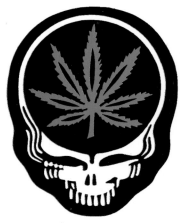

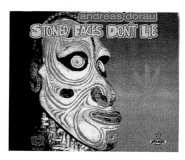

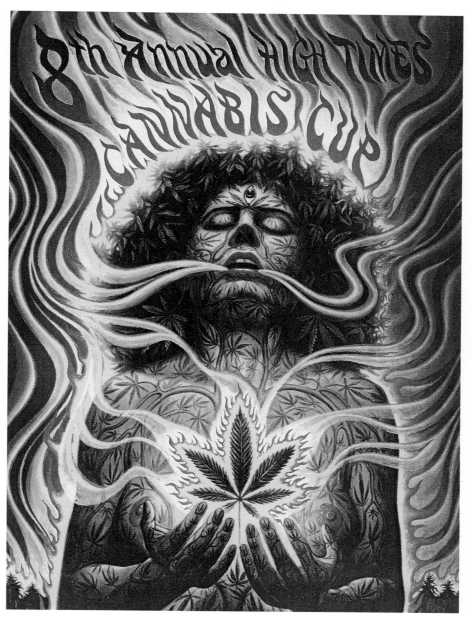

From top to bottom:
This anthology of punk bands from the German city of Hamburg makes a clear statement about hemp use. The text reads: "Hash stops hate, alcohol kills." (CD cover, EFA, 1994)

A wide variety of underground emblems elucidate the positive value and use of hemp to affect consciousness, as this American sticker shows (Grateful Dead "Space Your Face" motif).

On this cover, the German New Wave singer Andreas Dorau proclaims his opinion that hemp leads people to the truth. (CD cover, Motor Music, 1994)

In this painting, the American artist Alex Grey, renowned for his cycle *Sacred Mirrors*, reveals his vision of the goddess who lives in the hemp plant. In doing so, he harks back to an ancient shamanic tradition, in which the healer will ally himself with the spirit of the plant in order to do battle against disease.

73

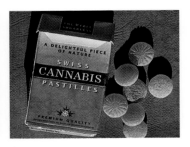

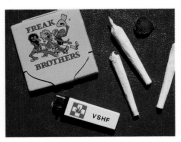

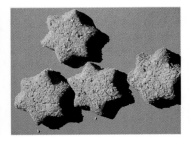

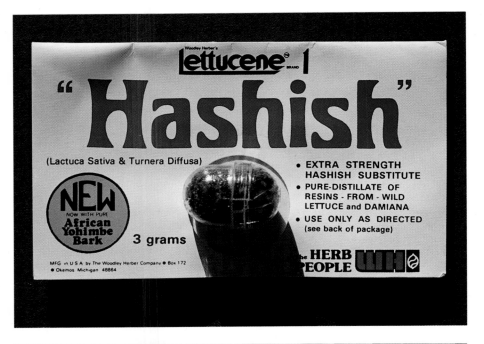

From top to bottom:
Pastilles with THC-free extracts of hemp are now widely available in Europe and the United States for the treatment of sore throats, hoarseness, and coughs.

Hashish or marijuana for smoking, sometimes mixed with other substances, may be rolled in cigarette papers into so-called joints.

When used medicinally, hemp is often eaten, for example, in the form of cookies.

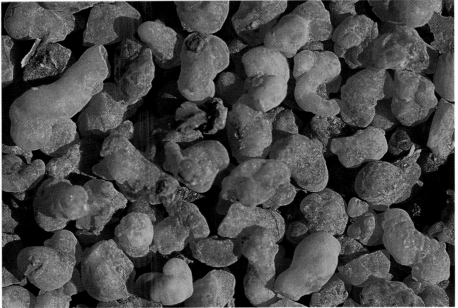

Above: Occasionally, legal hemp surrogates are offered for sale: An American product made from the dried juice (lactucarium or lettucene) of garden salad (*Lactuca sativa*) is marketed as "Hashish." In former times, lactucarium was used medicinally as an opium substitute.

Below: True frankincense, also known as olibanum, is the resin of the Arabian incense tree (*Boswellia sacra*). Since inhaling large amounts of the smoke will produce inebriating effects, it has been suggested that burning the resin yields THC.

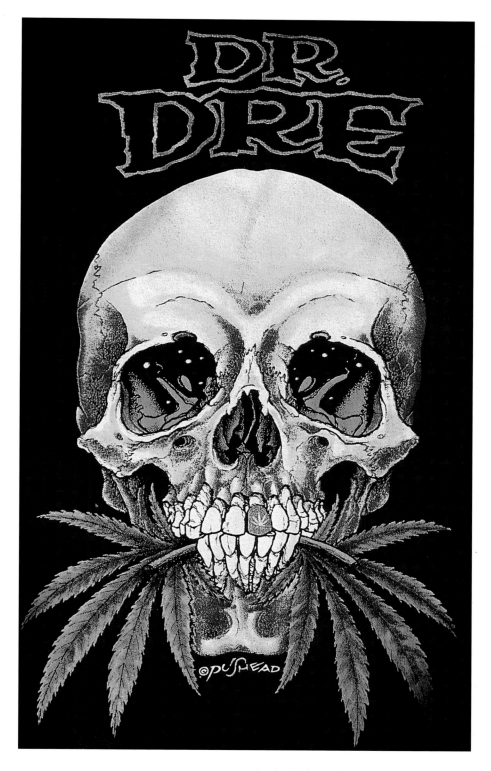

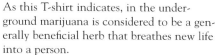

As this T-shirt indicates, in the underground marijuana is considered to be a generally beneficial herb that breathes new life into a person.

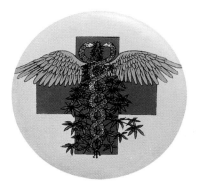

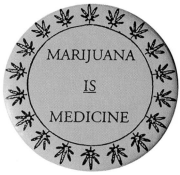

Above: This button from California clearly illustrates hemp's medicinal aspect.

Below: Many people today are openly expressing their opinion that marijuana *is* medicine. (button, ca. 1990)

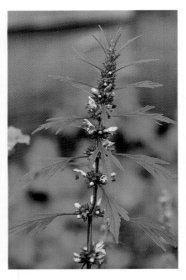

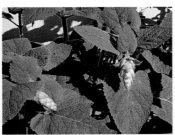

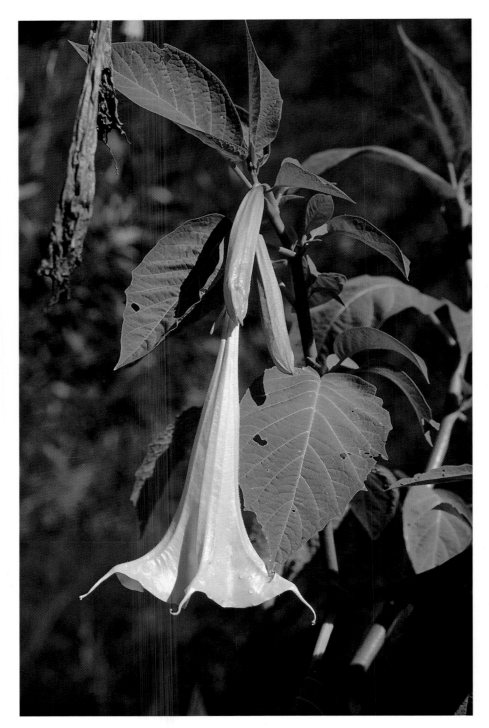

Above: Today, Siberian motherwort (*Leonurus sibericus*) is smoked in many parts of the world as a marijuana substitute. In Mexico, the herb is popularly known as *marijuanillo,* "little marijuana."

Below: Clary (*Salvia sclarea* L.) was formerly used to "cut" hashish, that is, it was mixed with hashish to increase the quantity, for illegal sale. When smoked, or when the essential oil is inhaled, clary can induce psychoactive effects somewhat like those of marijuana.

For medicinal purposes, hemp is often smoked in combination with dried leaves of angel's trumpet (*Brugmansia* sp.) as well as other members of the nightshade family.

Nascha

HEMP IN RUSSIAN FOLK MEDICINE

In Moscow and St. Petersburg, cities with millions of inhabitants, smoking grass has become a mass phenomenon among the Russian youth.

STEFAN HAAG
HANFKULTUR WELTWEIT
(1995:46*)

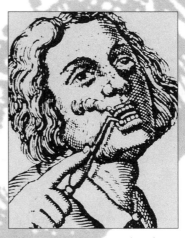

Before cocaine was introduced to Western dentistry as a local anesthetic, it was a common practice throughout Eurasia to pass smoke from henbane and hemp over a painful tooth. Special devices were developed for this purpose, as this old illustration shows. (engraving from Johannes Scultetus, *Armamentarium chirurgicum*, Ulm, Germany, 1665)

In an enormous country such as Russia, folk medicine has always played a significant role. For centuries it was the only type of medical care available for
large segments of the population in many isolated areas. The use of herbs is at
the center of Russian folk medicine. Many food plants are utilized medicinally, primarily dietetically, but plants that are pharmacologically active are also used,
including the oriental mandrake (*Mandragora turcomanica* MIZGIREVA), henbane
(*Hyoscyamus physaloides* L.), hellebore (*Helleborus* and *Veratrum),* and various
species of *Aconitum* (Khlopin 1980; Rowell 1978). The folk medical uses of these
plants are reminiscent of ancient traditions.

Hemp is probably one of the oldest healing plants in the Russian folk pharmacopoeia. Many botanists have localized the origin of hemp to the area around the
Caspian Sea, where the species *Cannabis ruderalis* still grows wild today. From there,
Scythian horse nomads may have carried the plant into all regions of central and
western Asia (Merlin 1972*).

Many Russians once believed that toothaches were caused by a "worm" (a conception that was also common throughout ancient Europe). Even today, one can
hear the expression "the worm's in there." For many centuries, hemp seeds and
flowers were one of the few known treatments for toothaches in Russia as well as in
Poland and Lithuania. A person suffering from a toothache would toss some hemp
onto a hot stone and inhale the rising smoke (perhaps this practice gave rise to the
expression "stoned"). A precise recipe has come down from the sixteenth century:

> For worms in the teeth, boil hemp seeds in a new pot and add hot stones to
> this. When the vapors are inhaled, the worms will fall out. (cited in Benet
> 1975:46*)

In the Ukraine, toothaches were treated by boiling a hemp gruel. Both the
vapors that arose during cooking and the gruel in the mouth were said to make the
"worm drunk," thereby driving it from the afflicted tooth.[1]

Hemp preparations are also used to treat other types of pains. The oil from
pressed seeds is applied to painful areas as a remedy for gout and rheumatism. In
Poland, wounds are dressed with a paste made from hemp flowers, wax, and olive
oil (Benet 1975:46*).

Hemp is even utilized in traditional veterinary medicine. When a house cat has
eaten *mukhomor* mushrooms (*Amanita muscaria, Amanita pantherina*)—cats often
exhibit an appetite for fly agaric mushrooms!—it is placed in a field of hemp so that
it may eat hemp until it is cured of its bemushroomed daze (Benet 1975:46*).

In the old Czarist Empire, hemp preparations were used ritually as well as medicinally. Hemp seeds, known as *semieniatka*, were made into a soup that was offered
on Christmas night as a food for the souls of dead ancestors (Benet 1975:43*).

The female, psychoactive flowers were attributed with magical and apotropaic
powers. In the Ukraine, flowers collected during Midsummer Eve were used in
amulets that could counteract witchcraft and protect cattle against the "evil eye."

---

1. The use of henbane smoke to treat toothaches was or is found throughout all of Eurasia
(Klein 1907). In some Oriental languages, hemp and henbane (*Hyoscyamus* spp.) even bear the
same name, for example, *benj, bhanj.*

The seeds were also used as an aphrodisiac love magic. Love-hungry girls would each carry several seeds in their belts, jump into a pile, and call out: "Andrei, Andrei, I plant the hemp seed in you. May God let me know with whom I shall sleep!" The girls would then undress, take water into their mouths in order to moisten the seeds, and frolic around the house three times while naked (Benet 1975:44*).

Shirts woven from hemp fiber could also have magical effects. A Ukrainian tale tells of a dragon that lived in Kiev, terrorizing the people and demanding great tribute. This dragon could only be killed by a man wearing a hemp shirt. A man wearing such a shirt killed the dragon, and the people of Kiev could now control their own destiny. Hemp contributed to the "political" freedom of the city.

In Tashkent, marijuana is affectionately referred to as *nascha*, and it is used with just as much affection. It can aid in the treatment of alcoholics (Antzyferov 1934), but primarily functions as a euphoric agent of pleasure and as a psychoactive aphrodisiac. Hashish dissolved in lamb fat is eaten as an aphrodisiac bread spread or massaged into the skin of the temples for headaches. This mixture is especially recommended for virgin brides. For one thing, it induces erotic sensations; it is also said to neutralize or minimize the pain of defloration. Similarly, the pains associated with a boy's circumcision are counteracted with a candy containing hashish (*guc-kand*). Some women prepare an ointment from hashish, tobacco, and fat. They smear this in their vaginas to make the passage narrower and more seductive. This procedure is also said to protect them from *fluor albus* or leukorrhea (Benet 1975:47*). But the most famous and most elaborate aphrodisiac is joy porridge, reminiscent of the ancient Oriental "joy pills" (Rätsch 1990b*). The men of Tashkent are crazy about the effects it produces.

Guc-Kand

Boil hemp leaves and/or flowers in water until a deep green extract results. Pour through a strainer. Sweeten the decoction liberally with sugar and add saffron threads and egg whites. Beat to a frothy paste. Form the mixture into little balls and place in the sun to dry.

Joy Porridge

Hemp flowers and seeds
Dried roses
Carnation petals
Pellitory root powder (*Anacyclus pyrethrum*)
Saffron threads
Nutmeg
Cardamom
Almond butter, melted
Honey
Brown sugar

Finely chop all ingredients and add to the melted almond butter. Add honey and brown sugar and stir to produce a paste. The dosage must be determined on an individual basis.

Hemp substitute: Inebriating mint (Lagochilus inebrians BUNGE; Labiatae) is a bushy mint species indigenous to the central Asian steppes of Turkestan and Uzbekistan; it is regarded as a substitute for hemp. Inebriating mint is typically gathered in the fall and hung on the rafters to dry over the winter. A tea, sweetened with honey, is brewed from the leaves. This produces a mild euphoria. It can also be used as a sedative (McKenna 1995:103). In Russian folk medicine and phytotherapy, this plant is also used to treat allergies, blood clots, and skin diseases (Schultes and Hofmann 1995:47). The dried leaves contain up to 17 percent lagochilin, a diterpene alkaloid (the average is around 3 percent; Tyler 1966:287). Numerous studies of this plant can be found in the Russian literature. The plant is or was even listed in the Russian Pharmacopoeia as a natural tranquilizer (McKenna 1995:103; Scholz; and Eigner 1983:78).*

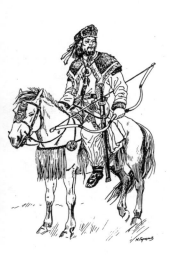

Scythian horse nomads are credited with spreading cannabis throughout Asia. Because of their activities, hemp became one of the drugs used in Russian folk medicine. (drawing by M. V. Gorelik)

REFERENCES

Antzyferov, L. V. 1934. Hashish in Central Asia. *Journal of Socialist Health Care in Uzbekstan* Tashkent [in Russian].

Golowin, Sergius. 1989. *Das Reich des Schamanen: Die eurasische Kultur der Spiritualität*. Munich: Goldmann.

Khlopin, Igor N. 1980. *Mandragora turcomanica* in der Geschichte der Orientalvölker. *Orientalia Lovaniensia Periodica* 11:223–31.

Klein, G. 1907. Historisches zum Gebrauche des Bilsenkrautextraktes als Narkotikum. *Münchener medizinische Wochenschrift* 22:1088–9.

McKenna, Dennis. 1995. Bitter Brews and Other Abominations: The Uses and Abuses of Some Little-Known Hallucinogenic Plants. *Integration* 5:99–104.

Rowell, Margery. 1978. Plants of Russian Folk Medicine. *Janus* 65:259–82.

Scholz, Dieter, and Dagmar Eigner. 1983. Zur Kenntnis der natürlichen Halluzinogene. *Pharmazie in unserer Zeit* 12(3):74–9.

Tyler, Varro E. 1966. The Physiological Properties and Chemical Constituents of Some Habit-Forming Plants. *Lloydia* 29(4):275–92.

Azallû-Qannapu

HEMP IN SOUTHWEST ASIA

In the ancient Orient, the belief in the magical powers of plants culminated in the idea of the herb of life. . . . A wide variety of plants with healing properties were characterized as the herb of life. For example, one Assyrian who had recovered from a serious illness said: "I drank the life herb of my mistress, the Goddess Gula, and I recovered."

VOLKERT HAAS
MAGIE UND MYTHEN IM REICH DER HETHITER
(1977:142F.)

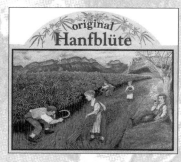

Label from a modern hemp beer, brewed in Switzerland. The Mesopotamians knew how to brew beer with hemp, as well as how to use it for medicinal purposes.

Among the cuneiform texts left by the Assyrians are a series of medicinal herbals. (excerpt from the herbal text from the library of the Assyrian king Ashurbanipal, Nineveh; from Thompson)

In Mesopotamian medicine, great value was placed on maintaining health and being free of diseases. The Sumerians had many magical and medicinal techniques at their disposal to stave off and avoid illnesses. They believed that diseases had their origins in the shadow world, the dark, unfriendly beyond, where they lurked in the form of ghosts and demons (Thompson 1903). Thus, "it seemed absolutely imperative to lead an enjoyable and cheerful life here on Earth for as long as one could. When a person was granted a life full of cheer, this was interpreted as an irrefutable sign of divine grace" (Zaragoza 1990:91). It is on this basis that we can understand the high esteem in which hemp was held. In the Sumerian city of Ur, a precious necklace was discovered that featured likenesses of hemp leaves in hammered gold (Emboden 1995:99).

The foundation of Mesopotamian therapy was exorcism, casting out the demons of illness from the afflicted. Physicians conducted exorcisms in accordance with ritual instructions (Haas 1977; Klengel-Brandt n.d.). Magically powerful, reality-changing songs accompanied fumigations, incantations, and the administration of medicines.

> He has cast out the demon of disease, who embraced him with his outspread wings. He has taken away the evil which wounded him. He has transformed the suffering of the man into jubilation. He has placed beneficent genies as watchers and protectors at his side. (cited in Zaragoza 1990:105)

The Mesopotamian Materia Medica was very similar to that of the Egyptians. Numerous fruits, grains, spices, vegetables, tree resins, minerals, and organic excrement ("pharmacy of filth") were utilized: "Among the medicines with strong effects were hellebore, henbane, mandrake, opium, and hemp" (Sigerist 1972:101; Pollak 1978:140*).[1]

Hemp was one of the most commonly used medicines in Mesopotamia (Zaragoza 1990:102). It was administered for bladder ailments, sleeplessness, rheumatism, and painful bronchitis (Thorwald 1985:170). Known as *azallû*, hemp was also called the "plant of forgetting worries" (Farber 1981:271). Seeds, roots, and branches were combined with beer or palm wine into various medicinal drinks to remedy disturbances of potency.[2] They were also used to produce magical incenses (Bennett et al. 1995:19*).

The Assyrians in particular used hemp (*azallû, qannapu,*[3] *ganzigunnu*) and hashish (*martakal*) in their medicine (Albright 1926; Thompson 1924). Numerous cuneiform tablets bear testimony to this fact. Hemp roots were prescribed for difficult births. The plant was boiled down and administered as an enema to treat

---

1. In other words, the most potent psychoactive substances were regarded as the best medicines, and this is why they were sacred and belonged to the "hierobotany" (Samorini 1996). Mandrake (*Mandragora* sp.) was used in Mesopotamia and neighboring areas in ritual and medicinal spirit conjurations and in exorcisms (cf. Emboden 1995).
2. "Their favorite magical arts consisted of causing fertility and infertility, potency and impotency" (Haas 1977:58).
3. It is uncertain whether the Babylonian name *qu-nu-bu*, which is documented from the rule of Esarhaddon (ca. 680 B.C.E.), did indeed refer to hemp, but it is a possibility (Emboden 1995:104).

abdominal pains. Similarly, hempseed oil or hemp in petroleum was rubbed onto a swollen stomach. The roasted seeds were administered to treat the *arimtu* disease (a type of trembling of the limbs). Mixed with flour, hemp was given as an antidote. Mixed with other plants, hemp with "pig oil" was applied as a small anal compress. Finally, hemp was also used in beer. This brew was consumed to treat illnesses caused by witchcraft (Thompson 1949:221). Beer was the most important carrier substance for medicines in Mesopotamia (Hartman and Oppenheim 1950; Röllig 1970). Hemp beer, in other words, has long been considered beneficial to health.

It is possible that the Assyrians learned of and adopted the practice of inhaling hemp smoke from the Scythians. The Scythians had a long history of trade with the Assyrians before contributing to their destruction (Pjotrowski 1980:178–82). The Assyrians inhaled the smoke to remedy worries, want, and sorrow (Thompson 1949:220). Since these afflictions often hide behind the masks of demons, it is very likely that hemp was also used in exorcisms. These were, after all, usually carried out in the temple, and they began with the burning of incense (Davies 1898). Some scholars have suggested that the Assyrian word *qunapu* did not refer to hemp alone, but also meant "incense" (Leipe 1997:131f.*).

It appears that the ancient Assyrians also made medicinal use of *dilbat*, their name for a species of the genus *Mesembryanthemum*, together with Indian hemp (*Cannabis indica*). The preparation was utilized to "suppress the spirits" (Thompson 1949:222).[4]

Hemp was known in the Promised Land as well. In the Talmud, it is referred to as *kanbus*, and is chiefly regarded as a source of fiber (Palgi 1975:209). It is also mentioned in the Bible (see, for example, Exodus 35:10, 17, and 18 and Ezekiel 27:19) as a source of fiber for clothing, ropes, nets, and so on. It was an important material for the tabernacle (Waal 1988:44), and was also used in the construction of Solomon's temple (Benet 1975:42*).

Although no explicit mention of medicinal hemp appears in the Bible (Rätsch 1991c*), in ancient Israel it was very likely used as an analgesic. A report from the Deutsche Presse Agentur, a German press agency, on June 4, 1992 noted:

> Israeli archaeologists are convinced of this. In a 1700-year-old family grave, they discovered the remains of a girl of perhaps 14, who was well advanced in her pregnancy. Alongside the skeleton, the researchers found the dried remnants of a brew of hashish, herbs, and fruits. The Israeli Office of Antiquities interpreted the find as providing proof that hashish was being used to alleviate the pains of labor. No agent of the time, however, would have been able to help this young woman. A Cesarean section would have been necessary.

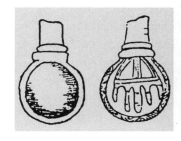

Archaeological excavations in the region between Palestine and Syria have yielded stone pipes dating to the period of 1000–600 B.C.E. These were probably stuffed with hemp, henbane, and other substances. (from C. Ernest Wright, *Biblical Archaeology*)

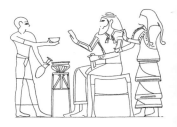

In ancient times Egyptian medicine was widely known for its effective treatments and medicines. This wall painting depicting the Egyptian physician Nebamun presenting a remedy to foreign patients illustrates this fact. (Grave 17, Thebes, eighteenth dynasty)

---

4. It is possible that this particular *Mesembryanthemum* sp. (*Sceletium?*) may have also been psychoactive (cf. Rätsch 1998:360f.*). In South Africa, species of this genus have found use as psychoactive substances even into the present day (Smith et al. 1996).

In the oldest story of humankind, the Epic of Gilgamesh, it is told how Gilgamesh went on a quest for the Plant of Life (also referred to as the Grass of Life). Using this wondrous plant, a person would become "rejuvenated like an eagle." During his adventurous search, which has striking resemblances to shamanic stories, Gilgamesh wanders though the various worlds. Along the way, he comes to the mighty mountain of Mâschu, "whose peak reaches to the vault of heaven and whose breast touches the underworld." This myth spread from Mesopotamia over the Himalayas and into China. There, numerous stories also tell of gods, heroes, or humans who undertook the search for the Plant of Life or the Drink of Immortality (Couliano 1995:78–86).

REFERENCES

Albright, W. F. 1926. Assyr. *martakal* "Haschisch" und *amurtinnu* "Sidra." *Zeitschrift für Assyrologie* 37:40.

Couliano, Ioan P. 1995. *Jenseits dieser Welt: Außerweltliche Reisen von Gilgamesch bis Albert Einstein*. Munich: Diederichs.

Davies, T. Witton. 1898. *Magic, Divination, and Demonology Among the Hebrews and Their Neighbours*. London: James Clark.

Emboden, William A. 1995. Art and Artifact as Ethnobotanical Tools in the Ancient Near East with Emphasis on Psychoactive Plants. In *Ethnobotany: Evolution of a Discipline*, edited by Richard Evans Schultes and Siri von Reis. Portland, Oregon: Dioscorides Press, pages 93–107.

Farber, Walter. 1981. Drogen im alten Mesopotamien—Sumerer und Akkader. In *Rausch und Realität*, edited by G. Völger. Vol. 1. Cologne: Rautenstrauch-Joest-Museum, pages 270–90.

Haas, Volkert. 1977. *Magie und Mythen im Reich der Hethiter: I. Vegetationskulte und Pflanzenmagie*. Hamburg: Merlin Verlag.

Hartman, Louis Francis, and A. Leo Oppenheim. 1950. On Beer and Brewing Techniques in Ancient Mesopotamia. *Journal of the American Oriental Society* Supplement No. 10 (Baltimore).

Klengel-Brandt, Evelyn. n.d. *Magie im Alten Vorderasien*. Berlin: Staatliche Museen zu Berlin, Vorderasiatisches Museum.

Palgi, Phyllis. 1975. The Traditional Role and Symbolism of Hashish Among Moroccan Jews in Israel and the Effects of Acculturation. In V. Rubin *Cannabis and Culture*, edited by V. Rubin. The Hague: Mouton, pages 207–16.

Pjotrowski, Boris. 1980. *Urartu*. Munich: Heyne (Archaeologia Mundi).

Röllig, Wolfgang. 1970. *Das Bier im alten Mesopotamien*. Berlin: GGBB.

Samorini, Giorgio. 1996. *Ierobotanica mesopotamica*. Altrove 4:13–28.

Sigerist, Henry E. 1972. *Der Arzt in der mesopotamischen Kultur*. Esslingen, Germany: Robugen.

Smith, Michael T., Neil R. Crouch, Nigel Gericke, and Manton Hirst. 1996. Psychoactive Constituents of the Genus *Sceletium* N.E.Br. and Other Mesembryanthemaceae: A Review. *Journal of Ethnopharmacology* 50:119–30.

Thompson, R. Campbell 1903. *The Devils and Evil Spirits of Babylonia*. London: Luzac and Co.

———. 1924. *The Assyrian Herbal*. London: The British Academy.

———. 1949. *A Dictionary of Assyrian Botany*. London: The British Academy.

Thorwald, Jürgen. 1985. *Macht und Geheimnis der frühen Ärzte*. Munich: Droemer-Knaur.

Waal, M. de. 1988. *Medicinal Herbs in the Bible*. York Beach, Maine: Samuel Weiser.

Zaragoza, Juan R. 1990. Die Medizin in Mesopotamien. In *Illustrierte Geschichte der Medizin*, edited by R. Toellner. Vol. 1. Salzburg: Andreas und Andreas, pages 91–107.

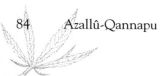

Šmšmt
HEMP AMONG THE PHARAOHS

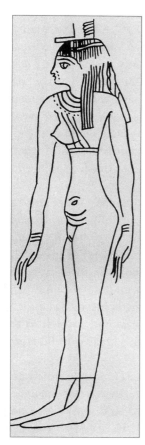

The Egyptian goddess Isis was known as "the Magically Powerful," "the Magically Abundant," and "the Great Magician." She was "great in magical abilities" and had the reputation of having "extraordinary cleverness, cunning, and endurance." Isis was primarily the Goddess of Magical and Healing Plants, and hemp stood under her protection. (drawing from an ancient Egyptian linen painting)

Death stands before me,
like the scent of lotus flowers,
as when one sits on the shore
of drunkenness.
FROM THE EGYPTIAN *BOOK OF THE DEAD*

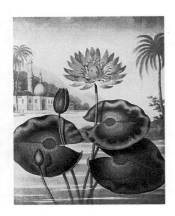

The ancient Egyptian name for hemp, *šmšmt*, as written in hieroglyphics. (from Manniche 1989)

In ancient Egypt, many psychoactive plants were known and used in both medicinal and ritual contexts. The blue lotus (*Nymphaea caerulea*) was probably the most important of these plants. (aquatint by Stadler, from Robert John Thorntons's *The Temple of Flora*, 1799–1801)

Homer (ninth to eighth century B.C.E.), the great Greek poet, had the following to say about Egypt: "A fertile soil which brings forth drugs in abundance; some are medicines, the others poisons. The home of the most scholarly physicians in the world" (cited in Leca 1990:119). Exuberant praise indeed, but also a statement that was accurate with regard to the situation at the time. The healing arts of Egypt were renowned well beyond its borders, and the Egyptians exerted a considerable influence upon ancient medicine in the eastern Mediterranean (Westendorf 1992).

The most important sources detailing ancient Egyptian pharmacology are the medical papyruses. The *Papyrus Edwin Smith* (2700–2400 B.C.E.) is essentially a treatise on treating wounds and performing trauma surgery. A number of medicinal recipes are contained in the somewhat more recent *Papyrus Hearst*. The *Kahun Papyrus* (ca. 1900 B.C.E.) lists a variety of medicines. The most comprehensive book of recipes is the *Papyrus Ebers* (1555 B.C.E.). There must have been a great many such medicinal texts, but only a few fragmentary scrolls have been recovered (Valette 1990:463). Unfortunately, most of the names of the plants used in the formulas contained in the papyruses cannot be botanically identified with certainty. The identification of hemp was always problematic as well, but this has changed as a result of modern archaeology and pollen analysis.

Pieces of hemp have been found in the grave of Amenhotep IV (Akhenaton) in el-Amarna, a site active between 1550 and 1070 B.C.E. Hemp pollen was detected on the mummy of Ramses II (Manniche 1989:82). Thus, the use of hemp in burial rituals has been demonstrated for dynastic Egypt (the New Kingdom) in the second millennium before Christ. As a result, it has also been possible to identify the ancient Egyptian word *Šmšmt* as hemp. The inscriptions on the pyramids and papyruses bear witness to diverse uses of marijuana as a medicine (cf. Manniche 1989:82f.): "A treatment for the eyes: celery; marijuana; is ground and left in the dew overnight. Both eyes of the patient are to be washed with it early in the morning" (P. Ramesseum II, 1700 B.C.E.).

This recipe, from the *Papyrus Berlin* (3038:81, 1300 B.C.E.), is interpreted as a treatment for glaucoma, a common disease in Egypt: "A remedy to treat inflammation: leaves [or buds?] of hemp; white oil. Use as an ointment" (cf. Westendorf 1992:74; Manniche 1989:82). From the *Papyrus Ebers* (821, 1550 B.C.E.): "A remedy to cool the uterus: hemp is pounded in honey and administered to the vagina. This is a contraction [of the uterus]." The *Papyrus Ebers* (618) also mentions a poultice for toenails made of hemp. In the *Papyrus Chester Beatty* VI:24 (1300 B.C.E.), hemp is used together with carob (*Ceratonia siliqua* L.) as an enema (Manniche 1989:82).

In addition to the alkaloid-rich and strongly inebriating mandrake (*Mandragora autumnalis*) and the opium poppy (*Papaver somniferum*), the Egyptians used Indian hemp as a sedative and as a spasmolytic agent (Valette 1990:468). Whether hemp was used as a ritual inebriant, as were mandrake, opium, and the water lily (*Nymphaea caerulea*) (Emboden 1978, 1981, 1989), is not known. It is possible that it was an ingredient in the brews that were administered to patients before they settled in for their curative temple sleep (Stetter 1990:127f.). It is very likely that hemp products rich in THC were used ritually and hedonistically in ancient Egypt.

High concentrations of cannabinoids have been measured in nine Egyptian mummies (Balabanova et al. 1992*). Hemp is sometimes combined with Egyptian henbane (*Hyoscyamus muticus* L.).[1]

The use of hemp resin (hashish) as an inebriant has been found in Egypt as early as the twelfth century C.E. It was brought to Egypt by Syrian mystics during the Islamic Ayyubid Dynasty and initially used for meditation, to increase intelligence, and to produce mystical visions (Khalifa 1975:199). In the sixteenth century, balls of pulverized hemp leaves, known as *assis*, were popular. In his book *De medicina Aegyptorum* (London 1719), Prospero Alpini noted that the mixture called *bosa*, which was made of hemp fruits and flour made from another psychoactive plant, the bearded darnel (*Lolium temulentum* L.), had especially potent psychoactive properties (Hartwich 1997:14*). Since that time, the use of hashish has spread enormously. Today Egypt, in contrast to its Islamic-Arabic neighbors, is literally a land of hemp users (Sami-Ali 1971).

---

1. The ancient Egyptians called the henbane indigenous to their land *sakran*, "the drunken one"; in doing so, they made use of a word borrowed from Aramaic (Kottek 1994:129). It is mentioned as a medicinal plant in a Greek papyrus from the first century C.E. This member of the nightshade family is still used in Egypt as a medicine and as an inebriant (Germer 1985:169).

Egyptian Smoking Blend

Combine equal parts of henbane (*Hyoscyamus muticus* L.) and female hemp flowers (*Cannabis* sp.). The mixture is best smoked in a water pipe. If no Egyptian henbane is available, any other species of *Hyoscyamus* can be used (all contain the same active ingredients, although they are most highly concentrated in the Egyptian henbane).

LITERATURE CITED

Emboden, William A. 1978. The Sacred Narcotic Lily of the Nile: *Nymphaea caerulea. Economic Botany* 32(4):395–407.

———. 1981. Transcultural Use of Narcotic Water Lilies in Ancient Egyptian and Maya Drug Ritual. *Journal of Ethnopharmacology* 3:39–83.

———. 1989. The Sacred Journey in Dynastic Egypt: Shamanistic Trance in the Context of the Narcotic Water Lily and the Mandrake. *Journal of Psychoactive Drugs* 21(1):61–75.

Germer, Renate. 1985. *Flora des pharaonischen Ägypten.* Mainz, Germany: Philipp von Zabern.

Khalifa, Ahmad M. 1975. Traditional Patterns of Hashish Use in Egypt. In *Cannabis and Culture*, edited by V. Rubin. The Hague: Mouton, pages 195–205.

Kottek, Samuel S. 1994. *Medicine and Hygiene in the Works of Flavius Josephus.* Leiden: E. J. Brill.

Leca, Ange-Pierre. 1990. Die Medizin im alten Ägypten. In *Illustrierte Geschichte der Medizin*, edited by R. Toellner. Vol. 1. Salzburg: Andreas und Andreas, pages 109–43.

Manniche, Lise. 1989. *An Ancient Egyptian Herbal.* London: British Museum Publ.

Sami-Ali. 1971. *Le haschisch en égypte.* Paris: Payot.

Stetter, Cornelius. 1990. *Denn alles steht seit Ewigkeiten geschrieben: Die geheime Medizin der Pharaonen.* Munich: Quintessenz.

Valette, Simone. 1990. Die Pharmakologie im alten Ägypten. In *Illustrierte Geschichte der Medizin*, edited by R. Toellner. Vol. 1. Salzburg: Andreas und Andreas, 463–79.

Westendorf, Wolfhart. 1992. *Erwachen der Heilkunst: Die Medizin im Alten Ägypten.* Zurich: Artemis und Winkler.

Kokain und Haschisch im alten Ägypten

In ägyptischen Mumien haben Wissenschaftler der Universitäten München und Ulm Spuren von Haschisch, Kokain sowie Nikotin nachgewiesen. Die Drogen fanden sich in Haaren, Knochen und weichem Körpergewebe aller neun untersuchten Proben. Das Material stammte von Mumien aus der Zeit von etwa 1070 v. Chr. bis 395 n. Chr. ("Naturwissenschaften", Bd. 79, S. 358). Der Befund läßt Rückschlüsse auf die Lebensführung der damaligen Bevölkerung zu und erlaubt Vergleiche mit heutigen Gewohnheiten. Offenbar haben die Ägypter sogar Drogen verwendet, um schreiende Kinder zu besänftigen. Das geht aus einem Papyrus hervor, auf dem ein Gebräu aus Mohnsamen und Fliegenexkrementen als verblüffend wirksamer Beruhigungstrank gepriesen wird. Auf Haschisch, Kokain und Nikotin waren die Forscher zuvor schon bei der Untersuchung mehrerer peruanischer Mumien gestoßen. F.A.Z.

Cocaine and Hashish in Ancient Egypt
(*Frankfurter Allgemeine Zeitung*, August 26, 1992) Scientists at the Universities of Munich and Ulm have found traces of hashish, cocaine, and nicotine in Egyptian mummies. The drugs were present in the hair, bones, and soft tissues of all nine mummies studied. The material was taken from mummies from the period of ca. 1070 B.C.E. to 395 C.E. (*Naturwissenshaften*, vol. 79, p. 358). The find makes it possible to draw conclusions about the lifestyles of the population of the time and make comparisons to present-day practices. Apparently, the Egyptians even used drugs to pacify crying children. This can be seen in a papyrus, in which a brew of poppy seeds and fly excrement is praised as a surprisingly effective sedative drink. The researchers had previously detected hashish, cocaine, and nicotine during investigations of several Peruvian mummies.

Kannabion— Cannabis

HEMP IN THE MEDICINE OF ANTIQUITY

I went secretly in a boat to the dragon's cave—
Three keffed-out persons were stretched out on the beach
Bátis, Artémis, and the lazy Strátos—
Prepare an argilé [water pipe] for us, Strátos;
Artémis is bringing us good stuff from the city
[Constantinople]—
The mángas can smoke dope from Persia with a clear
*   conscience.*

EFSTRATIOS PYIOYMIDZÍS
ZEÏMBÉKANO SPANIMID (1934)

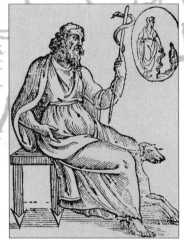

The Greek god Asclepius, a son of Apollo, was the Lord of the Curative Temple Sleep and of Medicinal Plants. His rod—the staff of Asclepius—which has now become the international symbol of physicians, is strongly reminiscent of the magical wands of ancient China, which were carved from woody hemp stalks. The snake seen winding itself around the staff recalls the Indian Kundalini serpent, which wraps itself around the phallus of the god Shiva. It is possible that Asclepius was originally an herbal healer or shaman who emigrated from Asia. Because of his healing abilities, he may have exerted a considerable influence upon ancient medicine, as a result of which he was elevated to divine status. (woodcut, sixteenth century)

In the *Odyssey* (eighth century B.C.E.), Homer speaks of the renowned *Pharmakon Nepenthes*, an Egyptian medicine that banished sorrow:

> But Helen, the daughter of Zeus, remembered something:
> and immediately put a magical agent into the wine which they drank,
> good against sorrow and bilious nature: for all evils
> it created forgetfulness. It was in the mixing jug: anyone who then drank of it,
> on that day would no tears flow down his cheeks,
> even when both his father and mother would die, yea even when
> his son, the beloved, or his brother
> would be slain with swords by the enemy directly before him,
> so that he would see it with his own eyes.
> Now the daughter of Zeus could avail herself of such
> skillful effects. . . . (IV, 219–28)

In the literature on the history of medicine and ancient philology, this magical agent has been variously interpreted as henbane (*Hyoscyamus niger*), mandrake (*Mandragora officinarum*), belladonna (*Atropa belladonna*), opium, and hashish (Baissette 1990:204; cf. Schmiedeberg 1918).

Democritus (460–371 B.C.E.), the "laughing philosopher," spoke of a plant called *potamaugis*, which should probably be construed as hemp. He said that when this plant is taken in wine together with myrrh it produces delirium and visions. He was particularly struck by the immoderate laughter that inevitably followed after someone had consumed this drink (Emboden 1990:219*).

Theophrastus (371–287 B.C.E.), the founder of scientific botany, described hemp using the name *dendromalache*. His description is still considered botanically correct (Emboden 1990:219*).

In the Dionysian tradition, consciousness-altering drugs were not only accepted, but were the very basis of the ecstatic worship services (Evans 1988:184). We can only conjecture whether hemp was mixed into the wine of Dionysus in order to heighten the mood at the Bacchanalian orgies (cf. Ruck 1982, 1995).

It is quite possible that the inhalation of hemp smoke was a part of the hierobotanical, that is, ritual practices. One classical Greek term is *cannabeizein*, "inhale hemp smoke" (Emboden 1990:219*). Another is *methyskesthai*, "become inebriated through the use of drugs" (Brunner 1977:222); Herodotus used this word to describe the inebriation of the inhabitants of the island in Araxes, an inebriation produced by smoke. It has frequently been suggested that the Pythia, the oracular priestess of Delphi, inhaled hashish smoke in order to enter her prophetic trance (Cooke 1860:149*; cf. also Rätsch 1987, and Stefanis et al. 1975:305).

In ancient times it was customary to visit oracular and sacred sites and submit oneself to a temple sleep, during which the gods and goddesses would reveal themselves and provide answers to questions or show ailing persons the ways in which they could become healthy once more. The shrine of the divine physician Asclepius of Epidaurus, located in Argolis, and the death oracle of Ephyra on the River Acheron in Asia Minor were especially renowned pilgrimage sites for those who sought to regain their health. The temple sleepers were placed into a

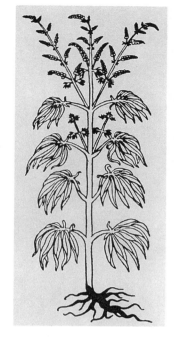

In the literature on cannabis, this illustration from a very early manuscript of the medical teachings of Dioscorides is usually considered one of the earliest depictions of the plant. In all likelihood, however, the illustration actually shows the chaste tree (*Vitex agnus-castus*), a plant common throughout Greece and that, on superficial examination, is indeed easily confused with cannabis. Chaste tree, which is also known as Monk's pepper, is used as a potent anaphrodisiac.

prophetic, healing sleep with such hierobotanical agents as opium, mandrake, the alkaloid-rich seeds of lupines (*Lupinus hirsutus*, *L. angustifolius*), and hemp. The Greek archaeologist Sotiris Dakaris, who began investigating the death oracle of Acheron in 1959, discovered "bags full of black clumps of hashish" in Ephyra (Vandenberg 1979:24). It is entirely possible that the temple sleepers on the Acheron were administered a preparation of hemp so that they would have especially intense dreams.

As many authors of antiquity (for example, Varro, Columbarius, and Gellus) have testified, hemp was known and esteemed as an excellent source of fiber and was planted on a large scale (Lenz 1966:432–4).

Gaius Plinius Secundus, usually referred to as Pliny the Elder (23–79 C.E.), was a Roman who drew his knowledge of nature primarily from Greek texts. He left us the thirty-seven-volume *Natural History*, the most comprehensive and significant nature writings of that time. He wrote about cannabis:

> Hemp is exceptionally useful for rope. Hemp is planted when the west winds of spring are blowing. The more closely together that it grows, the thinner are its stalks. The mature seeds are stripped off after the beginning of autumn and dried in the sun, the wind, or over a fire. The hemp plant is pulled out when fully grown. The peeling [of the stalks] and the cleaning are performed by candlelight. The best comes from Arab-Hissar; this is used especially to manufacture hunting nets. Three types of hemp fibers are produced at that place. Those types which come from just below the cortex are held to be of lesser worth, while that from the inside is highly esteemed. The second best hemp comes from Mylasa. As far as the height, the hemp from Rosea in the land of the Sabines grows as tall as a fruit tree. (*Nat. Hist.* 19.174)

Pliny had the following to say about hemp's medicinal properties:

> Hemp originally grew in the forest and had blacker and coarser leaves. Its seed is said to destroy the procreative powers of men. Its juice dispels the little worms from the ears and whichever animal has gotten in there, although it will give a headache; and so great are its effects that it is said that water in which it is poured becomes thicker; for this reason it also helps, when given in water, to treat diarrhea in beasts of burden. The root, boiled in water, softens joints that have become stiff, also from gout and similar fits. The root is placed raw on burn wounds, but should be changed frequently before it dries out. (*Nat. Hist.* 20.259)

Pliny's discussions are primarily based on the writings of his contemporary, Dioscorides, whose *Teachings on Medicines* was the most influential work of its kind (Baissette 1990), serving as a model for the Romans and Arabs as well as scholars writing during the Middle Ages and the Renaissance. Most of the time his work was simply copied and commented upon.

Pedanios Dioscorides lived during in the first century C.E., during the reign of Emperor Nero. A Greek from Anazarbas in Cilicia (Asia Minor), he served as a physician in the army, and his chief interests were in botany and pharmacology. He compiled his knowledge during numerous campaigns and tested out a number of medicines on the soldiers. His other sources were the treatises of the rhizotomist (root digger) Crateuas, the book of Andreas of Carystos, and the *Historia plantatum* of Theophrastus. In his five-volume *Teachings on Medicines*, written in Greek, Dioscorides had the following to say about cannabis:

> Cultivated hemp. Hemp —some call it Cannabium, others Schoenostrophon ["rope twisting"], Asterion ["star-like"]——is a plant which finds very great use in life to weave the strongest ropes. It has foul-smelling leaves like those of the ash; a long, simple stalk; and a round fruit which, when consumed in great quantities, destroys procreation. When green, made into juice, and trickled into the ears, it is a good remedy for ear ailments. (III, 156 [= 166])

The Roman physician Claudius Galen (131–201 C.E.) is regarded as the most important medical figure of antiquity (Debru 1997). Galen laid the foundation for a purely organically based medicine, but also recommended the use of dream interpretation and medical astrology for providing diagnoses (Villey 1990). Galen studied medicine in Smyrna (Izmir), Corinth, and Alexandria and collected medicinal plants and experiences during his travels to Syria, Phoenicia, Palestine, and Cyprus. It has been claimed that Galen wrote over five hundred medicinal and philosophical texts, although barely one-tenth of these have survived. Much of what he said is only known from the secondary literature of late antiquity. Galen was an admirer of Hippocrates who described himself as an eclectic (Villey 1990).

Aside from its purely medicinal use, which can be traced back to Dioscorides, Galen was the first to describe the hedonistic use of hemp. He compared it to the chaste tree *(Vitex agnus-castus)*, the sacred tree of Hera, which has a very similar appearance. Hemp seeds, however, were said to be difficult to digest or even indigestible, bad for the stomach, and able to produce headaches. The "seeds dispel the wind from the lower abdomen and dry the user to such an extent that—when eaten in excess—sexuality is extinguished. Some squeeze the juice from the green seeds and use it as a remedy to treat pains caused by blockages of the ear" (cited in Brunner 1977:223). He wrote that in Italy it was customary to serve small cakes containing marijuana for dessert. These increased the desire to drink; excessive use, however, had stupefying effects (Galen VI 549f.). Offering hemp to guests was considered a sign of good manners, for it was considered a "promoter of high spirits" (Brunner 1977:223; Merlin 1972:71*).

Following Galen, most medical authors characterized hemp as a remedy for earaches and attributed desiccant properties to the male seeds. Nothing new would be added until the Late Roman period, when Pseudo Apuleius would note that an ointment made from hemp herbage and fat could cause a swelling or enlargement of the breast to subside and that a mixture of crushed hemp seeds and nettle seeds (*Urtica* sp.) in vinegar was useful in treating herpes (*De Herbis* 116; Brunner 1977:224; Hunger 1935). The use of hemp to treat ear ailments is also described by Marcellus Empiricus (*De Medicamentis* 9.27/9.77–8) who, in another volume, added a medicinal-magical treatment for worms (treating worms was very important in the militaristic and imperialistic Roman culture) using hemp roots:

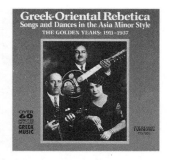

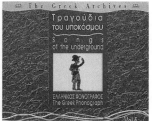

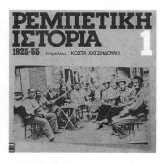

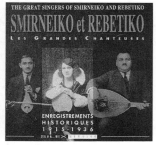

Tie the hemp root to your right arm: it is preferable that the entire arm be wrapped around with this root; if you have only a small amount on hand, then hang it around your neck with a thread from a weaving loom. In order to show you how strong this remedy is, when you utilize the root in the manner described, the flow of blood will immediately come to a stop. But when you untie and remove the root, the blood will flow again. (*De Medicamentis* 10.82, cited in Brunner 1977:224f.)

Hemp is listed as a medicine in a manuscript on ancient medicine written in the thirteenth century:

116. The name of the plant: *Cannabis silvatica.*

It grows in dry places, along the sides of paths, and near walls.

1. Cure: for nipple pains.

The application of ground *Cannabis silvatica* with fat dispels ulcers without delay and dissolves accumulations of (bad humors).

2. For frostbite.

Apply ground Cannabis fruits with Uertice seeds and vinegar; you will be amazed at the good effects.[1]

Very little is known about the Greek use of hemp in the period following antiquity; it does not appear again until the Rembetiko Movement, where it fertilized the consciousness of many people.

---

1. *Medicina antiqua*, fol. 108r/108v; cited in Zotter 1980:181; cf. *Medicina antiqua* 1996:53.

Hemp and the Greek Blues: PEMΠTΕΤΙΚΗ (Rembetiko)

Just as hemp has penetrated into every culture, it has also conquered every style of music. Marijuana smoke has permeated more than just early jazz and blues. Rembetiko* (also known as the "Greek Blues"), a musical style heavily influenced by Turkish music, developed in the early part of the twentieth century, from approximately 1910 to 1920 (Dietrich 1987). The anarchists (the "lumpen proletariat") and opponents of Fascism would meet in the harborside bars *(tekédes* or "Hashish Cafés"; *Cafés Amman, Café-aman)* of Piraeus and other places (Smyrna or Izmir, Volos, Thessaloniki, Athens) in order to forget the horrors of totalitarianism over coffee, ouzo, self-made music, and water pipes filled with hashish. They would inebriate themselves on the plaintive rhythms and yearning melodies of their own music, thereby strengthening their ability to resist.† Hemp's soothing effects promoted emotional solidarity among the rebels *(mangas, dais, koutsavakis)* and suppressed any hasty, rash, or aggressive behavior. In this case, hemp can be seen as a social remedy.

*Also written as Rebetiko, Rebetico, Rembetica, Rembetico, and other similar forms. Rebetes is the name for the musicians, who are also sometimes referred to as *mangas*. The word *rebetis* means "independent/unruly" or "rebel." The style from Smyrna is known as *smirneiko* or *zeibekiko*.
†During the Nazi occupation of Greece (1942), the Rebetika tis katochis, songs against German fascism, were written (for example, "Saltadoros," by Michalis Jenitsaris).

The lyrics of the Rembetiko songs speak primarily of hashish and its use, of ouzo and other drugs (including heroin and cocaine), and of worries and wants, loneliness and prison experiences, illness and suppression, sex and prostitution.

The Rembetiko scene was furnished with hemp products from Cairo, Turkey, and the Peloponnesus. In the highlands of the Peloponnesus, "hemp was planted on a large scale and made into hashish. The annual harvest amounted to some four million kilos" (Hartwich 1911:820*).

Just as the use of hashish was illegal in Greece, so too was Rembetiko. Even the use of the word *rebetika* was outlawed. The laws against Rembetiko were not lifted until after the fall of the Junta in 1974.

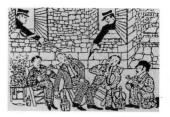

Police raid on a *teké*, a Greek hashish café, home of Rembetiko music. (contemporary newspaper illustration)

Selected Discography

Greek-Oriental Rebetica: Songs and Dances in the Asia Minor Style—The Golden Years: 1911–1937 (CD 7005 Arhoolie Productions 1991)

Rebettiki Istoria 1255–1955 (2 Vols., Minos/EMI 703642/703652)

Rembetica: Historic Urban Folk Songs from Greece (CD 1079 Rounder Records 1992). Historic original recordings from the legendary *tekédes* in the 1930s.

Rembetica in Piraeus 1933–1937 (Heritage Records HT CD 26 1994)

The Rebetiko Song in America 1920–1940 (The Greek Archives, Vol. 1, F. M. Records 627)

Songs of the Underground (The Greek Archives, Vol. 5, F. M. Records 631)

Woman of the Rebetiko Song (The Greek Archives, Vol. 6, F. M. Records 632)

Hemp Wine

(from Democritus)

Add a teaspoon of myrrh (resin of *Commiphora* spp.) and a handful of female hemp flowers to a liter of Retsina (white wine with resin) or dry Greek white wine and allow to macerate for a week. Strain before drinking.

REFERENCES

Aliotta, Giovanni, Danielle Piomelli, and Antonio Pollio. 1994. Le piante narcotiche e psicotrope in Plinio e Dioscoride. *Annali dei Musei Civici de Revereto* 9(1993):99–114.

Berendes, Julius. 1891. *Die Pharmacie bei den alten Culturvölkern*. Halle, Germany: Tausch und Grosse.

Baissette, Gaston. 1990. Die Medizin bei den Griechen. In *Illustrierte Geschichte der Medizin*, edited by R. Toellner. Vol. 1. Salzburg: Andreas und Andreas, pages 179–292.

Biedermann, Hans. 1972. *Medicina Magica*. Graz, Germany: Akademische Druck- u. Verlagsanstalt.

Brunner, Theodore F. 1977. Marijuana in Ancient Greece and Rome? The Literary Evidence. *Journal of Psychedelic Drugs* 9(3):221–5.

Debru, Armelle, ed. 1997. *Galen on Pharmacology, History and Medicine*. New York: Brill.

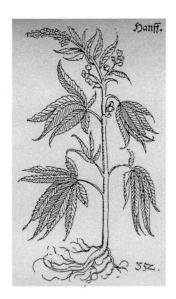

A male hemp plant, from the German edition of *Dioscorides*. (woodcut, 1610)

Dietrich, Eberhard. 1987. *Das Rebetiko: Eine Studie zur städtischen Musik Griechenlands*. 2 parts. Hamburg: Karl Dieter Wagner.

Dioskurides, Pedanios. 1902. *Arzneimittellehre*. Translated and with commentary by J. Berendes. Stuttgart, Germany: Enke.

Eliade, Mircea. 1992. *Schamanen, Götter und Mysterien: Die Welt der alten Griechen*. Freiburg, Germany: Herder.

Emboden, William A. 1977. Dionysus as a Shaman and Wine as a Magical Drug. *Journal of Psychedelic Drugs* 9(3):187–92.

Evans, Arthur. 1988. *The God of Ecstasy*. New York: St. Martin's Press.

Hunger, F. W. T. 1935. *The Herbal of Pseudo-Apulei: From the Ninth-Century Manuscript in the Abbey of Monte Cassino (Codex Casinensis 97) Together with the First Printed Edition of Joh. Phil. de Lignamine (Editio princeps Romae 1481) Both in Facsimile*. Leyden: Brill.

Kissling, H. J. 1957. *Zur Geschichte der Rausch- und Genussgifte im osmanischen Reiche*. Vol. 16. Munich: Südostasiatische Forschungen.

Krug, Antje. 1993. *Heilkunst und Heilkult: Medizin in der Antike*. Munich: C. H. Beck.

Lenz, Harald Othmar. 1966. *Botanik der alten Griechen und Römer*. Vaduz/Liechtenstein: Saendig Reprint (from 1859), *Medicina Antiqua*.

———. 1996. *Codex Vindobonensis 93 der Österreichischen Nationalbibliothek*. Commentary by Hans Zotter. Graz, Germany: Akademische Druck- u. Verlagsanstalt (Glanzlichter der Buchkunst, Vol. 6).

Plinius, Gaius [the Elder] 1950. *Natural History*. Translated by H. Rackham. Cambridge, Mass.: Harvard University Press.

———. 1973ff. *Naturkunde*. Edited, translated, and commentary by Roderich König and Gerhard Winkler. Munich: Heimeran, then Artemis and Winkler.

Pseudo-Apuleius 9th cen. *Herbarium* (cf.. Hunger 1935).

Rätsch, Christian. 1987. Der Rauch von Delphi: Eine ethnopharmakologische Annäherung. *curare* 10(4):215–28.

———. 1994. Die Alraune in der Antike. *Annali dei Musei Civici dei Rovereto* 10:249–96.

———. 1998. *Heilkräuter der Antike in Ägypten, Griechenland und Rom*. 2nd ed. Munich: Diederichs Verlag (DG).

Ruck, Carl A. P. 1982. The Wild and the Cultivated: Wine in Euripides' Bacchae. *Journal of Ethnopharmacology* 5:231–70.

———. 1995. Gods and Plants in the Classical World. In *Ethnobotany: Evolution of a Discipline*, edited by Richard Evans Schultes and Siri von Reis. Portland, Oregon: Dioscorides Press, pages 131–43.

Schmiedeberg, O. 1918. Über die Pharmaka in der Illias und Odyssee. *Schriften der wissenschaftlichen Gesellschaft in Straßburg* 36.

Stefanis, Coastas N., C. Ballas, and D. Madianou. 1975. Sociocultural and Epidemiological Aspects of Hashish Use in Greece. In *Cannabis and Culture*, edited by V. Rubin. The Hague: Mouton, pages 303–26.

Vandenberg, Philip. 1979. *Das Geheimnis der Orakel*. Munich: Orbis.

Villey, Raymond. 1990. Die Medizin in Rom: Galen. In *Illustrierte Geschichte der Medizin*, edited by R. Toellner. Vol. 1. Salzburg: Andreas und Andreas, pages 395–423.

Zotter, Hans. 1980. *Antike Medizin: Die medizinische Sammelhandschrift Cod. Vindobonensis 93 in lateinischer und deutscher Sprache*. Graz: ADEVA.

Hashish

HEMP IN ISLAMIC-ARABIC MEDICAL DOCTRINES

It is hashish that brings enlightenment to reason;
[but] he who devours it like food will become a donkey.
The elixir is moderation; eat of it just one grain, so that
it can permeate the being of your existence like gold.

AMIR AHMAD
MAHSATI-ROMAN
(TWELFTH CENTURY)

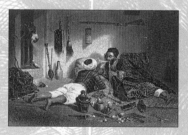

The smoking and enjoying of
hemp products is widespread and
culturally accepted in many parts
of the Islamic-Arabic world. The
medicinal use is also socially
approved. (copperplate engraving
from W. French, "The Kiafir,"
nineteenth century)

ctually, it is not possible to speak of either an Islamic or an Arabic medicine, even though it has become common to do so. It is a "medicine of the Arabic language," for all the literature is written in Arabic, the Eastern language of scholarship during the Middle Ages. Although most of the authors were Muslims, Jews (Moses Maimonides, for example) and Christians also contributed texts in Arabic. And while the majority of authors were Arabs, Spanish, Persian, and Greek authors also left a medicial literature written in Arabic (Sournia 1990).

Arabic medicine reached its zenith during the early Middle Ages. Not only were original works written, but classic works by such Greeks and Romans as Hippocrates, Dioscorides, Pliny, and Galen were translated into Arabic. In the Arabic literature, special emphasis was placed upon toxicology. Countless texts discuss the manufacture, use, and effects of *theriac*, a universal antidote, panacea, and tonic (Steinschneider 1971; Watson 1966). In addition to opium, snake meat, spices, and herbs, theriac often contained hemp. Theriac is sold in German pharmacies to this day, although it no longer contains opium and hemp. In modern folk medicine, theriac is an ingredient in the so-called Swedish drops, made famous by Maria Treben as a universal remedy (Treben 1980:67).

In the Arabic literature, hemp is almost always referred to as hashish. *Hashish* literally means "the herbs" and was originally a term used to designate all inebriating plants (Rosenthal 1971). Although the consumption of cannabis is tolerated today in some Muslim countries, such as Pakistan and Morocco, the use of hemp was once forbidden by all Islamic rulers; death was often the penalty for its use (Rosenthal 1971). During the Islamic Middle Ages, use of "the herbs" (also known as "the yeast of thought"), was typically associated with the secret order of the Sufis (Bakhtiar 1976; Gelpke 1982; Nahas 1982b:817*). This mystical order arose in the eighth century and quickly spread throughout the Islamic world, from Spain to the Himalayas. The Sufis, who were regarded as lawless, were always a thorn in the side of the rulers. Yet many Sufis were also part of the intelligentsia: a considerable number were alchemists, physicians, and druggists (Shah 1980:296).

The Sufis developed the dance of the dervishes, the heart meditation, and an ecstatic music and disseminated these throughout the Islamic world. They also discovered a number of psychoactive drugs, which they used both ritually and medicinally and also diffused throughout the world. The Sufis, for example, have been credited with popularizing the use of opium for producing mystical experiences and divine visions (Seefelder 1987:77). The stimulating qat bush (*Catha edulis*) and refreshing coffee (*Coffea arabica*) were discovered by Egyptian or Ethiopian Sufi monks as they were searching for agents that could help them stave off sleep during their long meditations (Ferré 1991:21f.; Schopen 1981:496; Shah 1980:51). But the Sufis also used wine, which is forbidden by Islam, and knew of *banj* or *bendsch* (henbane, *Hyoscyamus muticus*, *Hyoscyamus niger*),[1] thornapple (*Datura metel*), nutmeg, and saffron (Gelpke 1982:97). One of the founding fathers of Sufism, the

1. In the Arabic language, words such as *banj*, *bangh*, and *bendsch* mean "inebriating agent" in general but also refer to henbane in particular (Hartwich 1997:8*). Because the name is very similar to the name for hemp in Pakistan, India, Bangladesh, and Nepal, the secondary literature contains many false identifications.

druggist Fariduddin Attar (twelfth century), even knew about psychedelic mushrooms (Shah 1980:104–7). With such a supply of psychotropic drugs, it should not surprise anyone that the Sufis were also charged with discovering the inebriating effects of hemp (Anwari-Alhosseyni 1981:482).

Al-Ukbary, who lived in the twelfth century, told the story of how Sheik Haidar, the founder of the Haidari Sufi Order of Kharasan in present-day Iran and Afghanistan, discovered hashish. Haidar lived in a cloister in the Rama Mountains, where he practiced long meditations and spent his time in total seclusion. One day, while taking a walk in the searing midday heat, he noticed that the air was absolutely still. His glance fell upon a bushy plant whose leaves moved back and forth as if tossed by the wind. He interpreted this phenomenon as a sign of divine revelation. He ate some of the leaves or flowers and experienced enlightenment. Inspired by the amazing effects, he told his students: "You should ingest this gift of the Almighty God so that you may overcome the shadow sides of your souls and illuminate your spirits." Although the students were urged to keep the secret to themselves, hashish quickly became known throughout the Islamic world (Nahas 1982b:817f.*; Rosenthal 1971:48ff.)

The Sufi physician al-Razi (865–925) declared that hemp leaves could remedy ear ailments and prescribed them for dandruff and flatulence. He was also the first to describe the medicinal powers of hemp for treating epilepsy (Nahas 1982b:823*). In contrast, his contemporary, the physician Ibn Wahshiyah (early tenth century), warned against using hashish (especially when mixed with other drugs) in his *Book of Poisons* (Nahas 1982b:814*).

The Islamic author Ibn-al-Baytar (d. 1248) left behind a very influential work on nutritional and medicinal plants. He made an explicit distinction between fiber hemp and the inebriating Indian hemp. While he found that the Indian hemp was too potently inebriating, he prescribed fiber hemp for earaches, even though it could also cause headaches. He stated that the seeds were difficult to digest and had diuretic effects (II:327). The renowned Arabic physician Abu Ali Ibn Sina, also known as Avicenna (980–1037) did not add anything new, except to note that hemp could counteract headaches (Lib. II, trac. II, cap. 174). Another Arabic physician, al-Badri (1251) described hemp as an appetite stimulant. Hemp was often characterized as an aphrodisiac: it was said that it was able to open the "doors of desire." Excessive use, however, could diminish the desire for sexual intercourse (Nahas 1982b:823*; cf. Gelpke 1982:103f.).

The German explorer and naturalist Georg Eberhard Rumpf, also known as Rumphius (1627–1702), wrote in his *Herbarium* that the "Mussulmans" used Indian hemp as a remedy for asthma, gonorrhea, and constipation and as an antidote for poisonings (Nahas 1982b:823*).

In the Islamic world, which was influenced by the Arabic medical literature, when hashish is used for hedonistic purposes it is usually smoked in a water pipe. It is typically smoked alone or mixed with henbane or tobacco. When used for aphrodisiac or medicinal purposes, it is normally drunk (*bhang*) or eaten. Hashish is often mixed with honey and spices, and sometimes with mandrake root (Rosenthal 1971:34). The Egyptian author al-Maqrizi (thirteenth century) noted that physicians

Dervishes also love to use hashish: it heightens the enjoyment when listening to music, increases the exhilaration when dancing, and directs the ecstasy towards god. . . . In the Islamic Near East, hashish is considered to be the perfect instrument for accumulating and intensifying mystical experiences.

JÜRGEN FREMBGEN
DERWISCHE: GELEBTER SUFISMUS
(1993:198)

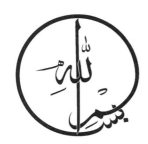

One of the calligraphic images used by the Sufis, "In the Name of God," refers to the mystical path. Many Sufis use the "Sacred Herb," hashish or hemp, as they travel on this path.

stipulated that hemp seeds or leaves only be ingested with sugar or honey, almonds, pistachios, or poppy seeds. In addition, hemp should be roasted before use. Otherwise, a demon might dwell within it that could make a person crazy (Rosenthal 1971:57).

In Pakistan, where the traditional use of hemp is socially accepted and culturally favored (Khan et al. 1975), and in the Islamic part of northern India, Unani medicine has been practiced since the Middle Ages. Essentially a method of healing with herbs, Unani medicine's origins can be traced back directly to Avicenna. Hemp is used medicinally in much the same way as recommended by Avicenna (Khan et al. 1981). It is prescribed especially for "headaches resulting from hot or cold temperaments without mucus" (Chisti 1988:195). It has also been observed that in Pakistan, regular users of bhang never suffer from dysentery, a very common disease in that country (Khan et al. 1975:348f.)

Today, hemp is still cultivated for medicinal purposes in Islamic Yemen, where it is known as *hasis*. The resin and the female inflorescences are used as a narcotic (Fleurentin and Pelt 1982:90f.). Hemp flowers are also mixed with dried qat (*Catha edulis*) leaves—which contain ephedrine—and smoked (Schopen 1981).

Symptomatic of the Islamic opposition to psychoactive drugs is the fact that hemp receives no mention in modern works on the Islamic healing arts of the Sufis (for example, see Moinuddin 1984).

Unani Headache Remedy

"This recipe is useful when the headache only appears on one side of the head and not on the other: 1 teaspoon of gummi arabicum [resin of *Acacia senegal*], 1/2 teaspoon hemp, 1/4 teaspoon saffron. Mix this with egg white or rose water. Spread this on a piece of paper and apply it to the temple of the affected side. It is especially useful when applied to a pulsing vein" (Chisti 1988:195).

Bhang (Pakistan)

Soften dried hemp leaves in water for 15 minutes. Heat the leaves in the same water, but do not boil. Pour water off. Wash the saturated leaves in running water for 15 to 20 minutes. Grind the treated leaves to a paste. Dissolve the paste in cold water and drink. The taste can be improved by adding ground almonds, sugar, and cardamom (Khan et al. 1975:352).

Duq-e wah-dat, "Buttermilk of the Divine Unity" (Iran)

Chop female hemp flowers. Mix with sugar, and stir into milk.

Hemp Coffee (Yemen)

Mix hashish with cardamom and stir into clarified butter (ghee). Add 1 teaspoon of this mixture to a cup of hot coffee. Sweeten according to taste.

REFERENCES

Anwari-Alhosseyni, Schams. 1981. Über Haschisch und Opium in Iran. In *Rausch und Realität*, edited by G. Völger. Vol. 2. Cologne: Rautenstrauch-Joest-Museum, pages 482–7.

Bakhtiar, Laleh 1976. *Sufi: Expressions of the Mystic Quest*. London: Thames and Hudson.

Chisti, Hakim G. M. 1988. *The Traditional Healer: A Comprehensive Guide to the Principles and Practice of Unani Herbal Medicine*. Rochester, Vermont: Healing Arts Press.

Ferré, Felipe. 1991. *Kaffee: Eine Kulturgeschichte*. Tübingen, Germany: Wasmuth.

Fleurentin, Jacques, and Jean-Marie Pelt. 1982. Repertory of Drugs and Medicinal Plants of Yemen. *Journal of Ethnopharmacology* 6:85–108.

Frembgen, Jürgen. 1993. *Derwische: Gelebter Sufismus*. Cologne, Germany: Dumont.

Gelpke, Rudolf. 1982. *Vom Rausch im Orient und Okzident*. Frankfurt am Main: Ullstein (Klett-Cotta).

Khan, A. B., M. Tariq, S. H. Afaq, and M. Asif. 1981. Poisons and Antidotes in Unani Systems of Medicine. *Indian Journal of History of Science* 16(1):57–63.

Khan, Munir A., Assad Abbas, and Knud Jensen. 1975. Cannabis Usage in Pakistan: A Pilot Study of Long Term Effects on Social Status and Physical Health. In *Cannabis and Culture*, edited by V. Rubin. The Hague: Mouton, pages 345–54.

Moinuddin, Abu Abdallah Gulam. 1984. *Die Heilkunst der Sufis: Grundsätze und Praktiken*. Freiburg i.B., Germany: Bauer.

Rosenthal, Franz. 1971. *The Herb: Hashish versus Medieval Muslim Society*. Leiden, Germany: E. J. Brill.

Seefelder, Matthias. 1987. *Opium: Eine Kulturgeschichte*. Frankfurt am Main: Athenäum.

Schopen, Armin. 1981. Qat in Yemen. In *Rausch und Realität*, edited by G. Völger Vol. 2. Cologne: Rautenstrauch-Joest-Museum, pages 496–501.

Shah, Idries. 1980. *Die Sufis: Botschaft der Derwische, Weisheit der Magier*. Dusseldorf, Germany: Diederichs.

Sournia, Jeans-Charles. 1990. Die arabische Medizin. In *Illustrierte Geschichte der Medizin*, edited by R. Toellner. Vol. 2. Salzburg: Andreas und Andreas, pages 585–625.

Steinschneider, Moritz. 1971. *Die Toxikologischen Schriften der Araber*. Hildesheim, Germany: Gerstenberg.

Treben, Maria. 1980. *Gesundheit aus der Apotheke Gottes*. Steyr, Germany: Ennsthaler.

Watson, Gilbert. 1966. *Theriac and Mithridatium: A Study in Therapeutics*. London: The Wellcome Historical Medical Library.

The intellect is not increased by eating hashish,
and the world (and its values) will not become different by not eating it.
Against sorrow (does it help) to eat a little;
but no one should eat himself full, so that
he will not be damaged by impudence.

MAHSATI
(TWELFTH CENTURY)
(CITED IN GELPKE 1995:65*)

Hanaf

THE HERB OF THE GERMAN LOVE GODDESS

Freyja is the Queen of the Valkyries (those who choose the slain). She is kindly disposed toward those who call upon her, and from her arose the name "Frau," which we use today for females. She loves the minnesong, and it is good to invoke her in matters of love. Freyja is the Love Goddess, the Goddess of the Night and the Night Sky, and therewith the Moon Goddess as well.

GÉZA VON NEMÉNYI
HEIDNISCHE NATURRELIGION
(1988:62)

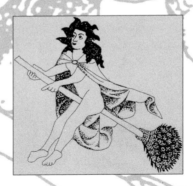

A painting on the inside wall of a vault in the Schleswig Cathedral in northern Germany depicts the Germanic love goddess Freia riding naked on a broom, like a witch. She is shown wearing the typical cloak of a Germanic seeress (known as *Völva* or *Alruna*). The witch's broom may be related to shamanic magical staffs that were made of hemp. Hemp was the sacred plant of Freia. (copy of the twelfth century original)

In his Romantic opera *Tannhäuser* (especially the 1861 Parisian version), Richard Wagner immortalized the legend of the singer and Venus. According to this legend, Venus—the Roman name of the goddess of love—lives in the interior of a mountain, in a pleasant grotto, a comfortable cave in the womb of the earth. There she is surrounded by frenzied bacchantes, lustful maenads, dancing nymphs, seductive sirens, lecherous satyrs, and potent fauns. In the Venusberg, every erotic dream comes true. Orgies, group sex, homosexual and heterosexual acts, even animals are allowed, such as Leda mating with the swan and Europa with the bull. Eroticism is an inebriation of sensual pleasure, a collective ecstasy, a sexual frenzy. Because Tannhäuser was a talented singer who could sing the praises of love and desire like no one else before him, Venus personally invited him to come to her realm of the senses. Like a shaman, he traveled to the mountain of the goddess. Once there, he discovered the wild activities and fell enraptured onto the thighs of the charming Venus, celebrating with her the festival of love, the sacred nuptials. He archetypically fulfilled the collective male fantasy: to unite with the goddess in the pinnacle of sexual ecstasy. And all of this occurred in a cave in Thuringia, Germany.

According to legend, the cave of Venus lies in Hörsel Mountain. While there is a Mount Hörsel on the map of Thuringia today, there are a number of possibilities about where it might have originally been located. Since Tannhäuser, no one has ever found their way into the grotto of Venus again, although many have tried. For humans are whipped through life by a fierce drive for desire, inebriation, and ecstasy. How wonderful it is that hemp was discovered along the way!

The people of Thuringia must have discovered hemp at a very early date, for hemp seeds were found in a cave near Eisenberg in deposits dating from the Band Ceramic period in the Late Stone Age; the deposits are some seventy-five hundred years old. The excavations do not tell us whether the Thuringian cave people used hemp for food, as a source of fiber, or as an agent of inebriation. But this may be the source of the legend of the Venusberg.

The oldest archaeological hemp find in Eisenberg/Thuringia thus far known dates to pre-Germanic times. But there is also archaeological evidence from the early Germanic period. Seeds of *Cannabis sativa* were discovered among the ashes in a funeral urn from Wilmersdorf (Brandenburg) that have been dated to the fifth century B.C.E. (Hartwich 1997:7*; Reininger 1941:2791* and 1968:14*).[1] Hemp seeds, fibers, and inflorescences have been recovered from graves in southern Germany that date to the same time (Kessler 1985:22). This supports the conclusion that the southern Germanic tribes were already using hemp ritually (as a grave offering) in prehistoric times. It must have been very highly esteemed indeed, for people only provide the dead with the very best and most important things for their journey into the next world.

Among the Germanic peoples, who were primarily farmers, hemp was known as *hanapiz*, *haenep*, or *hanaf*. The name *hanaf* or *hanef* was also used among the southern

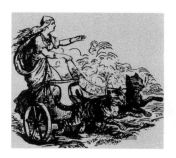

The Germanic love goddess Freia (or Freya) possessed "golden apples," the daily consumption of which maintained the immortality and the youthfulness of the gods and goddesses. Her "golden apples" were probably the fruits or inflorescences of the aphrodisiac hemp plant, which was sacred to her. (illustration, nineteenth century)

---

1. The find "consisted of leaves and fruits, those are the parts of cannabis that are still used today as agents of pleasure. . . .Thus, we may conclude that the marijuana buried near Wilmersdorf was intended to be used as an agent of pleasure" (Hartwich 1997:7*).

Germanic groups as a man's first name, and a certain Hanef von Othveginstunga achieved some degree of fame (cf. Grönbech 1997:55f.). Hemp was cultivated in fields together with grain, vegetables, and other useful plants (Derolez 1963:21). Only women could plant, cultivate, and harvest hemp (Storl 1986:324). Erotic rituals accompanied both sowing and harvesting (Rätsch 1992). During the harvest, people became very inebriated: "You can also get a good idea of this inebriation in the German hemp fields" (Tobler 1938:67). Hemp served as a source of fiber, as a food, and as an aphrodisiac and medicine. The stalks were used in the ritual banishment of winter: "You lay such a stalk flat on two garden stools and flick it into the air with a switch. . . . These flying hemp stalks represent the arrows of spring, by means of which the winter is shot away" (Perger 1864:197). After the winter had been banished, the earth would shine under the glow of May. The sun, climbing ever higher, would fertilize the forests, meadows, and fields. Easter is near. Easter, the Festival of Ostara, the goddess of love adorned in her spring garb. Her sacred animals, the hares (themselves products of erotic ecstasy) would be sacrificed and eaten in a communal meal. Within the flesh of the hare lies unbridled sexuality. It is best washed down with a good hemp beer. Unfortunately, the bacchanalian orgies that followed, through which fertility was transferred to the plants and animals by sympathetic magic, fell victim to the Christian liturgy. How wonderful it would be to celebrate an old Germanic Easter! A festival of erotic inebriation, a festival of joy, of nature, of hemp! Using pleasure to attain lustful rapture. Into the arms of the love goddess with hemp!

Among the Germanic peoples, hemp was a symbol of fertility:

> The hemp seeds also appear to serve as a fertility symbol. Hemp seeds, given to hens, cause them to lay eggs throughout the entire winter. On Christmas Eve, people eat hemp soup, poppy dumplings, fish, and dried fruit (called *Beuthen* in Upper Silesia). In Germany, there appears to be no evidence that the sowing of hemp seeds was used as a love oracle, as young girls will do in England. Hemp is also used in love oracles among the Slavic peoples. They use it the other way around: the man sows the hemp seeds, and his wife brings an egg dish ("hemp eggs") to the fields so that the hemp will thrive. In Transylvania, hemp pancakes are prepared on Epiphany for the same reason. . . . A childless Hungarian woman will eat Spanish fly and hemp flowers cooked in donkey's blood every Friday [the day of the love goddess Freia/Venus] before sunset." (*Handwörterbuch des Deutschen Aberglaubens*, 1931)

Hemp was the sacred plant of the goddess of love (Kessler 1985:22; Neményi 1988:94). The love goddess Frija—whom the Romans named Venus and was also known under the names Freia, Freyja, Holda, Frau Holle, Frau Venus—was the goddess of fertility, of spring, and of eroticism; she was the goddess who protected life and watched over marriage. Hemp, sacred to her, was used to promote desire, fertility, and health in humans. In a culture in which desire and eroticism were sacred, hemp was also a "plant of the gods," or more precisely, a plant of the love goddess.

It is possible that the Germanic peoples also regarded hemp as a symbol of fate, for the three Norns (the goddesses of fate, personified as the Past, the Present, and the Future) are said to have spun hemp fiber into their endless rope of fate (cf. Storl 1986:325).

Since the traditional method of obtaining fibers involved slowly burning the entire plant (Tobler 1938), it can be assumed that the ancient Germanic peoples also recognized that the fumes from flowers produced psychoactive effects when burned:

> From these hemp fumigations with narcotic effects follow the supposed effects of binding painful limbs with hemp tow, the "hair bath" of Upper German folk medicine (a replacement of the hemp baths [of the Scythians]), or using vapor baths of hemp leaves, an experience which may come from the Germanic nomadic period, during which hemp stalks may have occasionally been used to make fires inside the tent huts. The contemporary use of hemp oil to treat wheezing in horses is also derived from those hemp fumigations. During the Middle Ages, however, the hemp culture was expressed largely in the form of hemp oil, a Lenten soup (in Middle High German: *hanef-suppe*) made in one's own garden. This explains why the nutritious oil plant, like other nutritional plants which promote fertility, is used as a marriage oracle. (Höfler 1990:99)

What Was the Magical Plant of the Druids?

In the ancient literature, the most important plant of the Gallic Druids is often listed and described under the name *verbena* (see for example, Pliny XXV, 105f.). Today, this plant is usually interpreted botanically as vervain (*Verbena officinalis* L.). But vervain does not exhibit any of the effects listed in the ancient writings. For this reason, the botanical identification has remained in question.

The Gaul Marcellus (ca. 400 C.E.) served as a high government official under Emperor Theodosius I and wrote a recipe book in Latin for his sons entitled *De medicamentis* (Of the Medicines). This work is one of the most important sources of Gallic-Celtic ethnobotany. In this text, he wrote that verbena could heal goiter (which was known as the "royal malady") and was also a sympathetic agent for treating hemorrhages (X, 81; Höfler 1911:9, 277).

An Old High German gloss stated *verbena herba quam dicimus hanaf*, "vervain, which is called *hanaf*." The Gauls thus used the Germanic word for hemp to refer to the magical "vervain" of the Druids. There is archaeological and ethno-historical evidence for a Gallic-Celtic use of hemp as a fumigant: "even though the European hemp does not have the same power as the 'Indian hemp' it is still able to induce a trance state and was long used in rural areas for this purpose. With great likelihood, it can be assumed that the Druids also availed themselves of it" (Markale 1989:162).

Aphrodisiac decoction

Take 3 ounces of crushed hemp seeds; wild lettuce [Lactuca virosa], green purslane [Portulaca oleracea L.], 1½ handfuls of each, 2 ounces of four cooling grains, allow all to come to a boil in 6 pounds of water, continue boiling until only 4 pounds remain, strain off the decoction, sweeten this with fine sugar, and add 3 quintels of saltpeter.

NEU-VERMEHRTE, HEYLSAME DRECK-APOTHEKE (FRANKFURT AM MAIN, 1714: 79)

Germanic Incense
(from Olaf Rippe)

Laurel (bay) leaves (*Laurus nobilis* L.)
Henbane seeds (*Hyoscyamus niger* L., H. albus L.)
Mugwort herbage (*Artemisia vulgaris* L.)
Female hemp flowers (*Cannabis* spp.)

Combine equal parts of each ingredient. The mixture is strewn over glowing incense or wood coals. It is said to be suitable for oracular use.

Nordic Incense
(from Margret Madejsky)

Juniper needles (*Juniperus communis* L.)
Mugwort herbage (*Artemisia vulgaris* L.)
Spruce (*Picea abies* [L.] KARSTEN)
 or fir resin (*Abies alba* MILL., Abies spp.)
Yew needles (*Taxus baccata* L.)
Optional:
Ground amber
Female hemp flowers (*Cannabis sativa* L.)
Henbane (*Hyoscyamus niger* L.)

Combine equal parts of each ingredient. Strew the mixture over glowing incense or wood coals.

REFERENCES

Derolez, R. L. M. 1963. *Götter und Mythen der Germanen.* Einsiedeln, Germany: Benziger.

Grönbech, Wilhelm. 1997. *Kultur und Religion der Germanen.* Darmstadt, Germany: Primus Verlag.

Höfler, Max. 1911. Volksmedizinische Botanik der Kelten. *Archiv für Geschichte der Medizin* 5(1/2):1–35, 5(4/5):241–79.

———. [1908] 1990. *Volksmedizinische Botanik der Germanen.* Berlin: VWB.

Kessler, Thomas, ed. 1985. *Cannabis Helvetica.* Nachtschatten-Verlag.

Markale, Jean. 1989. *Die Druiden: Gesellschaft und Götter der Kelten.* Munich: Goldmann.

Neményi, Géza von. 1988. *Heidnische Naturreligion.* Bergen, Germany: Bohmeier Verlag.

Perger, K. Ritter von. 1864. *Deutsche Pflanzensagen.* Stuttgart, Germany: Schaber.

Rätsch, Christian. 1992. Die heiligen Pflanzen unserer Ahnen. In *Das Tor zu inneren Raümen,* edited by Christian Rätsch. Südergellersen, Germany: Verlag Bruno Martin, pages 95–103.

Storl, Wolf-Dieter. 1986. *Vom rechten Umgang mit heilenden Pflanzen.* Freiburg i.B.: Bauer.

Tobler, Friedrich. 1938. *Deutsche Faserpflanzen und Pflanzenfasern.* Berlin: Lehmanns Verlag.

De Hanff-Cannabus

HEMP IN HILDEGARD'S MEDICINE

Within himself, man holds Heaven and Earth, and all of the created world. And so the universe rests safely inside man.

HILDEGARD VON BINGEN

VON BINGEN

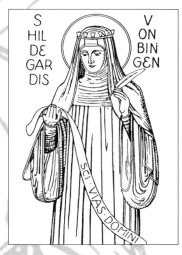

In addition to her medicinal works, Hildegard von Bingen also wrote a number of books about her cosmic visions as well as several musical compositions. Contemporary reports suggest that she was rather frail and sickly, but driven by a fanatical ambition. (woodcut, eighteenth–nineteenth century)

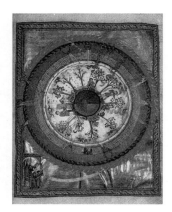

This medieval painting depicts Hildegard von Bingen (below left) and her vision of a calendrical course of the world that is divided into four sections. In her eyes, the "green power" pervaded through and animated the world. It is possible that Hildegard's visions were influenced by hemp. (from Hildegard von Bingen, *Scivias*, fol. 38r, twelfth century)

oday, Hildegard von Bingen (1098–1179) is often portrayed as "the first German visionary." But the Catholic mystic from the Rhine actually had a number of predecessors. During her lifetime, she assumed the ancient Germanic roles of seeress, saint, and physician, all of which originated in the pagan tradition. The special powers and abilities of the Germanic women had already been noticed by the Roman historian Tacitus in the first century C.E. who, in his *Germania*, had the following to say about these remarkable women:

> Indeed, they [the Germanic peoples] believe that there is even something inherently sacred and visionary about women; for this reason, they do not dismiss their advice, nor do they disregard their decisions. We have seen with the now departed Vespasianus how very many [Germanic people] long regarded a Velada as a divine being. But even before that, they venerated an Albruna[1] and many others, to be sure, not in submission (like us) and without making them equal to goddesses. (*Germania* VIII)

The power of the Germanic women was maintained into the Late Middle Ages (Rosenberg 1988:51). During the transition to the modern era, however, their pagan roots caused many of them to land on the pyre as "witches."

In the eyes of the Roman Church, Germania was completely converted to Christianity during the eleventh and twelfth centuries. But the twelfth century brought some confusion. Displeasure with the Church grew in all segments of the population. The Black Death spread throughout the land. "St. Anthony's fire" burned in many heads. There were widespread stories of witches and diabolical women. The dissatisfaction with the rulers and the Church led to the formation of numerous sects, for example, the Cathars and the Adamitae, whose heretical rituals were immortalized in Hieronymus Bosch's *Garden of Earthly Delights*. The apostasy of the population provoked the Church to take devastating steps, and the Church responded by launching the Inquisition and organizing the Great Crusades. In 1147, when Bernhard von Clairvaux "preached the cross and inflamed the masses with his passionate and spellbinding eloquence, the Valkyrie spirit was awakened in the secluded cells of nuns" (cited in Clausberg 1980:84).

This "Valkyrie spirit" was aroused particularly within the Rhenish prophetess, Hildegard von Bingen, visionary, nun, physician, scholar, and later abbess. The *prophetessa teutonica* from Rupertsberg was born in 1098, in the middle of a time of cultural uncertainty. She grew up a sickly, consumptive girl; her visionary experiences began early in life, but she did not dare to speak of them. It was only much later that she would dictate her visions and allow them to be recorded in Latin. In her prophetic work *Scivias* (Know the Ways), she provided a clear description of the manner in which her visions arose:

> The faces that I see, I do not receive in dreamlike states, not in sleep or in mental derangement, not with the eyes of the body or the ears of the outer per-

---

1. The German name for *Mandragora* (mandrake), *Alraune*, was borrowed from this name for a Germanic seeress, which means "the all-knowing."

son, and not in secluded places, but awake, calm, and with a clear mind, with the eyes and ears of the inner person, in generally accessible places, as God wills. How this happens is difficult for a man clad in flesh to understand. (Hildegard 1997)

This passage clearly shows her attempts to gain validation for the genuineness of her visions, as the Church has always viewed visionaries with great mistrust and has usually branded them as false prophets and heretics. Hildegard was also forced to fight for acceptance by the Church. Finally, during a synod in Trier (1147–48), a papal committee of investigation recognized her visionary gifts as having the "status of private revelations" (Clausberg 1980:89). Although the Rhenish visionary was widely regarded as a folk saint during her own lifetime, she has still not been formally canonized by the Vatican (Clausberg 1980:90).

Hildegard developed a visionary, mystical view of the world that combined animistic, ancient, Orphic, and early Christian elements. Her visions were intended to show the people of the Middle Ages a path through life and reveal to them the way to God; they were also aimed at bringing heretics back to the Church. Hildegard saw the *viriditas*, the "green power" that flows in all creatures and fills them with life and divinity, as the source of life (Metzner 1988). In her later work, *Liber divinorum operum*, the Book of Divine Operations, Hildegard developed an animistic-pantheistic, even alchemical, conception of the world:

I too am the fiery life of the divine substance, I blaze above the beauty of the fields and shine in the water and burn in the sun, moon, and stars; and with the airy winds, to some extent invisible, I am the life which maintains all, I excite all that lives. The air lives truly in the green and in the flowers; the waters flow as if they were alive; the sun lives truly in its glory, and the waning moon is enflamed by the light of the sun, so that he lives so to speak from anew; the stars too shine in their light as if alive. . . . And so I am the fiery power hidden in everything, and the things ignite through me as if of their own accord, as the breath ceaselessly moves men, and as the flickering flame is in the fire. All of these things live in their innermost being, and you can find no death in them, for I am life.

Her view of humans seems unusual: "Thus do both exist, body and soul, in spite of their different natures, nevertheless as a single reality. And so man also lives in his fully concrete state: above as below, outside as inside, he exists all and everywhere as corporeal. And that is the nature of man" (from Schipperges 1984:14).

Hildegard von Bingen has often been described as the "first woman scientist and physician of the Germans." In the cloister, she maintained a garden with food, spice, and medicinal plants. She also studied the ancient and Arabic texts on the doctrines of medicine and the healing arts of Dioscorides, Galen, Celsus, Avicenna, and the like. Because she was close to the people, she was also able to compile a great deal of indigenous Germanic knowledge about herbs. Her scientific and medical writings drew from these various sources (Rosenberg 1988:69). In her *Physica*, (Natural History) she described the medicinal properties and uses of indigenous and foreign plants, animals, and stones. In *Causae et curae* (Causes and Treatments of Diseases) she developed a coherent medieval medical system (Schipperges 1990). Both works contain much information about the medieval cloister and native uses of kitchen herbs and poisonous and healing plants (Müller 1982). Hildegard's time is often described as the "pinnacle of cloister medicine" (Kühnemann 1988). In chapters 1 through 11 of the *Physica*, it is stated:

> [*De Hanff-Cannabus*] *Of Hemp.* Hemp is warm, and when the air is neither very warm nor very cold, it grows, and so too is its nature, and its seeds contain healing power, and it is wholesome for healthy people to eat, and in their stomachs it is light and useful, so that it carries out the mucus from the stomach to some extent, and it can be easily digested, and it diminishes the bad humors and makes the good humors strong. But he who is ill in the head and has an empty brain and [then] eats hemp, this will easily cause him some pain in the head. But he who has a healthy head and a full brain in the head, it will not harm him. But he who is very ill, it will cause some pain in his stomach. But he who is moderately ill will not be harmed by eating it.
>
> But he who has a cold stomach, he should boil hemp in water and, after pressing out the water, wrap it in a small cloth. And he should lay it upon his stomach often while thus warm, and this will strengthen him and bring him back to his condition. And he who even has an empty brain and eats hemp, it will cause him some pain in the head. But it does not harm the healthy head and the full brain. A cloth made of hemp is good for binding ulcers and wounds, because the warmth in it is moderate.

Clearly, Hildegard von Bingen had discovered that the "green power" (which has been a synonym for hashish in Germany since the 1960s) is also present in hemp:

> Now in the discussion of Hildegard, who seldom provides information about the growing conditions of plants, her remark is striking that the plant thrives only under favorable climatic conditions, when the air is not too warm and not too cold, that is, in moderate climate zones. This unusual comment, together with her statement that cannabis could harm the head and cause headaches, could lead one to suppose that Hildegard had observed hemp plants which also occasionally produced small amounts of hashish. (Müller 1982:94)

Could we even go so far as to infer that the Rhenish sibyl herself partook of the resin, thereby strengthening her visions of the "green power"? After all, there is a direct link between the "green power" of the 1960s and the ecological Green Movement of the 1970s.

In recent years, the "medicine of Hildegard" has witnessed an astonishing renaissance in Neo-Christian, esoteric, and New Age circles. A number of books on herbs have appeared that are based upon her writings. In these works, Hildegard's recipes are often presented like the dogma of a new belief system. The physicians Hertzka and Strehlow (both men!), who are probably the most influential protagonists of Hildegard's medicine, believe that her recipes can only be truly effective when they are prepared and administered exactly as described in her original texts. "Dr.

Hertzka has repeatedly attempted to put together medicines following the saint's guidelines, which are now more than eight hundred years old. And so he managed to have one of the two very rare and highly protected white-headed vultures, which the Salzburg state government formerly allowed to be shot each year, 'approved for research purposes'" (Reger 1984:22). Hertzka proudly described the "vulture ointment" that he prepared from the protected bird, as only the original recipe was said to be able to cure cancer and paraplegia. In this case, the law was willfully violated for purely dogmatic reasons. At the same time, not one single mention of hemp can be found in Hertzka's writings (Hertzka and Strehlow 1987; see also the books by Reger 1984 and Schiller 1991). Clearly, this oversight has to do with the politics of medicine, which acts as if hemp was never a part of "Hildegard's medicine."

A great quantity of secondary literature on Hildegard's medicine was published during the so-called Year of Hildegard in 1998, the nine-hundredth anniversary of her birth, and hemp was omitted in all of them. The "rediscovery" of Hildegard's knowledge and the cloister medicine that surrounds it has been rightfully criticized:

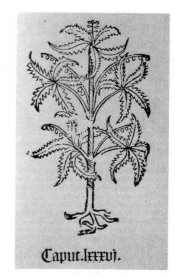

This woodcut from the medieval herbal *Hortus sanitatis* is probably the oldest German representation of hemp. (twelfth–thirteenth century)

> The medicine of Hildegard is a moralizing doctrine of medicine, firmly embedded in a medieval, Catholic view of the world: illness is the result of Original Sin. . . . Hildegard's medicine, as it is practiced today, seems old and venerable, but it is in fact a new literary creation, a risky modern interpretation. . . . Generally speaking, cloister medicine is overrated in esoteric-conservative, Eurocentric circles. Compared to the Chinese medicinal gardens or the Aztec garden of medicinal plants in Tenochtitlan, which contained over two thousand different species, the much-vaunted "Hortuli," that little cloister garden with its twenty-four pampered plants from foreign biotopes, appears rather modest. (Storl 1998:61)

A Hemp Cloth to Treat Stomachaches

Whoever has stomachaches, so that his stomach is suppurating or cold or hardened, so that he cannot digest the foods he eats, he should take tallow (from a deer) and add to this one-third as much oil of the fruit of the hornbeam or of the beech, and he should mix these at the same time, and then spread this on a hemp cloth, and this cloth he should place upon his stomach, and so should he wear it, and even when the pain in his stomach is strong, he will become better. But if he can obtain neither of the two oils, then he should spread tallow of deer onto the aforementioned cloth, as was stated, over his stomach.

Hildegard von Bingen
Physica VII, 11

Hemp, A Plant of the Midwives and Witches

It is very likely that medieval midwives were well acquainted with hemp and used it in their practices as both an aphrodisiac and an analgesic. Hemp has generally been regarded as a love drink and has been banned for that selfsame reason (cf.

Madejsky 1995; Lussi 1996*). In the same manner, midwives were increasingly demonized during the Late Middle Ages and were denounced as witches (Ehrenreich and English 1981).

An ordinance regulating midwives that was proclaimed in Württemberg in southern Germany in 1480, and that has been preserved in the *Crailsheimer Kirchenbuch* (Church Book of Crailsheim) describes an operation to perform a caesarean section in which hemp plays an almost magical role (Pfeilsticker 1928:97):

> Many mothers who notice during delivery that they are going to die will ask the midwife for a caesarean section, so that their child may be saved. In this case, a skilled midwife will cut open the left side of the woman's abdomen while she is still alive. It should be emphasized that it should not be the right side of the abdomen, for in women the heart lies on the right side, while in men it is on the left. The incision should be made in the area of the pubic bone and should be about as wide as a hand. The helpers should then lay the body of the woman on her back with the head in a lowered position. Using a hand that has been oiled, the midwife should carefully push the intestines aside and open the uterus. Now the body should be turned back onto its side and the child removed. If the mother stills shows signs of life, she should again be carefully laid on her back, and the wound should be stitched with a silken or other thread. A plaster made from three eggs and hemp cloth, and Armenian earth (*Bolus armenicus*) if it is available, should be fastened over this. To strengthen the woman after this, a little good wine should be given to her. (Kruse 1996:202)

Toward the end of the Middle Ages, poplar ointment, or *Unguentum populeum*, was one of the most commonly used painkillers and was widely known throughout the population. It has been listed in almost all herbals and pharmacopoeias since the fifteenth century. In addition to the resinous poplar buds, the *Gart of Gesundheit* (Garden of Health) from 1485 states that equal amounts of the following ingredients should also be used: poppy leaves (*Papaver somniferum* L.), houseleek leaves (*Sempervivum tectorum* L.), lettuce leaves (*Lactuca sativa* L. or *Latuca virosa* L.), orchid leaves (*Orchis* spp.), nightshade (*Solanum* sp.), henbane leaves (*Hyoscyamus niger* L.), and mandrake leaves (*Mandragora officinarum*). Grind all the ingredients and boil in lard. The use is also of interest: the ointment is applied to the temples and to the area around the navel. In later recipes, belladonna (*Atropa belladonna*) and hemp (*Cannabis sativa*) are also listed among the ingredients (Vries 1991).

During the sixteenth century, when the Inquisition was coming into its own, witches were often accused of using a flying or love ointment to practice the "forbidden arts" (necromancy). Consulting early modern physicians (all of them men) were of the opinion that the witches' ointment contained the same or very similar constituents as the medicinal poplar ointment (Kuhlen 1983; Vries 1991). All of the recipes that were made public included hemp or *Cannabis* among their ingredients. Not surprisingly, the "Witches' Bull" of 1484, in which Pope Innocent VIII declared war upon the witches, also forbade the use of cannabis (Amrein 1997). It should therefore come as no surprise that current drug laws still define hemp to be an illegal plant (cf. Müller-Ebeling et al. 1998*).

REFERENCES

Amrein, Josef. 1997. Verpöntes Medikament auf Schweizer Prüfständen. *Die Weltwoche* 15 (April 4, 1997):55.

von Bingen, Hildegard. 1985. *Ursachen und Behandlung der Krankheiten.* Heidelberg: Haug.

———. 1989. *Naturkunde.* 4th ed. Salzburg: Otto Müller Verlag.

———. 1991. *Heilkraft der Natur: Physica.* Augsburg: Pattloch. First text critical translation.

———. 1997. *Scivias—Wisse die Wege.* Augsburg, Germany: Pattloch (Weltbild Verlag).

Clausberg, Karl. 1980. *Kosmische Visionen: Mystische Weltbilder von Hildegard von Bingen bis heute.* Cologne, Germany: Dumont.

Ehrenreich, Barbara, and Deike English. 1981. *Hexen, Hebammen und Krankenschwestern.* Munich: Frauenoffensive.

Hertzka, Gottfried, and Wighard Strehlow. 1987. *Handbuch der Hildegard-Medizin.* Freiburg i.B., Germany: Bauer.

Kruse, Britta-Juliane. 1996. *Verborgene Heilkünste: Geschichte der Frauenmedizin im Spätmittelalter.* Berlin: de Gruyter.

Kühnemann, Antje-Kathrin. 1988. *Geheimnisse der Klostermedizin.* Augsburg, Germany: Pattloch.

Kuhlen, Franz-Josef. 1983. *Zur Geschichte der Schmerz-, Schlaf- und Betäubungsmittel in Mittelalter und früher Neuzeit.* Stuttgart: Deutscher Apotheker Verlag.

Madejsky, Margret. 1995. Von Liebestränken, gallsüchtigen Weibern und Sonnenbräuten. *Kraut und Rüben* 10/95:30–1, 35–9.

———. 1997. Hexenpflanzen—oder: Über die Zauberkünste der weisen Frauen. *Naturheilpraxis* 50(10):1552–63.

Metzner, Ralph. 1988. The Mystical Symbolic Psychology of Hildegard von Bingen. *ReVISION* 11(2):3–12.

Müller, Irmgard. 1982. *Die pflanzlichen Heilmittel bei Hildegard von Bingen.* Salzburg: Otto Müller Verlag.

Pfeilsticker, Walther. 1928. Eine württembergische Hebammenordnung von ca. 1480. *Archiv für Geschichte der Medizin* 20:95–8.

Reger, Karl Heinz. 1984. *Hildegard-Medizin.* Munich: Goldmann.

Rosenberg, Alfons 1988. *Die Frau als Seherin und Prophetin.* 2d abridged ed. Munich: Kösel.

Schiller, Reinhard. 1991. *Hildegard Pflanzen-Apotheke.* Augsburg, Germany: Pattloch.

Schipperges, Heinrich. 1984. *Hildegard von Bingen und ihre Impulse für die moderne Welt.* Eibingen: Buch- und Kunsthandlung St. Hildegard.

———. 1990. *Der Garten der Gesundheit: Medizin im Mittelalter.* Munich: deutsche taschenbuch verlag.

Storl, Wolf-Dieter. 1998. Die Wiederentdeckung der "Hexenmedizin." *Esotera,* 6/98:54–61.

Tacitus. 1988. *Germania—Bericht über Germanien.* Munich: deutsche taschenbuch verlag.

de Vries, Herman. 1991. Über die sogenannten hexensalben. *Integration* 1:31–42.

Hempe

HEMP AMONG THE FATHERS OF BOTANY

Hemp is a commonly known plant in all lands.

PIERANDREA MATTHIOLUS
KRÄUTERBUCH
(1627:315C)

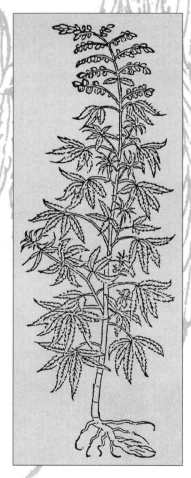

"Tame cannabis," *Cannabis sativa*,
male plant. (woodcut from
Fuchs, 1545)

With the beginning of the early modern period, radical changes were taking place in Europe. The invention of the printing press (ca. 1440) dramatically changed the sociology of knowledge. The discovery of the New World revolutionized the prevailing worldview that had been imposed by the Catholic Church. The Reformation occurred, the first major break within the Church. Scientists increasingly emancipated themselves from the rigid conceptions of the Middle Ages. Thought was increasingly oriented toward the future, as expressed in such books as *Utopia*. New inventions, new diseases (syphilis), and imported exotic drugs changed peoples' lives (Wilhelm 1984).

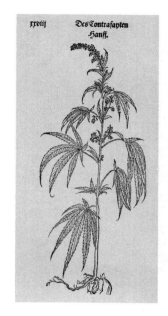

It was during this time of rapid cultural change that the "natural scientific" books were being written by authors who have gone down in the cultural history of Europe as the "Fathers of Botany": Otto Brunfels (ca. 1490–1534), Leonard Fuchs (1501–66), and Hieronymus Bock (1498–1554). Some of their students, including Johann Jakob Theodor, known as Tabernaemontanus (1522–90), and followers such as Adam Lonitzer, also called Lonicerus (1528–86), are sometimes numbered among their ranks (Gallwitz 1992:39ff.; Leibrock-Plehn 1992). The English author John Gerard (1633; cf. also Rohde 1971) and the Italian Pierandrea Matthiolus, whose work appeared in German in 1627, were part of this movement as well. German versions of Dioscorides' *De Materia Medica* were also published during this time (1610). Brunfels, Bock, and Fuchs all converted to Protestantism and initially worked in religious occupations before devoting themselves to their plant studies. Their "Herbals," as the works were known, all appeared during the first half of the sixteenth century, first in Latin, and later in a variety of German editions, and achieved a very wide distribution.

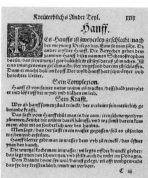

Facsimile of the chapter on hemp, together with the corresponding woodcut, from the *Teutschen Contrafayten Kreüterbuchs* by Otto Brunfels, published in Straßburg by Hans Schotten, 1532.

One of the significant innovations of these works was their inclusion of the first botanically useful illustrations (Heilmann 1973; Müller-Jahncke 1995:69; Rix 1989). While these illustrations marked an important step toward scientific botany, the texts themselves remained strongly bound to the Greco-Roman and Arabic traditions of Dioscorides and Avicenna. The German authors did move away from the elaborate composita used by the Arabic scholars, often including information that was clearly derived from German folk belief and folklore, and possibly even from the earlier Germanic tradition (Beckmann and Beckmann 1990:39; Leibrock-Plehn 1992:78).

The Fathers of Botany knew of hemp, and in fact they distinguished between "tame hemp," that is, the cultivated plant, and "wild hemp." Referring to the latter, Bock noted that: "the wild hemp is a weed in our land" (1577:126). Although the wild plant was considered to be of inferior quality, Bock still knew of a medicinal use: "Wild hemp crushed / and placed over the inflammation and wild fire / disperses the same when put upon the heat and pain" (1577:126f.)

Apart from Bock, the Fathers of Botany agreed that hemp had a warm and dry nature and could therefore dissipate wind and flatulence. All repeated the indications given by Dioscorides for ear ailments and warned: "But he who drinks too many hemp seeds / will lose his natural procreative power" (Brunfels 1532), that is, he will become impotent.[1]

---

1. Although there is no basis for this claim, this rumor has tenaciously persisted into the

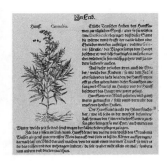

The German edition of the herbal from Pierandrea Matthiolus, which was adapted and expanded by Joachim Camerarius, describes numerous medicinal uses of German hemp. (facsimile, detail, 1626)

Brunfels mentioned a new and different treatment: using a boiled hemp root as a wrapping to treat limb pains. This information may have been derived from an ancient Germanic custom. Hiernonymus Bock describes a use from Franconia:

> In the land of the Franconians / and also in other places / they cook the hemp seeds for a daily dish / like the barley / but in truth such food used every time / makes a stupid cold stomach / wipes out the warmth and strengthens the natural works.

He gives two additional recipes that were clearly indigenous in origin:

> Hemp seeds boiled in milk and drunk when quite warm / stop and dispel the hot, oppressive cough.
>
> For the cramps in the abdomen take hemp seeds, as much as you wish / wash off the dust with water / pour good white wine over them / and boil until the grains burst / after this make a milk out of it / of this take a warm draught / so it will soothe the painful days / but you should not do this only once / but again and for a third time.

The most important new information is contained in the German edition of Matthiolus's work from 1627: "The women / who fall down from cramps in the womb / should have burning hemp held to the nose / then they will soon stand once more" (page 316). A similar description was recorded by Tabernaemontanus, whose *Kräuterbuch* (Herbal Book) is among the most comprehensive of its kind: "Those women who have cramps in the womb / for them hemp should be burned / and held to the nose" (1731:937). To my knowledge, this is the first written mention of medicinal hemp smoking in the German literature.

The works of the Fathers of Botany had a significant influence on folk medicine during the centuries that followed.[2] Thus, it comes as no surprise that some of their information concurs with the folk medicinal uses of recent and modern times. These herbals also made a significant contribution to the systematization of the plant kingdom in scientific botany.

---

present. In fact, the opposite is the case: hemp users enjoy an active sex life. After all, there must be a reason why hemp is regarded as a dependable aphrodisiac all around the world (cf. Amendt 1974*; Brodmann 1997*; Cohen 1982a*; Halikas et al. 1982*; Holmstrom 1991*; Lewis 1970*; Müller-Ebeling and Rätsch 1986*).
2. Similar works, often with the same contents, were written in England and Ireland. The most influential was the immense herbal by Gerard, in which hemp is described in great detail. An Irish herbal from 1735 (*Botanalogia Universalis Hibernica*) even lists the same medicinal effects as are found among the German authors (Scott 1991:81).

Against Hip Pains (from Bock)

Boil hemp seeds in milk; drink the entire mixture as hot or warm as possible.

According to Matthiolus (1926:316), this preparation is also effective against dry coughs.

Against the Stomach Worms of Horses (from Bock)

Pour a decoction of a hemp plant into the parasite-infested horse.

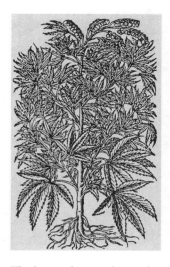

The hemp plant, as depicted in the most comprehensive herbal in European history. (woodcut from Tabernaemontanus, 1731)

REFERENCES

Beckmann, Dieter, and Barbara Beckmann. 1990. *Alraune, Beifuß und andere Hexenkräuter*. New York: Campus.

Bock, Hieronymus. 1577. *Kreütterbuch*. Straßburg, France: Josiam Rihel.

Brunfels, Otto. 1532. *Contrafayt Kreüterbuch*. Straßburg, France: Hans Schotten.

Dioskurides, Pedanios. [n.d.] *Kreutterbuch*. Frankfurt am Main: Bringern/Corthons.

Fuchs, Leonart. 1543. *New Kreütterbuch*. Basel, Switzerland: Michael Isingrin.

Gallwitz, Esther. 1992. *Kleiner Kräutergarten: Kräuter und Blumen bei den Alten Meistern im Städel*. Frankfurt am Main: Insel.

Gerard, John. 1633. *The Herbal*. London: Norton and Whitakers.

Hartlieb, Johannes. 1980. *Das Kräuterbuch des Johannes Hartlieb*. Graz, Austria: Akademische Druck- u. Verlagsanstalt.

Heilmann, Karl Eugen. 1973. *Kräuterbücher in Bild und Geschichte*. Munich-Allach: Verlag Konrad Kölbl.

Leibrock-Plehn, Larissa. 1992. *Hexenkräuter oder Arznei: Die Abtreibungsmittel im 16. und 17. Jahrhundert*. Stuttgart: WVG.

Lonicerus, Adamus. 1679. *Kreüterbuch*. [Frankfurt]: Matthäus Wagner.

Matthiolus, Pierandrea 1626. *Kreutterbuch*. Frankfurt am Main: Jacob Fischers Erben.

Müller-Jahncke, Wolf-Dieter. 1995. Herbaria picta: Zur Tradition der illustrierten Kräuterbücher des Mittelalters. *Pharmazie in unserer Zeit* 24(2):67–72.

Rix, Martyn. 1989. *The Art of Botanical Illustration*. London: Bracken Books.

Rohde, Eleanour Sinclair. [1922] 1971. *The Old English Herbals*. Reprint, New York: Dover.

Scott, Michael, ed. 1991. *An Irish Herbal—Botanalogia Universalis Hibernica (1735)*. Dublin: Anna Livia Press.

Tabernaemontanus, Jacobus Theodorus. 1731. *Neu vollkommen Kräuter-Buch* (BAUHIN-edition). Basel/Offenbach: Johann Ludwig König.

Wilhelm, Michael. 1984. *Das grüne Geheimnis*. Reinbek, Germany: Einhorn-Presse Verlag.

Distillates

HEMP IN ALCHEMY

Alchemy is a rainbow which bridges the gulf between the earthly and the heavenly realms, between matter and spirit. Like the rainbow, it seems close enough to grasp, but it will retreat if you pursue it solely so that you may find a pot of gold. . . . In all times, true alchemists, who despise riches and worldly honors, have searched tirelessly for the cure-all, the panacea, which in its highest sublimation becomes the fountain of youth, the elixir of life, and the key to immortality, both in a spiritual as well as in a mysterious physical sense.

STANISLAS KLOSSOWSKI DE ROLA
ALCHEMIE: DIE GEHEIME KUNST
(1974:7)

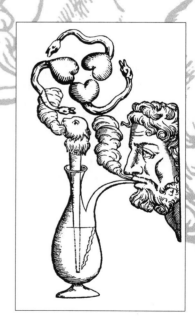

Alchemical illustration of a water pipe. The man shown drawing from the pipe sees a typical psychedelic vision in the ascending smoke. But what is the smoke pouring from the "lion's mouth"? (woodcut, Bibliothèque de Gèneve)

Alchemy is the doctrine of the inner connectedness of matter and its regularities during transformation or transmutation in the material and spiritual world, which is built from the four elements (air, water, fire, earth). Alchemy joins together natural scientific and spiritual methods. On the material plane, chemical techniques guide the search for elixirs that lead to immortality and enlightenment, to the "philosopher's stone," and to panaceas, or cure-alls. On the spiritual plane, efforts are made to achieve an expansion of consciousness, the so-called distillation of the spirit, the step-by-step clarification of consciousness and the initiation into higher spheres. Often, the complicated external, technical processes are simply symbolic representations of corresponding internal processes. Alchemy can be understood as a ritual through which activities in the laboratory are brought into harmony with one's own conscious processes (Hartlaub 1959; Metzner 1971:83–105, 1989).

The word *alchemy* is derived from the Arabic *al kimiya*, "the black." In ancient times, it was already a secret science based upon the Greek/ Egyptian god Hermes-Trismegistos (Fowden 1993; Luck 1990:443–65). The chemical/technical and philosophical/magical/astrological methods, which enjoyed enormous popularity during the European Middle Ages, both existed in ancient times. In addition to the desire to make gold from lead, the goal of the Egyptian and Greek alchemists of antiquity was to develop and improve medicines (Luck 1990:445f.). During the heyday of Central European alchemy (the fourteenth through seventeenth centuries), the improvement of medicines was a primary goal as well as the development of complex philosophical systems (such as that of the Rosicrucians): "The alchemists were concerned in part with imitating in the laboratory processes which occur in nature, while simultaneously accelerating and perfecting these. Their intention was to improve nature, to achieve the same results as nature but in a more rational manner" (Luck 1990:446). As part of this, the principle of distillation became a focus of alchemical interest. The beginnings of the distiller's art lie in darkness. The oldest known archaeological find of an apparatus for distillation comes from the ruins of Mohenjo Daro, in the Indus Valley, where the roots of the Arian/Vedic soma ritual and yoga also lie. The find consisted of a complete terra-cotta setup that dates to the third millennium B.C.E.; it was apparently used to distill essential oils and aromatic substances (Rovesti and Fischer-Rizzi 1995:10f.). During the Renaissance, many women worked as distillers. One of the women renowned in this area was Caterina da Forlì; one of her patrons was Giovanni de Medici:

> In addition to other wondrous pharmacological agents, Caterina da Forlì, a distiller of vital substances, prepared an "electuary to make lusty." To make this, skinks, shelled pine nuts, cinnamon, calamus roots, and hemp seeds were added to a kilo of honey (which "protects from spoiling" and "quickly transforms into blood"). As an experienced distiller, she concocted a proper recipe "to make the member stand stiffly the whole night through." After drinking the balsamic elixir, the effects of the astonishing liquid would quickly become apparent. And she encouraged them: "go to bed with the woman, and you will see that it stands stiffly, and you will be able to do it as often as you wish, and you will be able to celebrate. (Camporesi 1991:52f.)

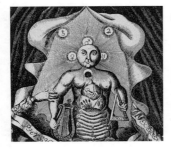

The planetary god Saturn, also known as Saturnus or Kronos, rules the element lead and all dark, poisonous, or magical herbs, including mandrake (*Mandragora officinarum*), henbane (*Hyoscyamus niger*), hemlock (*Cicuta virosa or Conium maculatum*), and hemp. The alchemists regarded Saturn as a symbol of life, death, and rebirth. (copperplate frontispiece from Johann Becher, Leipzig, 1738)

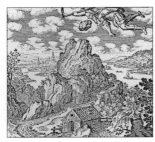

The god Saturn, shown here flying through the heavens like a shaman or a witch, spits out the *lapis philosophorum*, the "philosopher's stone." Since all psychoactive plants (mandrake, henbane, hemp, aconite, and the like) are assigned to Saturn, it can be assumed that his alchemical elixir is capable of effecting a movement of the spirit. (copperplate engraving from Michael Maier, *Atalanta fugiens*, 1618)

This is an example of a language whose directness is very rare in the alchemical literature.

The "art of distillation" was perfected especially by the Strassburger wound doctor Hieronymus Braunschweig (fifteenth century). His book, which appeared in German translation in 1610, had a great influence on the emerging fields of the apothecary arts and scientific chemistry (Gebelein 1991:196; Reichen 1964). In addition to very detailed technical information, the book also contains hundreds of medicinal recipes for manufacturing so-called waters, that is, distillates. In addition to "waters" made with other psychoactive plants (mandrake, henbane) that have generated a lively interest among alchemists since ancient times, he also included a recipe for "hemp water":

> Of hemp water. The best part and time for its distillation is when the umbels of the same are young and green / chopped and roasted.
>
> Hemp water is exceptionally good for the headache / which comes from heat / the head / temples and forehead are rubbed with it / and repeat from time to time. Hemp water extinguishes and dispels all heat / where it is / cloths moistened with it and laid on top / and this two times a day in winter / but in summer done three times daily. (Braunschweig 1610:73)

The renowned English physician, astrologist, and apothecary Nicholas Culpeper (1616–54) wrote *Culpeper's Complete Herbal*, the most influential work of its kind. In it he compiled the alchemical, astrological, and scientific knowledge of his time together with his own experiences as an attending physician and practicing apothecary. In England, his book was regarded as *the* standard work on the medicinal uses of herbs for more than three centuries. It had an enduring influence on entire generations of physicians and had a considerable impact on English folk medicine. Culpeper wrote the following about *Cannabis sativa*:

> It is a plant of Saturn. The seeds dispel wind, and too much use allows the seeds of reproduction to dry out; but if it is boiled with milk and ingested, this will help with a hot or dry cough. The emulsion from the seeds is good for jaundice when it increases, for it opens the stoppage of the gall bladder and effects the digestion of the bile. Emulsions or decoctions of the seeds have purgative and liquefying effects, soothe colic, calm the unpleasant bodily fluids of the intestines, stop bleeding in the mouth, nose, and other places. They kill worms in men and beasts; the juice, trickled into the ear, kills the worms that befall it and dispels earwigs and other living creatures. The decoction of the roots soothes inflammations of the head and other places. The herbage or the distilled water will do the same. The decoction of the roots relieves the pains of gout, the solidified humors of the nodules in the joints, the pains of the tendons and their shrinkage, and the pains in the hip. The fresh root, mixed with some oil or butter, is good for burns. (Culpeper n.d.:183)

Here, Culpeper brought together information provided by the ancient authors Dioscorides and Pliny while also adding knowledge he had accumulated on his own (cf. Rippe 1997).

In the alchemical tradition, hemp was assigned to the element water, the planetary god Saturn (Cunningham 1989:121), and the zodiacal sign Aries (Zalewski 1990:127). It was thus numbered among the Saturnian plants, together with mandrake *(Mandragora officinarum)*, henbane *(Hyoscyamus niger)*, the opium poppy *(Papaver somniferum)*, hemlock *(Conium maculatum)*, and aconite *(Aconitum napellus)*, all of which distinguish themselves because they are able to alter consciousness, that is, transform the spirit. It must thus be assumed that the alchemists of ancient and medieval times, for example, Agrippa von Nettesheim, were aware of the psychoactive effects of hemp. And so, hemp as an "elixir" approaches the ancient Chinese Taoists' drinks of immortality. Since hemp transcends time, the alchemist can have an experience of immortality (cf. Metzner 1989).

In the alchemical literature, *plants in and of themselves* have also been characterized as "alchemists," because they transform the light of the sun into matter and use the four elements to create vegetable life (Uyldert 1987:49ff.). By ingesting hemp, for example, the material ingredients of the plant can be transmuted into the illumination of the spirit. Richard Rudgley, the British drug researcher and winner of the Prometheus Prize, has characterized the influence of the psychoactive plant world upon human history as "the alchemy of culture" (1993).

Today, the expression *cannabis alchemy* is also used to refer to the manufacture of hashish and the refinement of hemp products (Gold 1994).

Of the operations of Saturn, when this planet would ascend, the ancients would depict on a so-called magnet stone an image of a man with the face of a stag and the feet of a camel, who sat on a stool or a dragon, and who held a sickle in the right hand and an arrow in the left. They hoped that this image would help them to live a long life, for Saturn is said to aid in prolonging life, as Albumasar has shown in his Book of Sadar, where he also describes that in some areas of India which are ruled by Saturn, the people live very long and only die when they have reached a very advanced age.

AGRIPPA VON NETTESHEIM
DIE MAGISCHEN WERKE
(1982:302)

REFERENCES

Agrippa von Nettesheim, Heinrich Cornelius. 1982. *Die magischen Werke*. Wiesbaden, Germany: Fourier.

Braunschweig, Hieronymus. 1610. *Ars destillandi oder Destillierkunst. . . .* Straßburg.

Camporesi, Piero. 1991. *Geheimnisse der Venus: Aphrodisiaka vergangener Zeiten*. New York: Campus.

Culpeper, Nicholas n.d. *Culpeper's Complete Herbal*. London: Foulsham.

Cunningham, Scott. 1989. *Cunningham's Encyclopedia of Magical Herbs*. St. Paul, Minn.: Llewellyn.

Fowden, Garth. 1993. *The Egyptian Hermes*. Princeton, New Jersey: Princeton University Press.

Gebelein, Helmut. 1991. *Alchemie*. Munich: Diederichs.

Gold, D. 1994. *Cannabis Alchemy: The Art of Modern Hashmaking*. Berkeley, Calif.: Ronin.

Hartlaub, G. F. 1959. *Der Stein der Weisen*. Munich: Prestel.

Klossowski de Rola, Stanislas. 1974. *Alchemie: Die geheime Kunst*. Munich: Knaur.

Lorber, Jakob. 1934. *Der Saturn*. Bietigheim, Germany: Lorber-Verlag.

Luck, Georg. 1990. *Magie und andere Geheimlehren in der Antike*. Stuttgart: Kröner.

Metzner, Ralph. 1971. *Maps of Consciousness*. New York: Macmillan.

———. 1989. Molecular Mysticism: the Role of Psychoactive Substances in the Transformation of Consciousness. In *Gateway to Inner Space*, edited by C. Rätsch. Bridport, Dorset, England: Prism Press, pages 73–88.

Reichen, Charles-Albert. 1964. *Geschichte der Chemie*. Lausanne, Switzerland: Editions Rencontre/Erik Nitsche Intern.

Rippe, Olaf. 1997. Pflanzen und ihre kosmischen Heilkräfte. *Naturheilpraxis* 10/97:1541–51.

Rovesti, Paolo (and Susanne Fischer-Rizzi, ed.). 1995. *Auf der Suche nach den verlorenen Düften*. Munich: Irisiana.

Rudgley, Richard. 1993. *The Alchemy of Culture*. London: British Museum Press.

Uyldert, Mellie. 1987. *Verborgene Kräfte der Pflanzen*. Munich: Hugendubel.

Zalewski, C. L. 1990. *Herbs in Magic and Alchemy*. Bridport, Dorset, England: Prism Press.

Home Remedies

HEMP IN FOLK MEDICINE

Crushed hemp seeds boiled in milk is one of the Dutch folk remedies. But in earlier times hemp seeds were already renowned for jaundice and drunk as a tea or emulsion. The good effect of this agent is said to have also been experienced in particular during an epidemic of jaundice in Göttingen.

JOHANN FRIEDRICH OSIANDER
VOLKSARZNEYMITTEL
(1826:154)

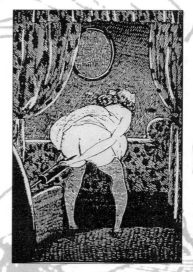

The use of enemas was popular in folk medicine, for both medicinal purposes and also for erotic ends. During the nineteenth century, smoke enemas were all the rage. Enema syringes were used to blow smoke from tobacco, or even better, from "strong tobacco" (also known as hemp), into the large intestine via the rectum. This must have quickly produced potent psychoactive effects. (illustration from *La vie de garçon*, nineteenth century)

In the nineteenth century folk medicine in Germany was largely shaped by the appearance of the so-called Doctor's Books. These books could be found in most households, especially in those of the middle, and upperclasses of society. Any time there was a little "boo-boo," a burn, vomiting, or a similar problem, people would consult the doctor in the book. The appropriate prescription would then be more or less precisely followed. The most influential Doctor's Book was the *Encyklopädie der gesammten Volksmedicin* (Encyclopedia of Complete Folk Medicine) by Dr. Georg Friedrich Most. Born in 1794, Most studied medicine in Göttingen, and ultimately became a Professor of Medicine in Rostock. He died in 1842. Most was a polymath with literary ambitions who left behind a wealth of medical and philosophical writings. But his main work was the *Encyklopädie der gesammten Volksmedicin*, which appeared a year after his death. He tracked down some of the recipes and procedures from German folk sources, discovered others himself, and adopted still others from friendly physicians, travel reports, and the medical literature of the time. With this text, he made a conscious effort to produce a popular book that would be useful for the general public. In 1849, this well-received work was republished under a new title: *Der Hausarzt. Ein vollständiges Handbuch der vorzüglichsten und wirksamsten Haus- und Volksarzneimittel aller Länder. Nach den besten Quellen und nach dreißigjährigen Beobachtungen und Erfahrungen gesammelt und herausgegeben von Georg Friedrich Most* (The House Doctor. A Complete Handbook of the Most Excellent and Effective Home and Folk Remedies of All Lands. Collected and Edited by Georg Friedrich Most from the Best Sources and after Thirty Years of Observations and Experiences). The title determined the role that the book was to play.

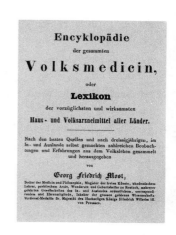

Title page of Georg Friedrich Most's influential and popular nineteenth century work on folk medicine. (F. A. Brockhaus, Leipzig, 1843)

Most devoted an exceptional amount of space to hemp as a medicine and an inebriant. As his texts demonstrate, he himself used the plant for many purposes:

> Small children in their early years often have difficulty urinating after catching a cold. . . . An old woman [taught me] a very effective home remedy against this, a half-cup of boiling water poured over a teaspoonful of crushed hemp seeds (*Semen Cannabis*). The tea is drunk warm, with sugar. (Most 1843:244)

Under the heading *Hanf*, he described the most effective way to use hemp for inebriating purposes:

> **Hemp** (*Cannabis*, from *Cannabis sativa* L.). The seed, as well as the entire plant, is used dried with effect in tea form as a gentle remedy for painful urination, urine retention in infants . . . In Morocco, dried hemp leaves are smoked instead of tobacco in order to make one cheerful and to dispel hypochondriacal moods. The Joy Pills of the Orient also have hemp as a main ingredient.— To treat whooping cough in children, Hufeland praises an extract of the entire plant. You can make this yourselves by collecting hemp before it blooms, crushing it, pouring some river water over it, then pressing it out and evaporating the fresh juice over a low fire until it reaches the thickness of an extract. Children ages two to six are given two to three grains three times a day, adults receive six to ten grains. This extract is also a well-known and often misused stimulant which is ingested as such in the following mixture:
> No. 89. Take: Hemp extract, two grains; water of bitter orange flowers, six

ounces; tincture of Spanish pepper, one-quarter ounce. Take one to two tablespoons full of this with wine one to two hours *ante actum*. Rubbed onto the afflicted area, pressed, fatty hemp oil *(Oleum cannabium)* is an old remedy for neuralgia, colic, stomach cramps, and induration of the uterus.

In nineteenth-century Germany, it was very common to use hemp as a psychoactive aphrodisiac in the manner noted or recommended by Most (Aigremont 1986:24; Hovorka and Kronfeld 1908/09). At the time, it was believed that this use had been introduced by Serbian gypsies. They were said to have ingested "the hemp flower pulverized and mixed with menstrual blood" (ibid). Hemp was also regarded as a love magic (Kronfeld 1981:40; Lussi 1996*). Most provides an even clearer statement under the heading *Semen Cannabis:*

Semen Cannabis. We add the following to the article on hemp: A very effective home remedy against spastic urine retention in infants (and adults) that I myself have tried often is one to three teaspoons full of crushed hemp seeds, infused in two cups of boiling water and drunk while warm.—According to Freudenstein (Diss. de cannabis sativae usu et viribus narcoticis. Marpurgi 1841), there is another species in addition to *Cannabis sativa* L.: *Cannabis indica* Lamarck (*sic*), whose effects are more narcotic than the former. According to Herodotus, the ancient Scythians were already aware of smoking hemp leaves as an inebriant,—in Egypt, the rogues also use this in order to make those persons fall asleep that they wish to rob, and Aubert (De la Peste etc. Paris 1840) has praised hemp extract especially for the plague, where he saw seven of twelve afflicted recover because of it. Dr. O'Shaughnessy used the resinous hemp extract as a narcotic agent, whereby it should be noted that in hotter climates than with us, the leaves and the stalk of hemp exude a resinous juice which has a sharp, narcotic scent and a bitter taste. The extract is obtained by boiling the dried plant in spirits and evaporating the fluid, whereby a tincture can also be made by dissolving three grains of extract in one dram of alcohol. The medicine is said to have been especially effective with tetanus, where one dram of tincture is given every half hour until the cramps have dissipated. (British and Foreign med. Review, July 1840.) In many regions of the Orient, hemp occupies the place of spirits, wine, and brandy as an inebriant.—Persons who take it for pleasure feel a special cheerfulness, merriment, and gaiety of disposition, a comfortable forgetting of all sorrow and every pain; they have a constant, gentle smile, even when no outer reason is present, all anger and hate is stilled, and after a few hours they fall into a mild and gentle sleep, during which they delight in the most pleasant of fantasy images, as they did while still awake.—All signs of hemp inebriation. According to the information provided by Sonnini, this disturbance of the thinking abilities, this type of mental sleep, is in no way comparable to the inebriation from wine or other spirituous drinks, and our language possesses no expression for alluding to such a feeling. Hemp inebriation also has the quality that its does not accelerate the circulation of the blood, does not increase the rate of breathing, and does not attack the head; but it may produce a veritable dog's hunger *(fames canina)*. By the way, this misuse of hemp, if it is continued for too long, results in stupidity, idiocy, and great bodily weakness.

There are a variety of ways to prepare hemp for use as an inebriant. In India, according to Ainslie, three are usual. One drink, called Banghie, is prepared from the leaves, the Mohammedans in particular use this. Another preparation is called Majum, for which poppy leaves, flowers of thornapple, crow's eye [*Strychnos nux-vomica*], sugar, and milk are used along with hemp leaves. An electuary made from these substances is very potent, but is used only by very debauched persons. There are also pills made from this, which Sanskrit writers refer to using the name Gandschakini.—The use of hemp is especially popular in Persia, where hemp seeds are mixed with tobacco leaves and smoked in special pipes, which are called *nardschihli,* or they make a drink from hemp, crows' eyes, potash, and wine, which the orthodox Mussulmans do not use; finally, they also make an infusion of hemp and poppy leaves with crows' eyes which is called Bangue, Baeng, or Beng, names which point to an Indian origin. According to the report of Olearius, who was in Persia in 1633, they also make pills there from the leaves and seeds of hemp with honey that are used as an aphrodisiac. In the Berber regions, they also use hemp powder or smoke the leaves in order to encourage and stimulate themselves *ad coitum;* but here impotence and sterility is also very common as a result of this misuse (see Dublin Journ. March 1841). Curious! Woyt (l.c.p.156) speaks much differently of hemp. "The seeds"—he says—"lessen the masculine nature, and are also used against semen flow (pollutions), pains, aches in the side, coughs, and yellow jaundice." Quite right! for everything which momentarily stimulates, quickly has inability as a result (see *Hemp*).

A very potent recipe is found under the heading *Joy Pills:*

> **Joy Pills.** To dispel bad moods and hypochondriacal temperaments, the Orientals, who are known to also amuse themselves with opium smoking and opium eating, find refuge in a mixture known as *Nepenthe,* consisting of the powder of the dried topmost leaves and flowers of hemp, in combination with opium, areca nut, spices, and sugar, which they swallow in pill form.

Since the recipes that Most provided were followed diligently, it can be assumed that wide segments of the population knew about hemp's effects. Other, similarly influential authors, such as the physician Johann Friedrich Osiander (1838), also wrote about the "wondrous effects of the Oriental Joy Pills" (cf. Rätsch 1990b:11*).

In addition to the widespread use of the Doctor's Books, it was also customary to make one's own collection of recipes for home remedies and to record these in House Books. One especially interesting and much respected House Book was penned by Rath Schlosser, a woman who was a close relative of Goethe's. She recommended hemp in several places. For treating the bites of rabid animals, she suggested laying a bandage of hemp fibers soaked in oil of vitriol over the wound (Bernus 1982:20). Herpes zoster, or shingles, is a disease that has long been treated with folk remedies and magical practices. Rath Schlosser knew of an especially good method:

> **Against shingles.** From 9 walnuts, remove the so-called cross, make a decoction of this like tea and drink while finely crushed hemp is placed on the inflamed area. (Bernus 1982:25)

How to obtain magical powers. On the evening before the Festival of Adalbert (June 1), kill a snake, cut its head off, place 3 hemp seeds in it, and bury everything in the ground: after the hemp has grown, make a string of it. When you have tied this around your body, then even the strongest will not overcome you.
DAS SECHSTE UND SIEBENTE BUCH MOSIS (STUTTGART 1849)

For treating hair loss, she even had two recipes with hemp:

Pomade for Growing Hair. Take chicken fat, hempseed oil, and honey, 4 ounces of each, allow everything to dissolve in a pot and mix thoroughly until it has the consistency of a pomade. Rub this into the head for eight days in a row. (Bernus 1982:52)

Medicine to Make the Hair Grow and Return Anew. Take the root of a white grapevine, root of hemp, and tender cabbage stalks, two handfuls of each, dry these, and then burn them. Make the ashes into a lye. Before washing the head with this lye, massage it with honey, and do this three times in a row, every second day. (Bernus 1982:57)

Who can say whether hemp will incite the hair to grow anew? But many such recipes were passed on and preserved among the people because they were found to be effective.

In Upper Bavaria, hemp, which was usually referred to as "Knaster"[1] or "strong tobacco," was used up until the nineteenth century, for example, "Allow juniper smoke to waft across hemp tow and apply the latter to swollen, arthritic feet" (Höfler 1994:124). "Wild growing hemp" was generally used to treat pain in areas where the skin has been lost as a result of leprosy (Höfler 1994:178). In Tübingen, the country folk would wrap "the painful limb in heated hemp tow" to treat gout and rheumatism (Osiander 1826:85). When the flow of milk was interrupted, the breasts were rubbed with "heated hemp oakum" (ibid:242).

Even into the twentieth century, hemp was a popular, even magical folk remedy:

In folk medicine, hemp is a febrifuge (Upper Silesia, Bohemia). Wrap a ball of hemp around three splinters of different sizes and ten lentils and allow to burn on a fire of coals and pass the smoke to the ears, or the woman of the house should make three balls of hemp, set these on fire, and blow these out of the window and into the courtyard or out onto the street, this will also cast the fever from the house. Against cramps and violent contractions, strings twisted from tow or hemp are placed, 1–2 around the body and 1 on each of the legs, arms, and the head; you may not slip these on and off, you should lose them "unthanked." Hemp tow is laid under women in labor so that they will not be afflicted with cramps. To treat exostosis, tow or hemp that has been placed around the "holy sheaf" [of herbs, a smudge stick] is tied around the wrist, for cramps in the calf of the leg, wrap *rystä* (hemp fibers) which were placed in palm branches and consecrated on Palm Sunday around the lower leg. A pregnant woman should avoid urinating on hemp. (Marzell 1931:1437f.)

In the literature on household medicine, the demonizing of the hemp plant began in the late nineteenth century. For example, the influential book *Kräutersegen* (Herbal Blessings) notes that hemp does indeed have "its well-earned place" in the healing arts, however:

Thus, while we are also unable to resist having a certain mistrust when look-

Flower oracle. They say in Franconia that if the cowslips have long stems, then the barley will also grow tall, in Swabian (in the area of Tuttlingen) this oracle pertains to the length of the hemp.
HEINRICH MARZELL,
VOLKSBOTANIK
(1935:25)

---

1. Osiander (1826:78) wrote that "knaster" was more effective than normal tobacco when used in a "smoking tobacco enema" in which the smoke was administered rectally.

ing at hemp and must say: "Here is a plant which has already caused much mischief and can and will cause much more," we must not avoid the fact that it is only an immoderate use of hashish, caused by passion and vice, that is guilty of the evils which lie like a curse over millions of people, while with proper use the bad principle here, like everywhere in general, can be made to be good. If we thus weigh the benefits of hemp against its harms, then the former exceeds the latter by far. With some care, hemp can be used to advantage even in our home medicine cabinet.

In its preparations, in small doses it has stimulating and invigorating effects upon the nervous system. This is why the doctor will prescribe it for severe fatigue and weakness following great physical exertion.

Larger amounts are sedating. This is why it is sometimes given in place of morphine.

Moreover, it is a good remedy for ailments of the urinary apparatus, for painful urination, dropsy, kidney stones, kidney and bladder infections, etc. (Zimmerer 1896:51ff.)

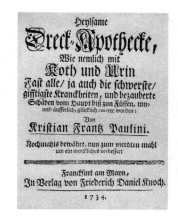

In German folk medicine, the so-called *Dreckapotheke* (Pharmacy of Filth) has always had great importance. In earlier times, the excrement of every conceivable animal including that of humans was made into medicaments (today, we speak of "auto-urine therapy"). In most of these recipes, the excrement was mixed with medicinal plants before being swallowed. Hemp appears in some of these recipes. For example, a hempseed cake that contained pigeon dung and spices was ingested as a remedy for dropsy. (title page of a book that was used for centuries)

To Treat Burning Urination
(from Osiander 1826:117)

　1 part ground hemp seeds
　1 part licorice

Mix the ingredients and use to make a decoction. Drink several times daily. Sweeten with syrup if desired.

Hemp Tea
(from Zimmerer 1896:53)

Pour 1 liter of boiling water over 30–60 grams of hemp seeds and steep for at least 10 minutes. The tea is drunk throughout the day for rheumatism, dropsy, eczema, urinary problems, and jaundice.

REFERENCES

Aigremont, Dr. [1917] 1986. *Volkserotik und Pflanzenwelt*. Reprint, Berlin: EXpress Edition.
von Bernus, Alexander. 1982. *Urgroßmutters Hausmittel: Aus dem Hausbuch der Frau Rath Schlosser*. Frankfurt am Main: Insel.
Höfler, Max. [1888] 1994. *Volksmedizin und Aberglaube in Oberbayern, Gegenwart und Vergangenheit*. Reprint, Vaduz/Liechtenstein: Sändig.
Hovorka, Oskar, and Adolf Kronfeld. 1908/09. *Vergleichende Volksmedizin*. Stuttgart: Strecker und Schröder.
Kronfeld, Moritz. [1898] 1981. *Donnerwurz und Mäuseaugen*. Reprint, Berlin: Clemens Zerling.
Marzell, Heinrich. 1931. Hanf. In *Handwörterbuch des Deutschen Aberglaubens*, edited by E. Hoffmann-Krayer, Hanns Bächthold-Stäubli et al. Vol. 3. Berlin: de Gruyter, pages 1435–8.
———. 1935. *Volksbotanik: Die Pflanze im Deutschen Brauchtum*. Berlin: Enckehaus.
Most, Georg Friedrich. 1843. *Encyklopädie der gesammten Volksmedicin*. Leipzig, Germany: Brockhaus.
Osiander, Johann Friedrich. 1826. *Volksarzneymittel und einfache, nicht pharmazeutische Heilmittel gegen Krankheiten des Menschen*. Tübingen (reprint, Heidelberg: Haug, n.d.).
———. 1838. *Volksarzneymittel und einfache, nicht pharmazeutische Heilmittel gegen Krankheiten des Menschen*, Tübingen (expanded edition).
Zimmerer, E.M. 1896. *Kräutersegen: Die Bedeutung unserer vorzüglichsten heimischen Heilkräuter . . . und ihre praktische Verwendung als Hausmittel*. Donauwörth, Germany: L. Auer.

Dagga

HEMP IN SUB-SAHARAN AFRICA

In many non-Western cultures, the ancestors are in an intimate and absolutely vital relationship with the world of the living. They are always available to provide counsel, instruction, and strength. They form a path between this world and the next. And most importantly—and most paradoxically—they embody guidelines for a fulfilling life—for everything which is precious in life.

MALIDOMA PATRICE SOMÉ
VOM GEIST AFRIKAS
(1996:20)

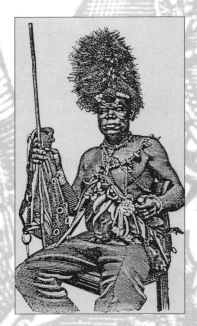

Many African medicine men use hemp and other psychoactive flora as oracular plants, aphrodisiacs, and medicines. (illustration from Max Bartels, *Medizin der Naturvölker*, Leipzig, 1893)

Of all the continents, Africa has given us the fewest psychoactive plants, or its people have only discovered and integrated a few into their cultures (de Smet 1996). In many parts of Africa, the Pygmies, the small and gentle people of the forest, are given credit for discovering psychoactive magical plants, including the psychedelic iboga root (*Tabernanthe iboga*) as well as the euphoriant hemp. The iboga root, which is eaten in a cultic context, is an endemic plant that occurs only in the rain forests of western Africa (Schultes and Hofmann 1995:112*). Hemp, in contrast, appears to have made its way to western and southern Africa from the Orient, via Egypt and eastern Africa (Du Toit 1975). Nevertheless, the Pygmies are enthusiastic hemp users. They also maintain that using the drug provides them with the strength needed for their dramatic elephant hunts (Du Toit 1975:101). They smoke the beneficent herb from large bamboo pipes (Reininger 1941:2780*).

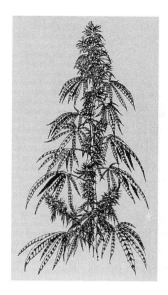

A typical female hemp plant from the Central Africa nation of Malawi. (from Clarke 1997:151*)

Today, hemp is known as *dagga* in wide parts of Africa. This word is either derived from the Arabic term *duXan* or from a Hottentot word *daXab*. During the early period of European contact (the seventeenth century), the word *dagga* (and its variations, such as *dacha*) appears to have been used to characterize psychoactive plants in general (for example, *Datura fastuosa* or *D. metel*)[1] and *Leonotis leonurus* in particular (Du Toit 1975:88; Watt 1961). *Leonotis* is a small plant that was already being smoked throughout southern Africa prior to the introduction of hemp as a stimulant and euphoriant (Du Toit 1980:58). Today, it is hardly smoked at all, as hemp has taken its place, most likely the result of the fact that the latter is better tolerated and has more pleasurable effects.

What is "Wild Dagga"?

"Two other plants which are also smoked are called dagga as well, namely *Leonotis leonurus*, 'wild dagga,' and *L. ovata*, 'rock dagga.' The English forbade its use in Cape Land, just as they forbade the use of hemp" (Hartwich 1997:8*).

The southern African bush *Leonotis leonurus* (L.) R. Br. (Labiatae)—lion's tail, or lion's ear—has orange-colored flowers and is said to be hallucinogenic (Schultes and Hofmann 1995:367*). In Africa, it is known as *dacha*, *daggha*, or *wild dagga*, "wild hemp." The Hottentots (Heusaquas) and bushmen smoke the buds and leaves as an inebriant (Schleiffer 1979:93ff.). The resinous leaves or the resin itself, scraped off or extracted from the leaves, may be smoked alone or mixed with tobacco (*Nicotiana tabacum*). In California, many people now smoke the leaves and inflorescences. Chemical studies are lacking (Ott 1993:411*). The bitter-tasting smoke of the inflorescences has mildly psychoactive effects reminiscent of those of *Cannabis* as well as *Datura*.

The leaves and flowers of one closely related species, *Leonotis nepetaefolia* (L.)

---

1. In Africa, *Datura metel* is used for criminal telepathy and in initiations. The seeds, however, are also misused to poison victims so they can be robbed. The hallucinogenic properties of the plant are well known in East Africa, where the seeds are added to the locally brewed beer in order to increase its potency (Weiss 1979:49). In the land of the Tsonga, which stretches across Mozambique and the Transvaal, *Datura metel* var. *fastuosa* is used as an hallucinogenic ritual drug (*mondzo*) when girls are initiated into womanhood (Johnston 1972).

R. Br., which is used in Caribbean folk medicine, have been found to contain bound oils, bitter constituents, diterpenes, coumarins, and resins (Puroshothaman et al. 1974a and 1974b). In Mexico, this plant is known as *flor de mundo*, "world flower," or *mota*. Mota is normally used to refer to marijuana; this usage indicates that *L. nepetaefolia* is used as a marijuana substitute. The extract has antispasmodic effects and appears to inhibit acetylcholine and histamine.

It has long been known that hemp is smoked in South Africa alone or with tobacco under the names D'Amba, Dakka, Dacha, Deijamba, Djamba, Congo-Tobacco. . . . The use of this plant appears to be very widespread in the south of Africa, where it is found especially in the land of the Hottentots and the Kaffir. You can find it cultivated here and there and also in a wild state near the huts. This plant is a variety of Cannabis sativa *and is the same that is so often grown by the Dongos, Domaras, and other tribal peoples south of Benguela. . . . Among the aborigines of Angola, the Ambondas, the plant is held in high regard not just for its narcotic effects, but also because of its healing powers.*

GEORG MARTIUS
PHARMAKOLOGISCH-
MEDICINISCHE STUDIEN
ÜBER DEN HANF
(1855:37F.*)

Hemp is cultivated as a source of fiber throughout Africa and is used to manufacture ropes, textiles, and carpets (Kokwaro 1995:222f.).It is considered to be an aphrodisiac throughout almost all of sub-Saharan Africa, especially in Mali (Du Toit 1980). Among the Mashona, it is said that hemp eroticizes and improves work effort and performance (Du Toit 1975:98). In Rwanda, the Twa say that hemp, which they call *injaga*, gives strength and courage and dispels exhaustion and rheumatism (Codere 1975:223). It is used to relax after a full day's work and smoked to relax cases of nervousness, even to therapeutically treat nervous breakdowns (Du Toit 1980:208).

Customarily smoked without additives in water pipes of enormous size, hemp is occasionally mixed with thornapple leaves *(Datura stramonium)* (Du Toit 1975:108; Watt 1961). The use of tobacco as a hemp additive is uncommon.

Hemp is also often used in ritual contexts. It is said that it establishes a connection to the ancestors, for they too delighted themselves with the plant. In order to invoke the ancestors, an incense made of cannabis flowers and the sweet-smelling resin of the evergreen *impepho* plant (*Helichrysum miconiaefolium*, an immortelle) is burned (Du Toit 1980:208).

It is possible that hemp may also be used to induce the shamanic ecstasy that is found in some parts of Africa (Chesi 1989:18). The plant, together with its ritual, magical, and medicinal uses, has even spread to the islands of the Indian Ocean. On Réunion, it is known as *zamal*, and is used to dispel injurious spirits and to treat vomiting (Benoist 1975:230).

A cult of hashish use was encountered by the German Africa explorer Hermann von Wißmann (1853–1905) among the Baluba, a Bantu tribe in the Belgian Congo, and among the tribes subservient to them. As Wißmann reported in 1888, Kalamba Mukenge, the chief of the Baluba, publicly burned the old fetishes of the individual tribes so that he could secure the kingdom that his conquests had established and tie together the various tribes he had subdued into one unified cult. In place of the fetish cult, he introduced hemp smoking as a ritual valid for all.

"From that time on, the Baluba smoked hemp at all important occasions, such as festivals, conclusions of agreements, and treaties of friendship. They usually smoked from large bottle gourds, some of which had a circumference of one meter. In addition, the men would gather at the main squares of the villages every evening for a common ceremonial smoke. But hemp was also used as a means of punishment. Miscreants were watched while they smoked an especially large amount, which often caused them to pass out. Soon, the subjects of Kalamba had become so unified as a result of their hemp use that they began to call themselves "Riamba," after the name for the drug, as well as "Bena Riamba" (sons of hemp). (Reininger 1941:2791*)

Hemp is also used for medicinal purposes in Africa, although the hedonistic use is predominant among many peoples and tribes (James 1970; Morley and Bensusian 1971). In many parts of Africa, it was once valued as a medicine for dysentery, malaria, anthrax, and all feverish diseases (Schultes and Hofmann 1995:97*). In Rhodesia, it was used as a medicine to treat a number of serious diseases: malaria, black water fever, blood poisoning, anthrax, and diarrhea (Du Toit 1980:58). In Tanzania, preparations of dried hemp leaves, *ubami* gum (a type of olibanum or frankincense), and a decoction of roots and bark of *Securidaca longepedunculata* Fres. were used to treat syphilis, typhus, and rheumatism (Neuwinger 1998:762).

Throughout Africa, hemp is a well-known asthma remedy, relaxing asthmatic spasms and even completely healing this strange disease (Du Toit 1980:59, 208). The medicinal use is found especially in South Africa, but has also spread to West Africa (Chesi 1989:232), where plants are addressed with magical formulae or prayers and conjurations before they are used. Only in this way will the plant acquire the necessary healing power (Ayensu 1978; Chesi 1989:164). Only by being addressed does hemp, the widespread agent of pleasure, become the highly effective medicine that bears the same name.[2]

The Hottentots, or Khoi, and the Mfengu, both of whom live in South Africa, remain convinced of the effectiveness of hemp for snakebites (Schultes and Hofmann 1995:97*). Hunters always carry some of the plant with them so that they can apply it immediately if they are bitten (Du Toit 1980:58). Among the South African pastoralist peoples, even cancer is treated with hemp. The patient ingests a brew made from the leaves of the cancer bush (*Sutherlandia frutescens*) and is rubbed with the oily remnants that collect in a water pipe after long, regular use (Du Toit 1980:58).

Among the South African Zulu, the flowers and the resinous exudate are smoked for pleasure, while the stalks and roots are used for medicinal purposes. Beverages made from the stalks and roots are drunk as an expectorant for diseases of the respiratory tract (Du Toit 1980:133). The Zulus also ingest hemp in the form of cold water extracts, infusions, steam baths, and enemas. They rub ground leaves into cuts purposely made in the skin so that the drug can work on painful areas, a type of subcutaneous application. Hemp is most frequently used for various "cold" illnesses caused by colds, asthma, and tuberculosis. Asthma is treated with a cold water infusion; flowers are smoked to treat attacks. Teaspoons full of the liquid are taken daily for a period of two months. For dry coughs, hemp flowers are mixed with other irritating herbs, rolled into a cigarette, and smoked. The patient is instructed to inhale deeply so that he will be forced to cough heavily. The procedure is repeated until the mucous secretions have been expelled from the lungs (Du Toit 1980:133). Decoctions are drunk to treat tuberculosis. In general, hemp is said to

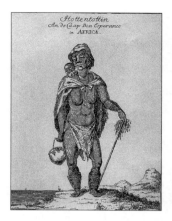

The first Europeans to encounter the Hottentots (Khoi), who live in South Africa, were surprised to find that they are serious smokers who utilize a variety of herbs for that purpose. It was even said that for good smoking wares, the women would gladly give themselves to the donor. (copperplate engraving from Georg Meister, *Der Orientalisch-Indianische Kunst- und Lustgärtner*, 1692)

2. In many traditional cultures, especially those that have been shaped by shamanism, plant drugs only become specific remedies through the word—in the form of spells, formulae, mantras, and so forth. The accompanying words do not appear to simply impregnate the drugs, but also program the mind of the user (the so-called set). In this way, those effects that are desired from the overall pharmacological spectrum of effects of the substance can be perceived and experienced more strongly.

cleanse the respiratory tract (Du Toit 1980:208). When they smoke the plant, the Zulus usually use water pipes made of large, curved ox horns (Reininger 1941:2792*).

The South African shaman and artist Percy Konqobe told me that in Zululand and Swaziland there used to be wise men, the "dagga smokers," who used hemp ritually. Twice a day, at sunrise and again at sunset, they would smoke female hemp flowers in water pipes that were up to ten meters in length. Because especially large lungs and a strong constitution are needed to smoke from these enormous devices, only a few were able to become a dagga man, but every village had at least one. These wise men were consulted when there were worries, needs, and problems to solve, or diseases to diagnose. They were also consulted during times of war, when they would contemplate strategy and try to find paths to peace while under dagga's influence. Even today, hemp is still regarded as the "plant of knowledge or insight" in South Africa.

Throughout southern Africa, hemp is used as a universal analgesic. As in Russia, it is smoked for toothaches and is drunk as a decoction for headaches. A brew of the roots, together with other medicinal plants, is used to treat "heart aches." Hemp extracts are used as anesthetics during minor surgical procedures, such as the ritual removal of finger joints. Moreover, the drug is regarded as generally invigorating, disease preventing, and life prolonging. Many people eighty to one hundred years old or more have reported that they have grown as old as they are and were largely spared serious disease because they had used cannabis for decades (Du Toit 1980:134). The Bantu in particular believe that hemp prolongs life and increases the body's own defensive abilities. Enemas and steam baths containing the plant are especially beneficial for adults as well as children. When smoking, the only concern is that the flowers be free of all seeds (Du Toit 1980:134, 208). The Tsongas even say that "dagga deepens knowledge and makes men wiser"; this is why hemp is known as the "grass of knowledge" (Du Toit 1980:209). Hemp is believed to be a *njengozifo zonke*, a "general therapeutic agent for all diseases" (Du Toit 1980:210).

Among the Sotho, women smoke copious amounts of hemp while in labor to soothe their pains, increase their desire to give birth, and to make the birthing process easier (Du Toit 1980:58; Schultes and Hofmann 1995:97*). It is generally thought that women should smoke frequently while they are pregnant so that the child will come into the world healthy and strong (Du Toit 1980:209). In Cameroon, crushed leaves are laid onto or rubbed into the abdomens of women in labor in order to alleviate the pains of labor.

The San or Bushmen know of a number of psychoactive plants, such as *gaise noru noru (Ferraria glutinosa)*, which they ingest during their nocturnal healing dances so that they may deepen the communal ecstasy (*!kia*) and produce a collective healing power *(n/um)* to heal the sick persons in the group. They often use hemp as well, as they have been for at least five hundred years (Katz 1985; Winkelman and Dobkin de Rios 1989). Today the Bushmen also smoke for recreation and relaxation, just as their neighbors do:

In the Yaéda Valley of Tanzania, the Hadzabe, relatives of the disappearing

Bushmen, have been able to preserve remnants of their archaic culture as hunters and gatherers. For men, boys, and women, a drilled stone pipe, filled with Cannabis, is part of the evening's relaxation. (Leipe 1997:133*)

Unfortunately, the drug laws of African countries have suppressed most of marijuana's traditional uses. In addition, the traditional cultures have been pressured to assimilate. Many, however, confront this pressure with a well-filled water pipe.

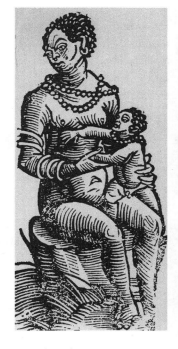

In Africa, hemp preparations are used to provide relief during childbirth, help in the mother's convalescence, and strengthen the child. ("Black Woman," woodcut, Italy, sixteenth century)

Ritual Entheogen (West Africa)

10 g pulverized iboga root (*Tabernanthe iboga*)
2 g dried marijuana flowers

This mixture should only be ingested in a ritual context, for it can evoke powerful visions and profound experiences.

South African Smoking Mixture

1 part dried marijuana flowers
1 part dried herbage of *Sceletium tortuosum* [L.] N.E. Br. (Kougoed)

Mix the ingredients together and smoke in a water pipe.

REFERENCES

Ayensu, Edward S. 1978. *Medicinal Plants of West Africa*. Algonac, Michigan: Reference Publications.

Benoist, Jean. 1975. Réunion: Cannabis in a Pluricultural and Polyethnic Society. In *Cannabis and Culture*, edited by V. Rubin. The Hague: Mouton, pages 227–34.

Chesi, Gert. 1989. *Die Medizin der Schwarzen Götter: Magie und Heilkunst Afrikas*. Vienna: Verlag Jugend und Volk.

Codere, Helen. 1975. The Social and Cultural Context of Cannabis Use in Rwanda. In *Cannabis and Culture*, edited by V. Rubin. The Hague: Mouton, pages 217–26.

de Smet, Peter. 1996. Some Ethnopharmacological Notes On African Hallucinogens. *Journal of Ethnopharmacology* 50(3):141–6.

Du Toit, Brian M. 1958. Dagga (*Cannabis sativa*) Smoking in Southern Rhodesia. *The Central African Journal of Medicine* 4:500–1.

———. 1975. Dagga: The History and Ethnographic Setting of *Cannabis sativa* in Southern Africa. In *Cannabis and Culture*, edited by V. Rubin. The Hague: Mouton, pages 81–116.

———. 1980. *Cannabis in Africa*. Rotterdam: A. A. Balkema.

Hall, James 1996. *Sangoma: Eine Reise zu den Geistern Afrikas*. Munich: Knaur.

Hartwich, Carl, and E. Zwicky. 1914. Über Channa, ein Genussmittel der Hottentotten. *Apotheker-Zeitung* 29:925f., 937-939, 949f., 961f.

Hien, Elie. 1997. *Afrika: Altes Wissen für Morgen*. Seeon: Ch. Falk-Verlag.

James, Theodore. 1970. Dagga: A Review of Fact and Fancy. *South African Medical Journal* 44:575–80.

Johnston, Thomas F. 1972. *Datura fastuosa*: Its Use in Tsonga Girls' Initiation. *Economic Botany* 26:340–51.

Katz, Richard. 1985. *Num—Heilen in Ekstase*. Interlaken: Ansata.

Kokwaro, John O. 1976. *Medicinal Plants of East Africa*. Nairobi: East African Literature Bureau.

———. 1995. Ethnobotany in Africa. In *Ethnobotany: Evolution of a Discipline*, edited by Richard Evans Schultes and Siri von Reis. Portland, Ore.: Dioscorides Press, pages 216–25.

Laidler, P. W. 1928. The Magic Medicine of the Hottentots. *South African Journal of Science* 25:433–47.

Meister, George [1677] n.d. *Der Orientalisch-Indianische Kunst- und Lustgärtner*. Reprint, Weimar: Kiepenheuer.

Morley, J. E., and A. D. Bensusan. 1971. Dagga: Tribal Uses and Customs. *Medical Proceedings* 17:409–12.

Neuwinger, Hans Dieter. 1998. *Afrikanische Arzneipflanzen und Jagdgifte: Chemie, Pharmakologie, Toxikologie*. 2d ed. Stuttgart: Wissenschaftliche Verlagsgesellschaft.

Puroshothaman, K. K. et al. 1974a. 4,6,7-Trimethoxy-5-methylchromon-2-one, A New Coumarin from *Leonotis nepetaefolia*. *J. Chem. Soc. Perkin Trans*. 1(1):2594–5.

———. 1974b. Nepetaefolinol and two Related Diterpenoids from *Leonotis nepetaefolia*. *J. Chem. Soc. Perkin Trans*. 1(1):2661.

Schleiffer, Hedwig, ed. 1979. *Narcotic Plants of the Old World: An Anthology of Texts from Ancient Times to the Present*. Monticello, N.Y.: Lubrecht and Cramer.

Sofowora, A. 1982. *Medicinal Plants and Traditional Medicine in Africa*. Chichester: John Wiley and Sons.

Somé, Malidoma Patrice. 1996. *Vom Geist Afrikas: Das Leben eines afrikanischen Schamanen*. Munich: Diederichs.

Watt, J. M. 1961. Dagga in South Africa. *Bulletin on Narcotics* 13:9–14.

Weiss, E. A. 1979. Some Indigenous Plants Used Domestically by East African Coastal Fishermen. *Economic Botany* 33(1):35–51.

Winkelman, Michael, and Marlene Dobkin de Rios. 1989. Psychoactive Properties of !Kung Bushmen Medicine Plants. *Journal of Psychoactive Drugs* 21(1):51–9.

Headache is a disease of thought, the brain is too small for all problems. You should keep your thoughts pure and practice thought hygiene!

PAPA ELIE HIEN
AFRIKA: ALTES WISSEN FÜR MORGEN
(1997:77)

Kif

HEMP IN NORTH AFRICA

*I knew how to make good kif, and I made it for
real smokers. . . .*

MOHAMMED MRABET
M'HASHISH
(1995:62)

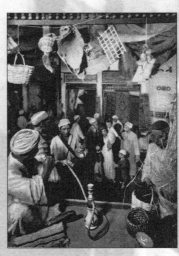

This old photo of a Moroccan
bazaar shows the central role of
the indigenous use of kif. (photo:
Hed Weisner, postcard from the
Übersee-Museum, Bremen,
Germany)

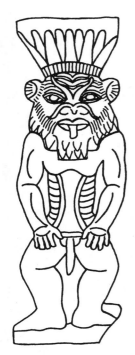

In ancient Egypt and in adjacent countries, and later in all of North Africa, Syrian rue (*Peganum harmala*) was the sacred plant of the fertility and bedroom god Bes. Like Bes fetishes, the psychoactive seeds have been used since ancient times to ward off demons, that is, as an antidepressant. They are still used today to treat depression and other illnesses in Morocco, where they are usually mixed with kif and either burned as a fumigant or smoked. (Bes statue, Eighteenth Dynasty)

n North Africa, hashish has been known since ancient times: "Recently, some hashish was recovered in an airtight container in the wreck of a Carthaginian warship, which is thought to have sunk off the coast of Sicily during the Second Punic War (218–201 B.C.E.). It was described as still being potent" (Stafford 1980:9*). Carthage was a Phoenician trade outpost on the peninsula near modern Tunis. Like all Phoenicians, the Carthaginians were seafaring merchants who essentially controlled the entire eastern and central Mediterranean. Since successful trade always seems to result in military confrontations, the Carthaginians became entangled in the Punic Wars with the Romans. Certainly, the Carthaginians contributed to the spread of various cannabis products in southern Europe and northern Africa.

The early history of hemp in North Africa has been poorly studied, and only fragmentary details have come down to us. In Egypt, hashish has been widely used since the thirteenth century. In Ethiopia, two ceramic water pipes were recovered from the Lalibela Caves, near Lake Tana, in the Begemeder Province. Chromatographic methods revealed that the residues contain cannabinoids. The pipes were carbon-14 dated to 1320–1380 C.E. (Van der Merwe 1975).

In the Er Rif Mountains, the main region in which hemp is cultivated today, the first written documentation of the plant comes from the nineteenth century. Since that time, its use in the area has been widespread. Almost all of the inhabitants of the Er Rif, who belong to various Berber tribes, partake of the herb. They call both the plant and the inebriating product *kif* (Barny 1997). The Moroccan government allows cultivation and indigenous use, but has prohibited trade, at least on paper. Of course, trade is still tolerated, for even the Moroccan police, the protectors of law and order, are traditional "kiffers." In Morocco, the use of kif is not seen as an offense against Islam, but is traditionally associated with the religion. In contrast, alcohol is prohibited (Barny 1997; Joseph 1975; Mikuriya 1967). In the nineteenth century—when the cannabis trade was still allowed—the growing areas around Ketama in the Er Rif Mountains covered 90 percent of the demand from French pharmacies (Behr 1982:81*).

In former times, hemp leaves and flowers were usually eaten in marmalade or syrup. Today, they are smoked in long pipes called *sibsa*. The kif that is manufactured in the Er Rif should not be confused with "Moroccan," the green hashish that is so well known in Europe. Kif is usually a mixture of 2 parts finely chopped female flowers and leaves with 1 part unfermented tobacco (Joseph 1975:187).[1] The Moroccans—both Arabs and Berbers—usually smoke kif alone, although they do sometimes mix it with commercial (cigarette) tobacco and occasionally with crushed poppy seeds (*Papaver somniferum*). They believe that the poppy seeds potentiate the effects of the kif (Mrabet 1995). Kif, mixed with seeds of Syrian rue (*Peganum harmala*), is said to stimulate the imagination.

Kif is regarded as a means for relaxing and for removing inhibitions. It is also often characterized as a "medicine" (Mrabet 1995:37).

Moroccan women are typically forbidden to use hemp; the men justify this by

1. Unfermented tobacco often retains a greenish or yellowish color and contains a much higher concentration of nicotine than fermented or "cured" tobacco.

arguing that while under the influence of the drug, the women would forget all shame and be perverted into adulterous nymphomaniacs (Palgi 1975:210f.). In contrast, the men allow themselves to continuously consume the aphrodisiac. To augment the effects, Spanish fly (*Cantharides*) may be added (Hartwich 1997:21*). But the woman do find that hemp can transport them to paradise:

> "I feel wonderful!" said the girl. "It can never be as beautiful anywhere else as where I am right now. The air blows by me like music—a music that is not of this world. I have no more connection at all with this world. I am in heaven! In heaven!" (Mrabet 1995:39)

Kif is frequently smoked to treat depression and states of anxiety (Joseph 1975:190). Some Berbers use kif from time to time in order to induce or increase transcendental experiences.

Kif is one of the main items offered by every *attar*, the herb dealers of Morocco (Boulos 1983; Vries 1984). When used medicinally, it is often mixed with opium, honey, and fat. It may also be combined with thornapple seeds and other nightshades (Vries 1989). Numerous recipes for *majun* (spice mixtures) contain kif. However, the medicinal use is not nearly as important as the daily use for relaxation and improving one's mood (Joseph 1973:235).

Aphrodisiac Blend
(from Venzlaff 1977:135f.)

1 part paradise grains (*Amomum grana paradisii* or *Amomum melegueta*)
1 part ginger root (*Zingiber officinale*)
1 part cloves (*Syzygium aromaticum*)
1 part nutmeg (*Myristica fragrans*)
1 part snakeroot (*Aristolochia longa*)
1 part wild lavender (*Lavendula* sp.)
1 part kif (*Cannabis indica*)

Mix all the ingredients and grind in a mortar until a paste results. Use as needed. Take care to avoid overdose (varies by individual).

This mixture is also recommended as a medicine to treat impotence (Venzlaff 1977:136).

In the opinion of North African mystics, the Heddâwa for example, a demon dwells in hemp which can enter into a person and make him crazy. It is known that they call the drug there that is prepared from the dried leaves and stalks of the hemp plant "kif," while the roasted and pulverized hemp seeds are called "hashish." A male demon is said to be active in the first, a female demon in the second. In order to find a cure, the possessed person must search out a hermit who has a saintly reputation and sacrifice an animal, a goat or also a black chicken, on his head.

RUDOLF GELPKE
VOM RAUSCH IM ORIENT
UND OKZIDENT
(1995:79F.*)

REFERENCES

Barny. 1997. Asilah: Dope Beats from Ketama. *HanfBlatt* 4(35):8–15.

Benabud, A. 1957. Psycho-pathological Aspects of the Cannabis Situation in Morocco: Statistic Data for 1956. *Bulletin on Narcotics* 9:1–16.

Boulos, Loutfy. 1983. *Medicinal Plants of North Africa*. Algonac, Mich.: Reference Publications.

Bowles, Paul, and Mohammed Mrabet. 1992. *El Limón*. Munich: Goldmann.

Joseph, Roger. 1973. The Economic Significance of *Cannabis sativa* in the Moroccan Rif. *Economic Botany* 27:235–40.

———. 1975. The Economic Significance of *Cannabis sativa* in the Moroccan Rif. In *Cannabis and Culture*, edited by V. Rubin. The Hague: Mouton, pages 185–93.

Mikuriya, Tod H. 1967. Kif Cultivation in the Rif Mountains. *Economic Botany* 21(3):231–4.

Mrabet, Mohammed. 1995. *M'hashish: Kiff-Stories aus Marokko*. Recorded by Paul Bowles, with a

Kif among the Gnâwa musicians, who act as healers and soothsayers while in trance: "In Morocco, the Gnâwa are regarded as extremely heavy kif smokers, and they themselves are proud of the fact that in spite of countless kif pipes, they appear to be unmoved by the hallucinogenic effects. . . . But the Gnâwa only smoke kif during their normal daily routine. As soon as the spirit rhythms are played at a hadra *[spirit conjuration], the smoking of kif and the drinking of alcohol is strongly prohibited, apart from a few ritual exceptions. . . . The trance of the Gnâwa thus has nothing to do with the hallucinogenic effects of kif, but rather with the withdrawal symptoms. . . . In addition to kif smoking, the Gnâwa are also heavy wine drinkers."*

FRANK MAURICE WELTE
DER GNÂWA-KULT
(1990:52F.)

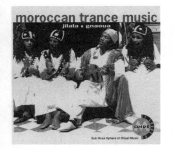

Moroccan trance music (Jilala, Gnâwa) is sometimes played under the influence of *kif*. (CD cover, Sub Rosa Records, 1990)

new afterword by Werner Pieper. Löhrbach: Werner Pieper's MedienXperimente (Der Grüne Zweig 49).

Palgi, Phyllis. 1975. The Traditional Role and Symbolism of Hashish among Moroccan Jews in Israel and the Effect of Acculturation. In *Cannabis and Culture*, edited by V. Rubin. The Hague: Mouton, pages 207–16.

Quedenfeld, Hr.M. 1887. Nahrungs-, Reiz- und kosmetische Mittel bei den Marokkanern. *Zeitschrift für Ethnologie* 19:241–84.

Van der Merwe, Nikolaas. 1975. Cannabis Smoking in 13th–14th Century Ethiopia: Chemical Evidence. In *Cannabis and Culture*, edited by V. Rubin. The Hague: Mouton, pages 77–80.

Venzlaff, Helga. 1977. *Der marokkanische Drogenhändler und seine Ware*. Wiesbaden: Franz Steiner.

de Vries, Herman. 1984. *Natural relations I—die marokkanische sammlung*. Stuttgart: Galerie Mueller-Roth.

———. 1989. *Natural relations—eine skizze*. Nuremberg: Verlag für moderne Kunst.

Welte, Frank Maurice. 1990. *Der Gnâwa-Kult: Trancespiele, Geisterbeschwörung und Besessenheit in Marokko*. Frankfurt am Main: Peter Lang.

Ganja
HEMP AND RASTAFARIANISM

Legalize Marijuana
Down here in sweet Jamaica
It's the only cure for glaucoma
I need a bush doctor, yeah
It's the only cure for asthma, yeah

PETER TOSH
"BUSH DOCTOR" (1978)

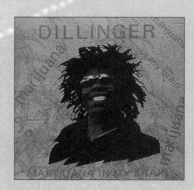

CD cover, *Burning Sounds*, 1996.

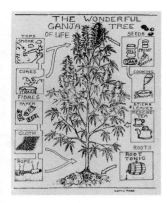

To the Rastas, "The Wonderful Ganja Tree of Life" is identical to the biblical Tree of Knowledge, and they use it in many ways. (illustration from the Rasta newspaper *Coptic Times*)

And God said, Let the earth bring forth grass, the herb yielding seed, and the fruit tree yielding fruit after his kind, whose seed is in itself, upon the earth: and it was so" (Genesis 1:11)—Yea, that is how it came to pass: God—known lovingly as *Jah*—created and presented humans with *de hola herb*, "the holy herb." The holy herb is none other than hemp, *ganja*, or *Cannabis indica*.

"In the midst of the street of the city, and on either side of the river, was there the tree of life, which bear twelve manner of fruits, and yielded her fruit every month: and the leaves of the tree were for the healing of the nations" (Revelations 22:2)—Yea, so indeed did it come to pass, that God gave humans the sacred plant, *de hola herb*, so that they might become healthy. The Rastafarians say, "*Healing of the Nations!*" This is how they interpret the Bible.[1]

On the picturesque Caribbean island of Jamaica, the Rastas, descendants of slaves brought from Africa, constitute a Messianic belief society know as the Rastafari or Rastafarians. This cult movement—which is not the first of its kind (Schuler 1980)—arose around 1930, and venerates Haile Selassie I of Ethiopia as the god-king Ras Tafari, the "head without fear." The Rastas hope that he will free them from "Babylon," the culture of the white and black suppressors. He will also make it possible for the Rastas to return peacefully to Africa, their true homeland. Haile Selassie is regarded as Christ returned and is said to be the 225th direct descendent of the enchanting Queen of Sheba and the wise King Solomon. The Rasta tradition of smoking hemp to honor God actually began with the progenitor of the god-king.

The plant first grew on the grave of Solomon, the "wisest of the wise," and for this reason it is considered to be the "herb of the wise" (Barrett 1988:219). Following the abolition of slavery, hemp (most probably *Cannabis indica*) was introduced to the islands of the Caribbean from Asia by Indians recruited to work on the sugar cane plantations (Lieber 1974; Witt 1995). The Rastas usually refer to their sacred plant simply as *herb*. Better qualities are known as *kali*, *callie*, or *cally*, and the best quality is known as *sensi* (from *sinsemilla*, cf. Mountain Girl 1995*). When referring to its medicinal uses, they speak of *weed* (Gebre-Selassie 1989:155). *Ganja*, the original Indian word, was re-etymologized: *gann-Jah*. *Jah* is a Jamaican adaptation of Jehovah, the vengeful God of the Old Testament. The Rastas, who are well versed in the Bible, find proof that God was a "head" in Psalms 18:8: "There went up a smoke out of his nostrils, and fire out of his mouth devoured . . ."

Ganja can be smoked in the form of a joint *(spliff)*, in a chilam, or in a pipe. The Rastas call the pipes in which they smoke the sacred herb *chalices* and see in them the Holy Grail, another chalice.

One Rasta leader summarized the cultural significance of hemp: "We use this herb as medicine and for spiritual experiences. It helps us to overcome illness, suffering, and death. . . . We use our herb in our church—as incense for God, as the Roman Catholics use incense in their church. We burn our incense in order to venerate our God through spiritual experience. . . . It gives us spiritual comfort, we praise God in peace and love, without force. . . . When we are depressed, when we are hungry, we smoke our little herb and we meditate on our God. The herb

---

1. In academic circles, the mention of hemp in the Bible remains the subject of debate; see Moldenke and Moldenke 1986:131; Rätsch 1991c*.

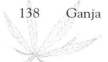

is a true comfort to us" (cited in Kitzinger 1971:581).

In the Rastafarian community, the first inebriation resulting from ganja smoking has the character of an initiation. The young smoker is supposed to receive a vision that will mark him as a full member of the community and reveal his path through life (Rubin 1975; Rubin and Comitas 1976). "Ganja is the most strongly shared experience among the brothers" (Gebre-Selassie 1989:156). The Rastas, it should be noted, largely eschew alcohol, which may only be consumed as a solvent for ganja and in tonics. Alcohol inebriation is considered objectionable, harmful, aggression-promoting, and antisocial (Blätter 1990*). Indeed, the Rasta communities do not have the problems with alcoholism that are typical in the Caribbean (Beaubrun 1975):

> On Jamaica, ganja is an agent of pleasure, like coffee, tea, or tobacco—only much more widespread. Because of reggae music and the Rasta cult, it has become a people's drug. Rasta is a religion, reggae is its mass, Bob Marley its prophet, and ganja its herb of wisdom—this more or less describes the ideology of the Rastafarian movement, which now numbers somewhere between 100,000 and 150,000 Jamaican men (total population = 2,300,000). (Körner 1989:3)

The Rastas see ganja as an agent that gives them strength and endurance to carry out their daily, often strenuous, work, and in fact even motivates them to do it at all (Comitas 1975; Dreher 1982). Ganja stimulates the appetite and is considered an "instant" aphrodisiac (Rubin 1975:265). Hemp also plays an important role in the Rasta menu, which is based on explicit nutritional guidelines. The resinous flowers are used as a spice for stews and cooking bananas, the stalks and leaves are used to produce an herbal tea, and the green leaves are boiled to a broth that serves as the basis for stewed vegetables (most Rastas are vegetarians). The fresh leaves are cooked like spinach; they are said to be very beneficial for children in particular (Kitzinger 1971:581).

Rasta medicine is rooted in the folk medicine of western and central Africa, but has also been influenced by the Ayurvedic medicine of India. Hemp, which the Indians first cultivated on Jamaica, was being used by folk healers ("bush doctors") before the Rastafarian movement (Barrett 1988:129). With the Rastas, the plant acquired the status of a cure-all. Ganja became a sacred thing that causes the life-giving grail to shine. A person who consumes enough ganja, whether smoked, as a tea, or in the form of a tonic, will always be healthy. The Rasta prophet Emanuel said: "Ganja is here . . . to promote the spiritual, mental, and physical health" (Gebre-Selassie 1989:158). This is why the Rastas say "the doctors who make money by treating the sick are against the legalization of ganja, because they are afraid that they would have to close their practices due to a shortage of patients if legalization were to occur" (Gebre-Selassie 1989:158). It is also why the musical Rastas loudly demand the legalization of the *international herb*.

The music of the Rastas, whether Niyabinghi drums, calypso-like Mento, swinging Blue Beat, pop Ska, rocking Rock Steady, foot-stomping Reggae, hard techno Psychedelic Dub, computer-controlled Dancefloor Ragga, the bass-rich Ragga-muffin, or Drum 'n Bass, is both a significant artistic medium for expressing the Rastafarian feeling and an important means of communication. Reggae, which has

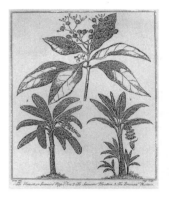

The Europeans first encountered the pimento (*Pimenta dioica* [L.] MERR.) on Jamaica as they were invading and colonizing the Caribbean islands. The plant soon became known in Europe as the "Jamaican pepper tree." Today, Jamaica is no longer associated with this plant, but primarily with ganja, or *de hola herb*. [plate from E. Silby, *An Appendix to Culpeper's British Herbal, being an Account of Foreign Plants*, St. Paul, 1821)

become a form of folk music, deals with folk medical knowledge. Many reggae lyrics sing of the medicinal qualities and uses of the sacred herb. Recalling the words of Hildegard von Bingen, who once wrote that hemp is good for those who have a healthy head, the reggae band Inner Circle, in its song *Mary Mary*, proclaims: "Smokin', smokin', smokin' is good for the brain . . . / I don't want no more of their cocaine."

Most reggae musicians, including Bob Marley and Dillinger, would likely agree. And the raggamuffin stylist Macka B raps: "If you smoke some good sinsemilla the inspiration just come!" and warns: "Don't drink too much . . . Legalize Marijuana!"

The ragga dancehall expert Dr. Alban also warns while he raps: "Cocaine will blow your brain, Ecstasy will mash your life . . ."

Apart from his compatriot Bob Marley, the most important idol of the worldwide Rastafarian reggae community was Peter Tosh, murdered in 1987 during a robbery. Tosh demanded that the sacred herb be legalized, as "it is good against flu / it is good against asthma / good against tuberculosis / even good against umara composis."

In the medicine of the Rastas, ganja is not merely regarded as a cure-all, an efficacious means for relaxing, and an invigorating tonic, but also as an analgesic. In Jamaica, it is used in much the same way that aspirin is used in Germany or the United States (Kitzinger 1971:581). The Zionistic-Coptic church of Ethiopia encourages the Jamaican Rastas in such use, declaring that "the herb may definitely be grown for its use as an asthma medicine, as a remedy for glaucoma, and for joint inflammations; also to aid in the treatment of cancer, as well as for economic use in the clothing industry and for producing paper, touse, for example, in the manufacture of Bibles" (Gebre-Selassie 1989:61).

Hemp is certainly the most important drug in Rasta medicine. Different ointments made from crushed leaves and fat are applied externally as analgesics (Comitas 1975:121). A poultice is used to treat open wounds and internal injuries. A mush is sometimes used to rub down newborns (Comitas 1975:125). Hemp tea is a popular drink for preventive use and is also consumed therapeutically for almost all ailments. Hemp preparations are often ingested for prophylactic purposes. The frequent use does not just protect from diseases, but also gives courage and strength, deepens spiritual inspiration, and improves vision.

The academic community of Jamaica is now taking the wisdom of the Rastas seriously. The November 1999 issue of the highly regarded German journal *GEO* reported on the research being carried out by a pharmacologist and an ophthalmologist, both on the faculty of Medical Sciences of the University of the West Indies in Kingston. The Jamaican scientists investigated and confirmed the claims of fishermen, who claimed that their copious use of ganja enables them to see better at night, allowing them to steer their boats. The fishermen drink an extract of hemp in rum one hour before their boats leave port. The two scientists, Dr. M. E. West and Dr. Albert Lockhart, discovered that the alcohol dissolves the active ingredient canasol from the ganja. They were also able to demonstrate that canasol lowers intraocular pressure. Since that time, many Jamaicans who suffer from glaucoma (which is marked by high intraocular pressure) have been officially treated with alcohol extracts of hemp. Dr. Lockhart also found that Rastas exhibit glau-

Why, the Rastas ask, should any government possess the authority to forbid a plant when its use is in principle allowed in the Bible. They protest not only against the harmfulness that the government is continuously attributing to ganja, but also point to its use as a medicinal plant. Finally, they also identify the plant with the "trees of life" that are described in the vision of "New Jerusalem" at the end of Revelations. . . . By referring to this Bible passage, the Rastas are alluding to the worldwide distribution of the plant for healing purposes. The reggae singer Bob Marley, who made the Rastafarian movement internationally known with his songs and made the veneration of ganja a topic of many of his songs, reiterates this reference.

KONRAD WITT *DIE BEDEUTUNG DER PFLANZE CANNABIS INDICA IN DER RASTAFARI-BEWEGUNG* (1995:81F.)

coma significantly less often than others (West 1991). The "sacred herb" appears to prevent this type of blindness.

When used medicinally, for example, to treat influenza and asthma, hemp is usually smoked (either as a joint or in a pipe). For these purposes, the female flowers are either smoked alone or (foolishly) mixed with tobacco. But there are other preparations as well:

Tonic I

Add 4 to 5 fresh female hemp flowers (ganja) to 1 liter of light rum or wine. The tonic is ready in about 1 week. It may be sweetened with honey. One glass taken once a day will improve health and elevate one's spirits.

Tonic II

Wash fresh hemp roots, chop, and cover with light rum. The tonic is ready for drinking in 3 to 4 weeks.

Night Vision Drink

Add fresh hemp leaves and stalks to light rum and allow to sit for several days. The more ganja that is added, the better, so that the resulting solution is as saturated as possible. Strain the mixture. To improve night vision, drink approximately one hour before sunset. The dosage varies greatly from person to person.

Ganja Tea

Boil leaves and stems. Strain. Add milk and honey or sugar to taste. Individual dosages can vary greatly.

SELECTED DISCOGRAPHY

Music plays a central role in the Rastafarian movement. The lyrics proclaim messages of worry, need, value, conviction, and worldview. Music is the most important cultural expression of the Rastas. Since they see cannabis as the world tree, it is referred to in numerous songs. Many of the songs describe medicinal effects and uses from the perspective of folk medicine. A number of record and CD covers feature hemp leaves or plants.

This discography lists the most important albums for understanding the perspective of the Rastas and their use of ganja medicine.

Culture, *International Herb*, Shanachie Records, 1990
Dillinger, *Cocaine*, Charly Records, 1986
———. *Marijuana in My Brain*, Burning Sounds, 1996
Dub Syndicate, *Stoned Immaculate*, On-U Sound Records, 1991
Grounation, *The Mystic Revelation of Rastafari*, VP Records, no date
The Inner Circle, *Everything is Great*, Island Records, 1979
The Jolly Boys, *Joy Bells (The Roots of Reggae)*, Lyrichord Records, no date
Macka B, *Looks Are Deceiving*, Ras Records, 1990
Mad Professor, *Psychedelic Dub*, Ariwa Records, 1982
Bob Marley, *Songs of Freedom* (4-CD compilation), Island Records, 1992
Mighty V., *So Mighty (Raggamuffin Shock Attack)*, Indigo Records, 1994

Johnny Osbourne, *Nightfall Showcase*, Munich Records, 1997

Ras Abraham and the Irie Vibes, *Smaddy Pickiney*, Picasso Records, 1996

Rastafari Elders, (self-titled), Ras Records, 1990

The Tassili Players, *The Wonderful World of Weed in Dub*, Universal Egg Records (EFA), 1995

Peter Tosh, *Legalize It,* Virgin/CBS, 1976

————. *Bush Doctor*, Rolling Stones Record/EMI Electrola, 1978

VARIOUS ARTISTS OR COMPILATIONS

Big Blunts: Smokin' Reggae Hits (3 vols.), Tommy Boy Records, 1996

Jamaican Ritual Music, Lyrichord Records, no date

Legalize de Erb: 12 Smoke Filled Reggae Classics, Kick Records, 1997

Spliff Relief: Reggae from the Yard, Mesa Records, 1994

The Story of Jamaican Music: Tougher Than Tough (4 CDs), Island Records, 1993

United Colors of Music: Reggae, M.A.C. Developments, 1996

REFERENCES

Barrett, Leonard E. 1988. *The Rastafarians: Sounds of Cultural Dissonance*. Boston: Beacon Press.

Beaubrun, Michael H. 1975. Cannabis or Alcohol: the Jamaican Experience. In *Cannabis and Culture*, edited by V. Rubin. The Hague: Mouton, pages 485–94.

Bender, Wolfgang, ed. 1984. *Rastafari-Kunst aus Jamaika*. Bremen: Edition CON.

Bilby, Kenneth 1986. Vom Kongo bis zur Karibik. In *Schwarze Rhythmen*, edited by G. Hayson and D. Marks. Munich: Knaur, pages 199–236,.

Comitas, Lambros. 1975. The Social Nexus of Ganja in Jamaica. In *Cannabis and Culture*, edited by V. Rubin. The Hague: Mouton, pages 119–32.

Dreher, Melanie C. 1982. *Working Man and Ganja: Marihuana Use in Rural Jamaica*. Philadelphia: ISHI.

Epp, Rainer. 1984. The King's Music: Über die Musik der Rastafaris. In *Rastafari-Kunst aus Jamaika*, edited by Wolfgang Bender. Bremen: edition CON, pages 49–56.

Epp, Rainer, and Klaus Frederking, eds. 1982. *Dub Version: Über Jamaikas Wirklichkeit*. Berlin: Rotbuch Verlag.

Gebre-Selassie, Girma. 1989. *Babylon muß fallen: Die Rasta-Bewegung in Jamaika*. Raymond Martin Verlag.

Haus der Kulturen der Welt, ed. 1992. *Rastafari-Kunst aus Jamaika*. Berlin: CON Verlag.

Kitzinger, Sheila. 1971. The Rastafarian Brethren of Jamaica. In *Peoples and Cultures of the Caribbean*, edited by Michael M. Horowitz. Garden City, New York: The Natural History Press, pages 580–8.

Körner, Peter. 1989. "Wanna have a good smoke?"— Ganja in Jamaika. *EPK* 1/89:3–4.

Lieber, Michael. 1974. The Economics and Distribution of *Cannabis sativa* in Urban Trinidad. *Economic Botany* 29:164–70.

Moldenke, Harold N., and Alma L. Moldenke. 1986. *Plants of the Bible*. New York: Dover.

Rubin, Vera. 1975. The "Ganja Vision." In *Cannabis and Culture*, edited by V. Rubin. The Hague: Mouton, pages 257–66.

Rubin, Vera, and Lambros Comitas. 1976. *Ganja in Jamaica*. Garden City, New York: Anchor Press/Doubleday.

Schuler, Monica. 1980. Myalism and the African Religious Tradition in Jamaica. In *Africa and the Caribbean*, edited by M. E. Crahan and F. W. Knight. Baltimore: The Johns Hopkins University Press, pages 65–79.

West, M. E. 1991. Cannabis and Night Vision. *Nature* 351(June 27, 1991):703–4.

Witt, Konrad. 1995. *Die Bedeutung der Pflanze Cannabis indica in der Rastafari-Bewegung*. Tübingen: Master's Thesis.

Zahl, Peter-Paul. 1995. *Teufelsdroge Cannabis*. Berlin: Verlag Das Neue Berlin

Kinnickinik

HEMP AMONG THE INDIANS OF THE AMERICAS

Europe's encounter with the New World was a confrontation with the exotic—with a nature and with peoples that shattered their horizon of experience.

WOLFGANG MÜLLER
DIE INDIANER AMAZONIENS
(1995:15)

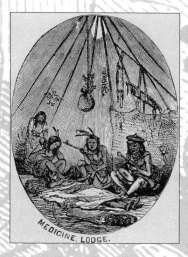

MEDICINE. LODGE.

The smoking of different blends of herbs is one of the essential medicinal-ritual practices of the North American Indians. In this medicine lodge, a patient is being treated by a shaman, who is using smoke, rattles, and drumming. When hemp was introduced into North America, the Indians enthusiastically greeted it as an herb to be smoked. (engraving from "Life of an Indian," *Harper's Illustrated Weekly,* June 20, 1868)

The so-called Indian hemp (*Apocynum cannabinum* L.) is a plant indigenous to North America that served the Indians as a source of fiber and as a medicinal plant.[1] In the early literature, Indian hemp was often confused with true hemp, the cannabis of Europe (Vogel 1970:319). Cannabis was not present in the New World until the arrival of the Europeans, but became widespread throughout the eastern coast of North America by the sixteenth century (Schultes and Hofmann 1995:99*). During the past four centuries, the cannabis introduced into and cultivated in North America has developed into a variety that grows very tall and produces good fibers and potent marijuana. In the botanical and pharmaceutical literature, this variety is referred to as either *Cannabis americana* or *Cannabis sativa* var. *americana* (Millspaugh 1974:615–7).

Just as the early settlers learned many things from Native Americans, the Native American medicine people and shamans investigated the plants intentionally and unintentionally brought to North America by the Europeans. They followed empirical criteria. When their experiences with a particular plant were good and desirable, they assimilated its use into their own culture. Amazingly, the Native Americans recognized the same powers in the European plants that modern pharmacology later found (Rätsch 1991:53–4).

Of all the plants introduced from Europe, the Native Americans were especially interested in hemp. Some members of the Lakota, Blackfoot, and Cherokee have told me that hemp was the only good thing that the White Man brought with him.

The settler Minnie Susan Decker, who compiled Native recipes in an old House Book (*Indian Doctor Book*) and used them quite successfully, said of hemp:

> This plant is good for things other than merely making rope. Soaked and softened, the seeds are very good against wind in the stomach; they open the blockage of the gall, they are good against the flows, and they are very good for killing worms in men and beasts. The juice, when dripped into the ear, kills the worms in there and dispels the earwigs. A decoction of the root is good for inflammations in the head or other areas, gout, joint or hip pain, and muscular atrophy. (Doane 1985:46)

Smoking herbs is an ancient Native American practice; Europeans were surprised to see smoke emanating from the mouths of their new acquaintances (Schroeter 1989). A large number of herbs were set aglow in the peace pipes of the various tribes. In many North American Indian languages, smokable herbs or herb mixtures are known as *kinnickinik*. In the languages of the peoples of the eastern forests, this term referred to the dried leaves of the bearberry (*Arcostaphylos uva-ursi*). Almost all Native American "tobacco mixtures" have bearberry leaves as their base (Emboden 1976:161).

The Iroquois traditionally used a number of psychoactive herbs in their "tobacco mixtures": stimulating lobelia leaves (*Lobelia inflata*), hallucinogenic thornapple

Among the South American Indians, there is no medicine without spirit-moving plants.
RICHARD EVANS SCHULTES

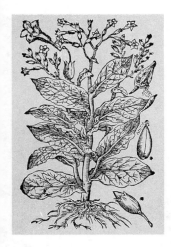

Tobacco, which was introduced into Europe from the New World, was initially referred to as *Hyoscyamus peruvianus*, "Peruvian henbane." Not only did the European authors recognize the botanical relationship between the two plants, they also compared the American smoking herb (*Nicotiana*) to the smoking herb common in Europe at the time, henbane (*Hyoscyamus*). (woodcut from Tabernaemontanus)

---

1. The plant, which is (confusingly) also known as dogbane, was used by the Iroquois to treat diarrhea in motherless children, as an emetic, and as a blood purifier (Herrick 1995:198).

leaves (*Datura stramonium*) (Rutsch 1973:31–3), and of course the narcotic farmer's tobacco (*Nicotiana rustica*).

The Iroquois adopted the name "marijuana" for *Cannabis sativa* (Herrick 1995:132). They regard the herb as a stimulating agent and a psychological aid. Hemp is used after a sick person has gotten well but does not believe that he has recovered. It is said that "this plant will get you going" (Moerman 1986 I:99).

Today, in the prairie states, marijuana smoking is widespread among the Lakota and other tribes. Many young Indians recognize that this plant is much better for them than the devastating firewater. Primarily smoked as an agent of pleasure and to intensify social contact, hemp's effects are an excellent fit with the concept of the peace pipe. Those who smoke together make peace. It has often been claimed or speculated that the great visionaries of the Dakota, such as Sitting Bull and Black Elk, stuffed hemp into their sacred pipes in order to increase the intensity of their visions (Andrews and Vinkenoog 1968:47–64*), but I have been told many times that under no circumstances was the plant allowed to be smoked during the Sun Dance, the most important ceremony in the lives of the Plains tribes. Using the drug would compromise the ceremonial purity that is necessary for the self-inflicted ordeals and would undermine the courage of the Sun Dancers, who prepare for the dance for four years.

Some healers among the Dakota, the *pejuta wicasa*, or "men of herbs," use hemp as a medicine. It is usually mixed with other herbs and smoked for asthma and bronchitis. Among the Lakota, hemp is known as *peji*. This term is a play on the Lakota name for the psychedelic peyote cactus (*Lophophora williamsii*), which they refer to simply as *pejuta*, "medicine" (Anderson 1996).[2]

Hemp also made its way into a number of Central American Indian cultures (Heffern 1974:131). The Cora Indians of Mexico, who live in the Sierra Madre Occidental and are related to the Huichol, smoke hemp at their most sacred ceremonies and communal rituals (ibid). Among the neighboring Tepehuan Indians, whose ancestry can be traced back to the pre-Spanish Totonaken, the plant has acquired the status of a true "plant of the gods." The flowers are called *Santa Rosa*, and are consumed by the community in syncretic rituals that combine pre-Spanish, Indian, colonial, and Catholic elements in order to obtain mystic visions of the divine Earth Mother. During these rituals, it is not uncommon for the participants to speak in tongues (glossalalia). The words that are spoken while under the influence of hemp have a divinatory character and show people the proper way to live (Emboden 1972b:229–32*; Williams-Garcia 1975). The Tepehuan venerate hemp as something very precious. They use it only in rituals and warn against misusing it outside of the ceremonies (Heffern 1974:131).

The Lacandon of Chiapas, Mexico, who are related to the ancient Maya, became acquainted with hemp only a few years ago. They call it *huntul k'uts*, "an other tobacco." But they use the plant almost exclusively as a medicine, usually in the form of an alcohol extract to treat strains, muscle pains, and rheumatic ailments (Rätsch 1994:57f.).

---

2. Interestingly, anhalonium (*Lophophora williamsii*) is listed as a substitute for cannabis in homeopathy (see the chapter on dilutions).

The Cuna Indians, who live on the San Blas Islands of Panama, venerate hemp as a sacred plant. It is communally smoked from pipes during meetings of their council (Schultes and Hofmann 1995:99*).

Hemp was brought to South America by slaves that had been taken from Angola (Partridge 1975:148f.). The ritual smoking of tobacco (*Nicotiana tabacum, Nicotiana rustica, Nicotiana* spp.) was and still is very widespread among South American Indians (Wilbert 1987). Some tribes, such as the Tenetehara, who live in Brazil, have adopted the practice of smoking hemp (Wilbert 1987:108). It is possible that shamans in the Amazon may have snuffed hemp powder in ceremonial contexts (de Smet 1985:80).

Today, hemp is one of the most popular agents of pleasure in the Amazon basin. It has also found a place in the store of medicines used by the shamans and ayahuasqueros. In his jungle clinic near Iquitos, the renowned Peruvian ayahuasquero Don Agustín Rivas uses marijuana to treat crack and basuco addicts. Basuco is the cocaine base that is produced in jungle labs, crack is cocaine hydrochloride "cooked" with baking powder; both products are cheaper than the pure "snow" and are usually smoked by socially subordinate persons with disturbed personality structures. Since their effects are euphoric and cause a person to lose his fear, both substances are extremely attractive, especially for anxious and dissatisfied individuals. Those who undergo hemp therapy come to Don Agustín's jungle clinic, Yushintaita, near Tamishiacu, for three months. During this time, they receive ayahuasca, a potent psychedelic and emetic healing drink, some four times. They are also frequently given marijuana in ritual contexts. No withdrawal symptoms appear during this treatment, and the patients report that they experience a steadily increasing satisfaction and peace. When these patients are released, they typically no longer have an appetite for basuco or crack, and they usually take with them a new perspective on life.[3] But if they smoke basuco again (it is frequently mixed with hemp) the addictive behavior can manifest itself anew.[4]

Don Agustín also uses cannabis, which is planted as a cultigen in the Amazon region, as a spiritual medicine in other ways. In a ritual setting, large amounts are smoked from a pipe, with each participant taking a total of nine deep puffs. The Peruvian marijuana is very potent and can even induce visionary experiences.

---

3. According to clinical studies and the experiences of physicians, using psychedelics (such as LSD, psilocybin, DMT, ayahuasca, ibogaine, and cannabis) to treat addictions to alcohol, cocaine, and opiates is very effective (cf. Grimm 1992*).

4. In Colombia, one of the major cocaine-producing countries, it is common to take a break from using the drug. Large amounts of Colombian grass may be smoked to help overcome any withdrawal symptoms that may appear (Nicholl 1990).

The following three recipes are from different healers in South Dakota.

Smoking Mixture I

 1 part bearberry leaves (*Arcostaphylos uva-ursi*)
 1 part white sage leaves (*Salvia apiana*)
 1 part female hemp flowers (*Cannabis* sp.)

Smoking Mixture 2

1 part silky dogwood bark *(Cornus amomum)*
1 part sweet grass *(Hierochloe odorata)*
1 part prairie sage/western mugwort *(Artemisia ludoviciana)*
1 part marijuana leaves *(Cannabis* sp.)

Smoking Mixture 3

1 part prairie sage/western mugwort *(Artemisia ludoviciana)*
1 part thornapple leaves *(Datura innoxia, Datura stramonium)*
1 part female hemp flowers *(Cannabis* sp.)

This smoking mixture is especially recommended by some medicine men for use in treating asthma, bronchitis, and other diseases of the respiratory tract.

REFERENCES

Anderson, Edward S. 1996. *Peyote: The Divine Cactus.* 2d ed. Tucson: The University of Arizona Press.

Doane, Nancy Locke. 1985. *Indian Doctor Book.* Charlotte, N.C.: APS.

Emboden, William A. 1976. Plant Hypnotics Among the North American Indians. In *American Folk Medicine: A Symposium,* edited by Wayland D. Hand. Berkeley: University of California Press, pages 159–67.

Heffern, Richard 1974. *Secrets of the Mind-altering Plants of Mexico.* New York: Pyramid Books.

Herrick, James W. 1995. *Iroquois Medical Botany.* Syracuse, N.Y.: Syracuse University Press.

Millspaugh, Charles F. 1974. *American Medicinal Plants.* New York: Dover.

Moerman, Daniel E. 1986. *Medicinal Plants of Native America.* 2 vols. Ann Arbor: University of Michigan, Museum of Anthropology, Technical Reports, No. 19.

Müller, Wolfgang. 1995. *Die Indianer Amazoniens.* Munich: C. H. Beck.

Nicholl, Charles. 1990. *"Treffpunkt Café Fruchtpalast": Erlebnisse in Kolumbien.* Reinbek, Germany: Rowohlt.

Partridge, William L. 1975. Cannabis and Cultural Groups in a Colombian Municipio. In *Cannabis and Culture,* edited by V. Rubin. The Hague: Mouton pages 147–72.

Rätsch, Christian. 1991. *Indianische Heilkräuter: Tradition und Anwendung.* 2d rev. ed. Munich: Diederichs.

———. 1994. *Ts'ak:* Die Heilpflanzen der Lakandonen. *Jahrbuch für Ethnomedizin und Bewußtseinsforschung* 2(1993):43–93.

Rutsch, Edward S. 1973. *Smoking Technology of the Aborigines of the Iroquois Area of New York State.* Rutherford, N.J.: Fairleigh Dickinson University Press.

Schroeter, Willy. 1989. *Calumet—Der heilige Rauch.* Wyk auf Föhr, Germany: Verlag für Amerikanistik.

de Smet, Peter A. G. M. 1985. *Ritual Enemas and Snuffs in the Americas.* Amsterdam: CEDLA.

Vogel, Virgil J. 1970. *American Indian Medicine.* Norman: University of Oklahoma Press.

Wilbert, Johannes. 1987. *Tobacco and Shamanism in South America.* New Haven, Conn.: Yale University Press.

Williams-Garcia, Roberto. 1975. The Ritual Use of Cannabis in Mexico. In *Cannabis and Culture,* edited by V. Rubin. The Hague: Mouton, pages 133–45.

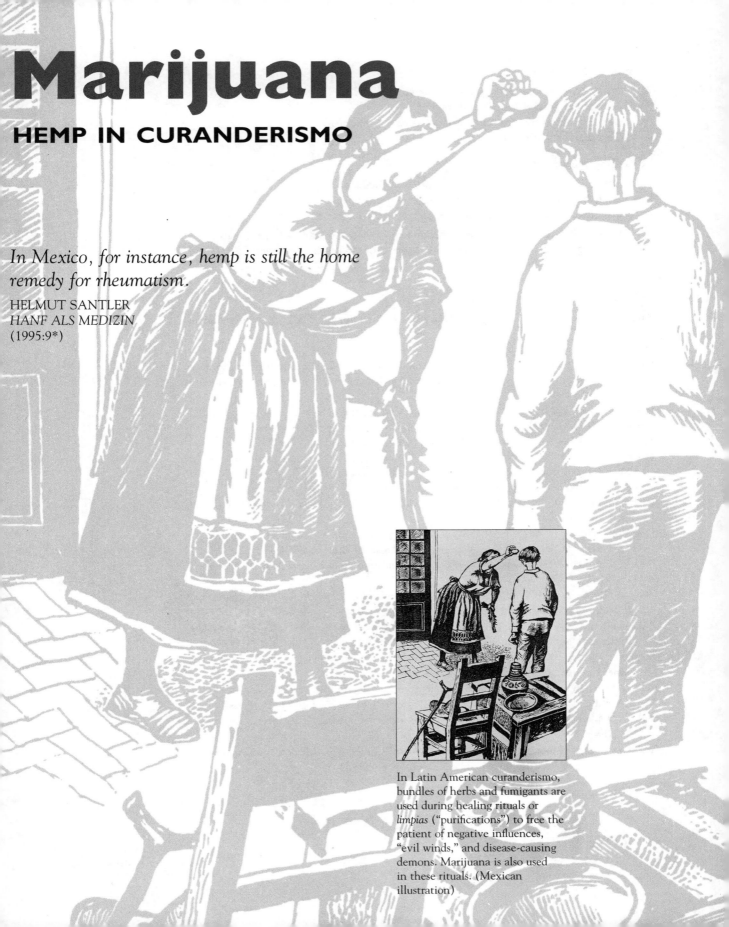

Marijuana

HEMP IN CURANDERISMO

In Mexico, for instance, hemp is still the home remedy for rheumatism.

HELMUT SANTLER
HANF ALS MEDIZIN
(1995:9*)

In Latin American curanderismo, bundles of herbs and fumigants are used during healing rituals or *limpias* ("purifications") to free the patient of negative influences, "evil winds," and disease-causing demons. Marijuana is also used in these rituals. (Mexican illustration)

The Spanish word *curandera* means "female healer"; the corresponding *curandero* means "male healer." The practices of the *curanderas* and *curanderos* are known as *curanderismo*. The main focus of this practice is a specialized knowledge of herbs, which goes far beyond the typical knowledge of home remedies, combined with a knowledge of the ambulatory treatment of such afflictions as broken bones, and so forth (Devine 1982:108f.). The herbal knowledge is based on Native American, European, and African traditions. While curanderismo is embedded in Latin American folk Catholicism, it also contains many elements of Mesoamerican shamanism (Madsen 1955). Curanderismo differs from *brujería*, the traditional folk magic, an amalgamation of the magical techniques of the Indians, voodoo traditions, and tarot practices (Sepulveda 1983). In Mexico and Colombia, these two systems are the most important regulators of national health. There are curanderas in every marketplace. Sick persons consult them much more frequently than they do the physicians trained in Western medicine. They are the basic unit of Mexican and Colombian folk medicine.

The name *marijuana* appears to have first been used in Mexico. It is a contraction of the name *María Juana* (Mary Jane). The word alludes to the female flowers as well as to their use as an aphrodisiac (cf. Reko 1936:64). The names *Rosa-María* and *María Rosa* are also used. During the early Colonial period, hemp was also known as *pipiltzintzintli*, an Aztecan name that means "the honorable little children." In pre-Spanish times, this name was used to refer to an Aztecan magical plant, the botanical identity of which is unknown. Curiously, a folk etymological explanation of marijuana in Mexico traces the name back to the Aztec words *mali*, "bundle of grass," and *ha huana*, "inebriating" (Diaz 1979:78).

Usually, either the female flowers (*marijuana* or *bota*) or the resin that has been rubbed off of them (*marijuana pura*) is smoked; the leaves (*la hoja*) are smoked less frequently. Both water and alcohol extracts are also employed. Often, the flowers and upper stems are ground, mixed with cane sugar or molasses and chilies, and drunk in a glass of milk or tequila (Reko 1936:64). Marijuana is drunk primarily for medicinal purposes.

In Mexico, marijuana has a number of uses in curanderismo. Early evidence of the folk medical use comes from the nineteenth century. In San Luis Potosí, cannabis herbage was mixed with *aguardiente*, "firewater" (an inexpensive liquor made from sugar cane) and used both internally and externally for tarantula bites and scorpion stings (Bye 1979:145). Patients suffering from tuberculosis or leprosy smoked copious amounts of marijuana to deal with their afflictions (Reko 1936:67).

Today there are many folk medicinal uses. Marijuana cigarettes are smoked for asthma and other muscle spasms in the respiratory tract. Alcohol extracts are ingested for all types of cramps, including those resulting from maniacal frenzy, delirium tremens, and tetanus, as well as for colic, tuberculosis, and diarrhea, and for sleeplessness and nervousness (Cabrera 1981:144–5). Marijuana is also used to lower fevers and as a laxative (Diaz 1979:78). In Guadalajara, alcohol extracts of marijuana are massaged into areas of the body affected by muscle pains, tension, and rheumatism.

In Mexico, marijuana is also seen as a remedy for social grievances. In the secret national anthem, the revolutionary song *La Cucaracha*, it is said:

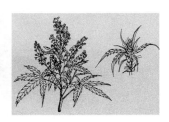

The hemp that is cultivated in Mexico is usually characterized as *Cannabis sativa* var. *indica*. It is very rich in THC and is consequently a highly esteemed euphoriant and agent of pleasure. In Mexican folk medicine, curanderos consume marijuana during *limpias*, magical purification rituals, in order to attract the gods and saints. In folk medicine, hemp is used for a variety of ills. (Mexican illustration, from M. Hernandez and J. Gally)

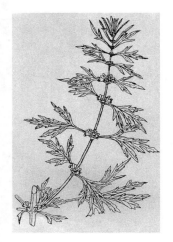

In Mexico, Siberian motherwort (*Leonurus sibiricus* L.) is commonly known as *marijuanillo*, "little hemp." It is smoked as a marijuana substitute. The plant, originally from Asia, is called *ganchaa-tade* in Thailand, a word that is derived from *gan-chaa*, cannabis. (old illustration, Thailand)

La cucaracha, la cucaracha	The cockroach, the cockroach
Ya no puede caminar	Still it cannot go
Porque la falta, porque la falta	Because there is no, because there is no
Marijuana que fumar	Marijuana to smoke

As in Mexico, the folk medicine of Colombia has also been shaped by curanderismo. Although Colombia is now generally regarded as a land of cocaine, it is actually a "marijuana land" (Elejalde 1975:327). The dried female flowers are known as *la mona, la armarilla, ella,* and *marijuana.* Large segments of the population use hemp as a regular means of inebriating and relaxing, and strengthening themselves during physical labor. But there are also countless folk medicinal applications. Alcohol extracts are applied externally as liniment for rheumatoid arthritis. For asthma, the extracts are taken internally (Elejalde 1975:341). Hemp is smoked for sleep disorders and exhaustion, for sexual validation, and as a general means of preserving health. Fresh leaves are ground to a paste and rubbed into the skin over painful areas of the body. Children who cry too much are given sweetened hemp decoctions to drink. One reason that hemp is so widespread and has so many medicinal uses in Colombia may be that during the pre-Spanish and in the early Colonial period tobacco had many of the same medicinal uses that hemp has today. Tobacco was already smoked to induce altered states; it was an easy transition to using hemp (Partridge 1975).

Hemp is a component of numerous herbal mixtures that are manufactured by professional curanderos. It is usually contained in preparations that are used to treat chronic disorders. It is also an ingredient in alcohol extracts (usually rum or *aguardiente*) that are taken internally for pain, snakebites, bleeding, and asthma (Partridge 1975:161). Unfortunately, the curanderos keep the precise composition of their remedies secret, for reasons that are easily understood (Elejalde 1975:341).

Many Colombians consume hemp on a daily basis without suffering any harmful effects. This was demonstrated in a study that found that "long-term cannabis use (more than 10 years) leads neither to apathy, parasitism, nor backwardness, rather, the oldest and most experienced consumers often improved their social and economic situations during their lifetimes" (Partridge 1975).

Hemp also plays an important role in the Peruvian San Pedro cult (Davis 1983), in which the Peruvian curanderos ingest a drink made from the sacred cactus *Trichocereus panchanoi* BRITT. et ROSE during their nocturnal *mesa* rituals and may also administer the drink to other participants. The *mesa* (Spanish for "table") is an altar with numerous objects (sticks, shells, ceramics, images of saints, and so forth) whose structure dates back to pre-Spanish times. The drink, which also contains mescaline, is ingested by the curanderos during their night ceremonies so that they may recognize the cause of a disease. Before this, however, an alcohol extract of farmer's tobacco (*Nicotiana rustica*), which is very rich in nicotine, must be "drunk" through the nose from a dish made from the shell of a snail or a mussel. This purifies and protects oneself from negative forces.

For certain purposes, other plants may also be added to the San Pedro drink (Davis 1983): "To increase 'seeing' in the altered state of consciousness, some 'maestros'—according to Don M. A. (Huancabamba)—have recently begun adding marijuana to their 'remedio'" (Giese 1989:229).

Marijuana Extract
(from Dr. Luis Cabrera)

Cover 100 g of female hemp flowers with pure grain alcohol. After 48 hours, strain. Carefully heat the liquid. When enough of the alcohol has evaporated so that only 7 to 10 g remains, dilute with distilled water until a homogeneous, green solution results that smells of hemp. Add 20 ml of this solution to a tea made from orange leaves or flowers. For medicinal use, drink three times a day for three days.

Marijuana Tincture
(recipe from Guadalajara)

Steep female flowers in 70 percent alcohol for three days.

Tequila Fuerte

Steep fresh hemp roots in tequila together with a dried chili pepper. Add a pinch of salt and lemon juice according to taste.

Mexican Asthma Cigarettes

Mix 2 parts chopped hemp with 1 part chopped cinnamon bark. Roll into cigarettes and smoke.

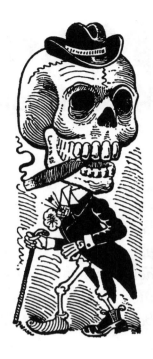

In Mexico, even the dead smoke everything from tobacco to marijuana. (A *calavera*, or death's head; single-page print from José Guadalupe Posada, Mexico, ca. 1911)

REFERENCES

Argueta Villamar, Arturo, Leticia M. Cano Asseleih, and María Elena Rodarte, eds. 1994. *Atlas de las plantas de la medicina tradicional mexicana.* 3 vols. México, D.F.: INI.

Bye, Robert A. 1979. An 1878 Ethnobotanical Collection from San Luis Potosí. *Economic Botany* 33(2):135–62.

Cabrera, Luis. 1981. *Plantas curativas de México.* México, D.F.: Libro-Mex Editores.

Davis, E. Wade. 1983. Sacred Plants of the San Pedro Cult. *Botanical Museum Leaflets* 29(4):367–86.

Devine, Mary Virginia. 1982. *Brujería: A Study of Mexican-American Folk-Magic.* St. Paul, Minn.: Llewellyn.

Diaz, José Luis. 1979. Ethnopharmacology and Taxonomy of Mexican Psychodysleptic Plants. *Journal of Psychedelic Drugs* 11(1–2):71–101.

Elejalde, B. R. 1975. Marihuana and Genetic Studies in Colombia: The Problem in the City and in the Country. In *Cannabis and Culture,* edited by V. Rubin. The Hague: Mouton, pages 327–43.

Giese, Claudius Cristobal. 1989. *"Curanderos": Traditionelle Heiler in Nord-Peru (Küste und Hochland).* Hohenschäftlarn: Klaus Renner Verlag (Münchner Beiträge zur Amerikanistik, Vol. 20).

Hernandez Maga a, Rafael, and Mireya Gally Jorda. 1984. *Plantas medicinales.* México, D.F.: Arbol Editorial.

Madsen, William. 1955. Shamanism in Mexico. *Southwestern Journal of Anthropology* 11:48–57.

Martínez, Maximino. 1994. *Las plantas medicinales de México.* 6th ed. México, D.F: Ediciones Botas.

Partridge, William L. 1975. Cannabis and Cultural Groups in a Colombian Municipio. In *Cannabis and Culture,* edited by V. Rubin. The Hague: Mouton, pages 147–72.

Reko, Victor. 1936. *Magische Gifte.* Stuttgart: Enke.

Sepulveda, María Teresa. 1983. *Magia, brujería y supersticiones en México.* México, D.F.: Everest Mexicana.

Maconha

HEMP IN BRAZILIAN FOLK MEDICINE

Bahia, along with Pernambuco (maconha de pernambuco), is one of the most important hemp-growing areas in Brazil. Grass is distributed throughout the gigantic Amazon basin, between Boa Vista in the extreme north, Rio Branco on the border to Peru, and Manaus in the heart of what remains of the primeval South American forest.

STEFAN HAAG
HANFKULTUR WELTWEIT
(1995:114*)

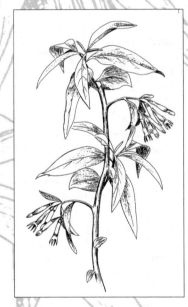

In Brazil, a number of night jessamines (*Cestrum* spp.) are known as *maconha brava*, "wild hemp," and are smoked as marijuana substitutes. Several psychoactive species of *Cestrum*, a member of the nightshade family, also serve as tobacco and hemp substitutes in other South American countries. (Chilean illustration)

Brazil is the country in which paramedicine has brought forth enormous fruit. People possessed by the spirits of deceased physicians carry out operations under unhygienic conditions. Fanatic cult followers proclaim somber oracles; demons are exorcised with bloody sacrifices. Alongside all of these manifestations, there is also a folk medicine that combines indigenous, African, and European elements and in particular uses herbs for self-treatment.

Hemp has been at home in Brazil for more than four hundred years. During that time, it has been used as a source of fiber, an agent of pleasure, and a medicine (Hutchinson 1975:173). Primarily used by those groups that invaded from Europe or were abducted from Africa, it plays a definite, albeit largely unknown, role among such African-Brazilian cults as Candomblé, Xango, Macumba, and Umbanda (Bucher 1995; Hutchinson 1975:179). It is smoked or otherwise ingested for the divinations and religious rites of the Catimbó cult (De Pinho 1975:294). In contrast, among the indigenous peoples, only the Tenetehara Indians are known to smoke it (Hutchinson 1975:174).

Hemp was originally known by the names *diamba* and *pito do Pango*; today, it is commonly called *maconha*, the name used for the plant in Angola (De Pinho 1975:294). South Brazilian fishermen and other coastal dwellers call *Cestrum laevigatum* SCHLECHT., a nightshade rich in alkaloids that has psychoactive properties, *maconha* or *maconha brava*, "wild hemp." They smoke the dried leaves as a marijuana substitute (Schultes and Hoffman 1995:38*). Other *Cestrum* species are also used as marijuana substitutes (Rätsch 1998:162ff.*).

In the past, the hemp known as maconha was usually smoked in water pipes; now it is smoked almost exclusively in cigarette form, sometimes mixed with tobacco. The leaves and flowers may also be chewed as a quid (Hutchinson 1975:179). A decoction of hemp leaves in water is usually prepared when the plant is used for medicinal purposes. These decoctions are drunk for rheumatic ailments, women's disorders, colic, and other painful afflictions. For toothaches, female flowers are placed on or wrapped around the afflicted tooth and retained in the mouth for a prolonged time. A *licor* of hemp flowers and *cachaça* (sugar cane liquor) is often made (Hutchinson 1975:180). In rural areas, it is especially common to use hemp to ease menstrual pains and cramps (De Pinho 1975:295). Among the people of the Amazon, it is smoked or drunk as a tincture for asthma, dysentery, cramps, and nervous disorders (Carneiro Martins 1989:77). Maconha is also used to relax after strenuous physical labor and is often referred to as the "opium of the poor" (De Pinho 1975). But the wealthy have also developed a liking for the herb.

Hemp is used to accompany people on the journey into death. One famous story tells of Queen Carlota Joaquino, who returned to Lisbon after spending six years in the Portuguese colony, taking her favorite slave, Felisbino, with her. As she was dying, she bade Felsibino to give her *diambo do amazonas*. The slave obeyed, preparing a tea of hemp and arsenic. After his mistress had gently slipped into sleep, he too drank a final tea so that he could rejoin her in heaven (Hutchinson 1975:175).

In Brazil, the past several decades have witnessed the rise of Santo Daime, a syncretic church in Brazil headquartered in Mapia, a village in the Amazon. This community utilizes an ayahuasca recipe stolen from Indian shamans to produce their

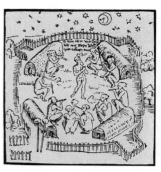

Smoking tobacco for hedonistic, medicinal, and ritual reasons was very common among indigenous people throughout Brazil. For this reason, hemp was introduced from Europe was quickly accepted as an alternative smoking herb and held in high regard by all. (smoking ritual of the Tupinamba; woodcut from Hans Staden, *Brasilien*, 1548–55)

sacrament, known as Santo Daime, or simply Daime. During their worship services, in which they carry out "healing work," they drink ayahuasca and smoke marijuana, which they call Santa María. The Santo Daime community believes that hemp is a medicine and represents a sacred sacrament for the believers (Fischer-Fackelmann 1996).

Licor de Maconha

Steep a handful of female hemp flowers in a liter of light rum or cachaça for 2 weeks. The flowers should remain in the bottle until it has been emptied.

REFERENCES

Bucher, Richard. 1995. La marihuana en el folklore y la cultura popular brasileña. *Takiwasi* 2(3):119–28.

Carneiro Martins, José Evandro. 1989. *Plantas medicinais de uso na Amazônia.* 2d ed. Belém-Pará, Brazil: CEJUP.

De Pinho, Alvaro Rubin. 1975. Social and Medical Aspects of the Use of Cannabis in Brazil. In *Cannabis and Culture*, edited by V. Rubin. The Hague: Mouton pages 293–302.

Fernández Chiti, Jorge. 1995. *Hierbas y plantas curativas, para curar el cuerpo, para elevar la mente.* Buenos Aires: Condorhuasi.

Fischer-Fackelmann, Ruth. 1996. *Fliegender Pfeil.* Munich: Heyne.

Hutchinson, Harry William 1975. Patterns of Marihuana Use in Brazil. In *Cannabis and Culture*, edited by V. Rubin. The Hague: Mouton, pages 173–83.

Leibing, Annette, ed. 1997. *The Medical Anthropologies in Brazil.* Berlin: VWB. *curare* special edition, December 1997.

Dilutions

HEMP IN HOMEOPATHY

In every discussion about homeopathy, when debating the effectiveness of the substances, after just a few sentences a debate usually develops about the substance of homeopathy itself. Here, more than anywhere else, the extent to which we tend to mistrust personal experience when it contradicts that which is considered scientific knowledge becomes clear.

MANFRED BRINKMANN AND MICHAEL FRANZ
NACHTSCHATTEN IM WEIßEN LAND
(1982:149)

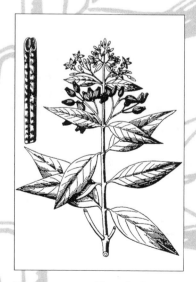

The antipyretic China bark tree (*Cinchona pubescens*) is not from China, but Peru. Samuel Hahnemann discovered homeopathy as he was experimenting with China bark.

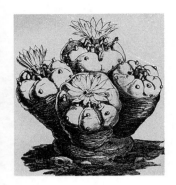

After it was introduced to Europe, the entheogenic peyote cactus (*Lophophora williamsii*) from Mexico was tested as a homeopathic medicine (Anhalonium lewinii hom.) and used as a substitute for Cannabis indica hom. (engraving from 1847)

Hemp: use leaves and seeds. Take 1 to 2 tablespoons with ¹/₂ liter of milk. If you drink a small cup of this several times a day, the jaundice will certainly be cured. Also use for severe constipation and a diseased liver. For chronic rheumatism, boil 1 to 2 tablespoons of leaves in ¹/₂ liter of water for 4 to 6 minutes to make a tea and drink two cold cups of this daily. Boiled seeds are an excellent remedy for rheumatic pains.

NIKOLA GELENČIR
NATURHEILKUNDE DES BALKANS
(1983:221F.)

Homeopathy is a medical system based on both material causes and on metaphysical aspects. It regards itself as an experiential science. Homeopathy was founded by the physician Samuel Hahnemann (1755–1843). Hahnemann experimented with a number of remedies. When testing the China bark tree from Peru (*Cinchona pubescens* Vahl),[1] he discovered the rule *Similia similibus curentur*, "let like be treated by like." The healthy Hahnemann drank a tea made from cinchona bark and suddenly experienced feverlike symptoms. This led him to conclude that a plant is able to cure precisely those symptoms that it evokes in healthy persons. He wrote:

> Every efficacious medicine provokes a kind of disease of its own in the human body. One should imitate nature, which occasionally heals a chronic disease by means of another which comes along, and utilize for that (preferably chronic disease) which is to be healed that drug which is capable of provoking another, artificial disease which is as similar as possible, and so it will be healed: Similia similibus. (Hahnemann 1796)

Hahnemann also assumed that every substance actually has two qualities of activity: one that is healing in weak or low dosage, and one that is toxic in high dosage. Every substance has within itself a "good, divine principle," the "vital energy," which acts as a counterpole to matter. If a solution of a substance is diluted, only the matter is watered down, while the spirit ("vital energy") of the substance remains. In the greatest dilution, only the vital energy, the "good, divine" remains in the agent that, purified of "evil matter," simultaneously develops its greatest abilities to heal. This is why the process of diluting (Dilution, abbreviated as D) a dissolved substance ("mother tincture") dilutes the matter while potentiating the healing power, and in fact to the tenth power.

Following Hahnemann's rule, numerous substances were dissolved and tested in various dilutions. During the past two hundred years, this has resulted in a quite uniform picture of the medical effectiveness of homeopathic preparations. In the large standard references on homeopathy, the medicinal descriptions of the individual substances are compiled according to the symptoms that they produce in healthy persons, so-called symptom pictures. When a patient exhibits one or more symptoms that correspond to the medicinal description, the homeopathically oriented physician will turn to that medicine which corresponds to these symptoms (Gäbler 1965).

Hemp has been a part of the homeopathic Materia Medica from the very beginning (Anonymous 1998). Hahnemann himself had the following to say about hemp:

> **Cannabis sativa.** Until now, hemp has been usefully applied for acute gonorrhea and several types of jaundice. This organotropic tendency is found again

---

1. For more on the influential pharmacological and cultural history of the cinchona bark tree (*Cinchona pubescens* VAHL, syn. *Cinchona succirubra* PAV. ex KLOTZSCH; also the species *Cinchona calisya* WEDD., syn. *Cinchona ledgeriana* MOENS ex TRIM.), see, for example, Dethloff 1944; Hobhouse 1992:14–66.

in testing the symptoms of the urinary organs. In Persian inns, the herb is used to alleviate tiredness among those who are traveling on foot. Here too, there are suitable symptoms for testing. For a long time, I administered hemp juice in the mother tincture, in the dosage of the smallest portion of a drop. But now I find that the dilution 30c is able to more highly develop these medicinal powers. (cited in Buchmann 1983:19f.)

Over the years, the experiences with hemp have become so comprehensive that Allen's encyclopedic standard reference now lists over forty printed pages of symptom pictures for it (Allen 1975:464–505). In the homeopathic doctrine of medicine, it has become customary to distinguish between *Cannabis sativa* and *Cannabis indica*. And indeed, the medical descriptions and symptom pictures of the two species vary considerably. Perhaps this is another indication of the fact that there are indeed two different species of the hemp plant.

The homeopathic remedy *Cannabis indica* is primarily used as a mother tincture and in low dilutions. The mother tincture is obtained from pure resin (hashish) and alcohol. The mother tincture must be prescribed, and the relevant drug laws taken into consideration. Only high dilutions can be bought in a pharmacy without a prescription. The effects of *Cannabis indica* are characterized as follows:

> Invokes highly remarkable hallucinations and concepts, **exaggeration of the sense of time and space are extremely characteristic.** No longer able to conceive of time, space, and place. Is extraordinarily happy and content, nothing disturbs. Thoughts bombard him. Has a very calming effect upon many nervous ailments, such as epilepsy, mania, dementia, delirium tremens, and exaggerated reflexes. Morbus Basedow. Catalepsy. (Boericke 1992:187)

Cannabis indica (Cannabis indica hom. *HAB34*, Cannabis indica hom. *HPUS78*) is prescribed for many ailments, including asthma, impotence, lack of appetite, sexual exhaustion, nightmares, and nervous disorders (Schmidt 1992:644*). Comparable homeopathic agents (correlations) are *Belladonna* (belladonna), *Hyoscyamus* (henbane), and *Stramonium* (thornapple), in other words, the witches' herbs of old. *Anhalonium lewinii*, the extract from the Mexican peyote cactus whose botanical name is *Lophophora williamsii*, is a substitute (Boericke 1992:188; Gäbler 1965:199–204).

The homeopathic agent *Cannabis sativa* is obtained by making an alcohol extract of the fresh herbage. It is used in the mother tincture to the third dilution (D3), but for stuttering, in the thirtieth dilution (D30).

Cannabis sativa "appears to especially influence the urogenital and respiratory tracts. It has characteristic sensations as from dripping water. Great tiredness as from overexertion; tiredness after eating. Sense of suffocating when swallowing; the swallowed material goes down the windpipe. **Stuttering.** Confusion of thought and speech. Shaking tongue, hasty and unconnected speech" (Boericke 1992:188).

Cannabis sativa is prescribed primarily for urine retention as well as diseases of the urinary tract (gonorrhea, inflammation of the penis) and the respiratory organs. A substitute is *Hedysarum ildefonsianum*, a Brazilian species of sweet clover (Boericke 1992:190).

As with all homeopathic medicaments, it is not easy to assign cannabis to a particular set of symptoms. Nevertheless, Hahnemann already crystallized out the use of cannabis for various diseases of the urinary tract, the chest (bronchus), and the sensory organs.

MANFRED FANKHAUSER
HASCHISH ALS MEDIKAMENT
(1996:216*)

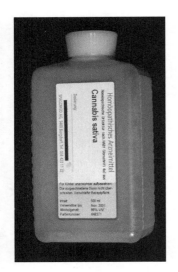

The mother tincture of *Cannabis sativa* is still used today—or is being used again—as a versatile medicament in homeopathy and in natural healing practices.

Parallel to specialized homeopathy, whose standards are as rigorous as those of scientific medicine, a folk homeopathy has also developed that is regarded as somewhat controversial. Folk medical books often contain uses and information that have been borrowed from homeopathy. In *Kölbl's Krauterfibel*, with the appropriate subtitle *Eine Fundgrube alter und moderner Heilkräuter- und Hausmittel Rezepte* (Kölbl's Herbal Fable: A Treasury of Old and Modern Recipes for Medicinal Plants and Home Remedies) the healing effects of hemp are described as follows:

> Hemp, in homeopathic dilutions (D1–D2) is only administered under doctor's orders for hysterical conditions, swelling of the liver, colic, and heart palpitations. Boiled in water, it is good for severe cough; it remedies a raw voice. Boiled in milk, it is recommended for dropsy. In essential form, it is also prescribed to treat lung inflammations with confused speech, for vomiting with bile, and for pains when breathing and speaking, also for chronic urine retention, especially when urine is excreted only drop-wise as a result of inflammation of the urethra. (Kölbl 1983:72)

In Europe, homeopathy is now a generally recognized natural healing method that is taken seriously by many physicians trained in scientific medicine. In Germany, there is even an official *Homöopathisches Arzneimittelbuch* (Homeopathic Drug Book) that regulates the procedures for manufacturing and testing products. The precise instructions for producing the "good, divine" spirit of the hemp plant can still be found in this work.

The German *Betäubungsmittelgesetz* (Drug Law) forbids the therapeutic use of *Cannabis* as a medicine in Germany (Körner 1994:56).[2] This even applies to hemp preparations that are free of active substances: "The homeopathic drugs and preparations fall under the purview of the Betäubungsmittelgesetz and are therefore not open to traffic" (Schmidt 1992:653*). An example of a typically absurd law:

> Although there are over two centuries of good experiences with homeopathic agents based on cannabis, these can not be obtained in our country: All of the manufacturers we spoke to had to pass, for cannabis is simply forbidden in Germany, even when it is only the spirit of the plant that has been immortalized in the solvents. The reason for this appears to be a downright pathological fear of an ominous power which might be inherent in the spirit in the bottle. (Anonymous 1998:15)

---

2. In the *Kommentar zum* [Commentary on the] *Betäubungsmittelgesetz* (BtMG 1994), it is stated: "The use of Cannabis plants to manufacture Cannabis cigarettes, to manufacture medicaments and Cannabis tinctures (cough agents, sleeping agents, asthma and migraine agents) is forbidden."

Migraine Oligoplex
(Dr. Madaus und Co., Radebeul Dresden; 1933)

A mixture of the following dilutions is made into tablets:

Homeopathic remedy	*Derived from*
Cannabis ind. D2	Indian hemp
Valerianae D2	Valerian
Chinin. hydrochlor. D2	Chinin HCL
Extract Hypoph. D5	Pituitary extract (from cattle)
Dimethyaminophenozon D1	

For migraine headaches, take 2 to 3 tablets (cf. Fankhauser 1996:178*).

Plantival
(Dr. W. Schwabe, Leipzig; 1933)

Mix together the homeopathic mother tinctures (Ø or = D1) of the following substances (presumably equal portions of the each):

Homeopathic remedy	*Derived from*
Aeth.	[probably] Dog parsley (*Aethusa cynapium*)
Valer.	Valerian
Avena sat.	Oats
Cannabis sat.	Hemp (*Cannabis sativa*)
Passiflora inc.	Passion flower (*Passiflora incarnata*)

This compound was sold as a sedative and hypnotic (sleeping aid) (cf. Fankhauser 1996:179*).

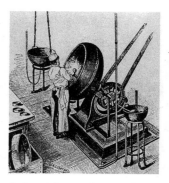

Industrial manufacture of homeopathic medicaments in the late nineteenth century. (engraving from Richard Haehl, *Samuel Hahnemann, his Life and Work*)

LITERATURE CITED

Allen, Timothy F. 1975. *The Encyclopedia of Pure Materia Medica*. New York: Boericke and Tafel.

Anonymous. 1998. Der Geist in der Flasche: Cannabis und Homöopathie. *Hanf!* 6/98:14–5.

Boericke, William 1992. *Handbuch der homöopathischen Materia medica* (translated from American English and revised by D. J. Beha, R. Hickmann, and K. F. Scheible), Heidelberg: Haug.

Brinkmann, Manfred, and Michael Franz, eds. 1982. *Nachtschatten im Weißen Land: Betrachtungen zu alten und neuen Heilsystemen*. Berlin: Verlagsgesellschaft Gesundheit.

Buchmann, Werner. 1983. *Hahnemanns Reine Arzneimittellehre*. Heidelberg: Haug.

Dethloff, W. 1944. *Chinin*. Berlin: Verlag Chemie.

Gäbler, Hartwig. 1965. *Aus dem Heilschatz der Natur*. Stuttgart: Paracelsus.

Gelenčir, Nikola 1983. *Naturheilkunde des Balkans*. Steyr: Verlag Wilhem Ennsthaler.

Hahnemann, Samuel. 1796. *Versuch über ein neues Prinzip zur Auffindung der Heilkräfte der Arzneisubstanzen nebst einigen Blicken auf die bisherigen*.

Hobhouse, Henry 1992. *Fünf Pflanzen verändern die Welt*. Stuttgart: dtv/Klett-Cotta.

Kölbl, Konrad. 1983. *Kölbl's Kräuterfibel. Eine Kompilation*. 20th ed. Grünwald: Reprint Verlag Konrad Kölbl.

Körner, Harald Hans. 1994. "Betäubungsmittelgesetz, Arsneimittlegesetz" *Beck'sche Kurz-Kommentare,* vol. 37, Munich: C. H. Beck.

Dope

HEMP IN MODERN SELF-MEDICATION

High, Stoned, and Wasted
sat around a table
a pipe they tasted.
GALAN O. SEID
GRASLAND-HYMNE 2

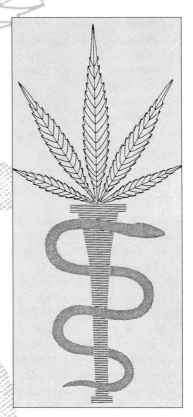

A modern variant of the staff of
Aesclepius, symbol of the healing arts: the Kundalini serpent
wound around a chilam filled
with hemp.

It is a sign of our times that there has been an enormous loss of faith in our political laws. Many people are no longer able to take seriously governments that collect disproportionately high taxes, conduct wars, and suppress the efforts of those who would protect the environment. These people consciously violate certain laws because they consider them to be wrong. The fact that many now disregard drug laws is nothing new. The people that are affected, for example, the "stoners," see nothing criminal about using hemp products and are not conscious of doing anything wrong. Rudi Gaul, a psychologist from Munich, hits the nail on the head:

> If politicians are able to decide which drugs are good and which are bad for the people (and thus for me), then I can do that as well, for I consider myself to have at least the same ability to decide and the same intelligence as many, if not most politicians. And so I too will make my own decision. (cited in Schuldes 1995:10)

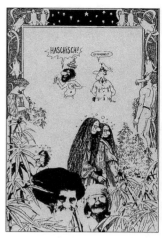

This caricature by the German cartoonist Gerhard Seyfried portrays both the medicinal side of hemp and the official government's lack of understanding about cannabis products. (from Gerhard Seyfried, *Wo soll das alles enden*, Rotbuch Verlag, Berlin, 1978, p. 45)

Unfortunately, studies on modern self-medication with hemp products have not yet been undertaken. While occasionally a newspaper article appears that reports on a cancer patient who illegally smokes hashish or marijuana to alleviate her suffering, reports such as these are typically written with the attitude that "a person who already has cancer can't make it any worse by using dope."

Recently, Dr. Lester Grinspoon (1992) described a dramatic case of self-medication with hemp. Kerry Wiley, thirty-five years old, was arrested in Kuala Lumpur, the capital of Malaysia, with over 500 grams of cannabis. Malaysian law dictates that the possession of such an amount be punished by hanging. Kerry used the hemp for purely medicinal purposes: As a twelve-year-old, Kerry had fallen from a ledge. While he miraculously survived the fall, he has suffered from exceedingly painful muscle spasms since that time. He tried all kinds of drugs and therapies in his efforts to come to grips with his pain and ultimately discovered that hemp was the only thing that provided relief. Through his own testimony, statements from international medical experts and other intervention, his capital sentence was reduced to a prison sentence.

Dr. Grinspoon, a physician, and James Bakalar, a lawyer, have repeatedly pointed out that increasing numbers of patients are turning to illegal drugs for self-medication (Grinspoon and Bakalar 1987). Patients suffering from quadriplegia (paralysis of all four extremities), paraplegia (paralysis due to severing of the spinal cord; spastic paralysis of both legs), and multiple sclerosis (hardening of the tissues and organs) often treat themselves with hemp products. The most common form of administration involves smoking marijuana cigarettes ("joints") or pure hashish:

> Many multiple sclerosis sufferers also report that their episodes occur less frequently, are not as severe, and disappear more rapidly when they use hashish. (Rieth and Heiler 1995:46)

In addition, many patients suffering from AIDS or cancer have learned or heard from others that using hemp can help them deal with the "wasting syndrome." There are even a few courageous physicians in Germany who now recommend the

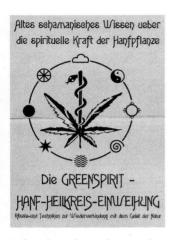

Altes schamanisches Wissen ueber die spirituelle Kraft der Hanfpflanze

Die GREENSPIRIT - HANF-HEILKREIS-EINWEIHUNG

Rituale-und Techniken zur Wiederverbindung mit dem Geist der Natur

A flyer from the underground announcing the inauguration of a hemp healing circle.

Drink the wine of Aluqah and breathe the Secret Smoke of God. / Intoxicated by the Green Shadows of the Paradise. / Know that nothing's true and that everything is permitted.

THERION, *VOVIN*
(NUCLEAR BLAST, 1998)

use of cannabis to their patients. One of them is Dr. Gölz, a physician who practices in Berlin:

> In my practice, I primarily treat HIV and patients with tumors. During the terminal stages of their diseases, these patients suffer from the so-called wasting syndrome, in which they no longer feel any urge to consume calories. I exploit the ability of cannabis to stimulate the appetite. After consuming THC, the patients often have a ravenous hunger for sweets, which has the effect that weight increases of up to 1 kilo per month can be attained. (Gölz, interviewed in *Hanfblatt* No. 5:7, 1994)

Several women who delivered their babies at home have told me that they smoked or ate hemp products to ease the painful contractions and the birth process in general.

Many people who use hemp have told me that they have found both it and hashish to be the best remedy for migraine headaches. I have even heard of cases in which persons who had suffered from migraines for years were freed entirely of this chronic affliction as soon as they began smoking the herb. Other stories report similar effects in treating asthma. One acquaintance suffered terrible asthma attacks in his youth. Since he began occasionally smoking hashish, his ailment has completely disappeared. It would certainly be worthwhile to conduct research into these modern folk medicinal uses.

I have often heard of successful self-medication for hepatitis, epilepsy, colds, bronchitis, and tension in general. One enthusiastic hemp user told me: "Dope is the best thing for knots in the brain. One joint can have the same effect as Alexander's sword."

In recent years, a ritualized use of hemp has emerged in underground circles (Rätsch 1996a*). Here, supervised healing circles heighten the plant's spiritual healing powers by utilizing shamanic techniques. Hemp is esteemed as a "plant teacher," analogous to the manner in which it is used by the ayahuasca shamans of the Amazon. This ritually controlled use helps the participants to restore their health, further their spiritual development, and establish a new relationship to nature.

> Under the influence of the shamanic power songs and special breathing techniques, embedded in a ritual context, hemp produces a more profound, more comprehensive, and more focused effect. Therapeutic and spiritual elements can combine to produce a situation in which the space is opened for holistic experience and a reconnection to the core of our being. . . .
>
> These initiations purify, strengthen, and rebuild the energy body anew and also open a way for hemp, as a plant sacrament, to continue to develop and unfold the human potential, to heal our relationship with nature, and to improve participation in our society. The respect that we bring to a plant as teacher also determines the quality of that which it is able to reveal to us. (Christof 1995:13)

Many people have now concluded that it is precisely the spiritual dimension and use of the plant that produces the actual healing effects (cf. Bello 1996*; Bennett et al, 1995*; Rätsch 1996a*).

But hemp is most frequently consumed for reasons having more to do with social health and is celebrated among young persons in rituals that have arisen more or less autochthonously:

> Central to the use of cannabis, however, is the motivation to more easily enter youth-specific cliques. By participating in the ritual of smoking cannabis, it becomes possible to more easily make contact and avoid the "outsider position." In addition to the emotional need to be recognized and accepted by other youths, cannabis consumption also implies an affirmation of "being grown up" and is regarded as a supporting element in making the most of the sense of community and belonging—the same thing that we also find with alcohol use. (Schneider 1996:22)

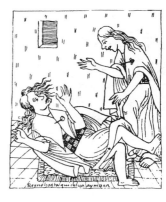

Epilepsy was once known as the "holy illness" or the "falling sickness." Epileptics were often treated with fumigations and aromatic substances. In Islamic medicine, European folk medicine, and in the self-medication of today, hemp smoke is sometimes used to revive a person after a seizure. (woodcut from a New Spanish Chronicle, sixteenth/seventeenth century)

Cough Therapy

Ingest opium internally, in one form or another. Along with this, a cannabis product is smoked (leaves, flowers, or pure hashish). Codeine can be used in place of opium.

Antidepressive Smoking Mixture

1 part female hemp flowers or hashish (kif)
1 part seeds of Syrian rue (*Peganum harmala* L.)

This mixture is best smoked from a pipe.

Asthma Smoking Mixture

1 part hemp (*Cannabis* sp.)
1 part henbane leaves (*Hyoscyamus* sp.)
1 part dried fly agaric caps (*Amanita muscaria*)

This mixture is best smoked from a pipe.

Warning!

In Central Europe, and recently in India as well, hashish is most often consumed mixed with tobacco. Because of the interactions between the principle active substances, mixing cannabis and tobacco can have very adverse pharmacological effects. Nicotine suppresses the effects of THC, while THC simultaneously potentiates the effects of nicotine. This means that a person would need to smoke many more joints with tobacco in order to produce a positive THC effect. In addition, many people who were originally nonsmokers have become addicted to nicotine by smoking tobacco-laced joints. According to Timothy Leary, nicotine is a "reality drug," that is, a substance whose use enhances the experience of everyday reality. This means in turn that nicotine brings a person "down" from their hemp high. Moreover, users who are interested in natural products would do well to consider what they are actually smoking when they consume the industrial tobacco produced by the tobacco companies.

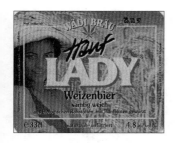

"The beer from Hamburg is usually made from wheat / and is preferred to other wheat beers / that are made in Germany / it has a good and charming taste / is strong and potent from the wheat malt / it nourishes very well / brings forth good moisture and a healthy and flowering appearance / and gives / to those who drink it / a beautiful and lovely color / as can be seen on the young fellows / maidens and women of this place / who are all well colored / and have a tender and soft skin."

These words can be read in the version of Tabernaemontanus's *Herbal* that was prepared by Hieronymus Bauhin and published in Basel (1731:639).

Today, many people still believe that wheat beer is healthy and gives one a beautiful complexion. If this is true, then a wheat beer with hemp would be even better; this at least is what the label of this Swiss beer suggests.

Many people who self-medicate with hemp often prefer to ingest hemp products orally. There are now a large number of books on cooking and baking with hemp that contain recipes. Interested readers can consult: Behr (no date), Buck 1998, Gebhardt 1997, Gottlieb (no date), Rippchen 1995, and Rathbun 1993*.

REFERENCES

Behr, Hans-Georg n.d. *Das Haschisch-Kochbuch*, Darmstadt: Melzer Verlag.

Buck, Ralf 1998. *Das Hanfbackbuch*. Göttingen, Germany: Verlag Die Werkstatt.

Christof, Helmut. 1995. Die heilige Pflanze: Der spirituelle Gebrauch einer alten Kulturpflanze. *Wege* 95/4:13.

Gebhartd, Kathrin. 1997. *Berauschend gut Backen mit Hanf*. Aarau, Germany: AT Verlag.

Gottlieb, Adam. n.d. *Kochen mit Cannabis*. An underground publication available in headshops and at festivals.

Grinspoon, Lester. 1992. A Brief Account of My Participation as a Witness in the Trial of Kerry Wiley. *Jahrbuch für Ethnomedizin und Bewußtseinsforshung* 1:199–202.

Grinspoon, Lester, and James Bakalar. 1987. Medical Uses of Illicit Drugs. In *Dealing with Drugs*, edited by Ronald Hamowy. San Francisco: Pacific Research Institute for Public Policy.

Rieth, Petra, and Hannes Heiler. 1995. Hilft Haschisch heilen? *Paraplegiker* 3/95:46.

Rippchen, Ronald. 1995. *Die Hanfküche: Gesund—traditionell—exotisch—psychoaktiv*. Löhrbach: Werner Pieper's Medienexperimente (Edition Rauschkunde).

Schneider, Wolfgang. 1996. *Der gesellschaftliche Drogenkult*. Berlin: VWB.

Schuldes, Bert Marco. 1995. *Psychoaktive Pflanzen. 2. verbesserte und ergänzte Auflage*. Löhrbach: MedienXperimente and Solothurn: Nachtschatten Verlag (Der Grüne Zweig 164).

Worman, Simon. 1993. *The Joint Smoking Rules*. Westmoreland, KS: 100 Flowers Publishing Co.

From a Portrait of the Hemp Culture

Unfortunately, there have not yet been any statistical studies of modern self-medication with hemp products. However, a questionnaire written by the Swiss Arbeitsgruppe Hanf und Fuss (Working Group Hemp and Foot) found that the majority of hemp users consider it to be a valuable medicine for many illnesses (Arbeitsgruppe Hanf und Fuss 1994:78f.*; cf. Giger 1995b*). In addition, many users utilize hemp products to treat pain (ibid:92*) and as a sleeping aid (ibid:159*). The following reasons were given for using cannabis:

I use cannabis, because . . . it is healthy/the brain needs it . . . it is the most peaceful and healthy drug.

. . . it is a natural product and medicine.

. . . it makes me almost innocuously happy.

. . . it doesn't make you fat.

. . . I have a clear head the next day.

. . . it makes me tolerant and takes away the pains.

. . . it is guaranteed that there will be no hangover.

. . . it is healthier than alcohol.

. . . I love my liver.

. . . there are no known deaths, whereas there are many with alcohol. (ibid:165*)

Results of a Questionnaire on Folk Medicine

A questionnaire on the folk medical use of and self-medication with cannabis products was circulated in the German-speaking area of Switzerland and in Germany between June 1995 and 1997. It was distributed via the "snowball system" and returned to me anonymously or sent to me by mail. Most of the people with whom I spoke about filling out this questionnaire expressed a great interest in the survey as well as in the findings that it produced. Even the very first questionnaires that were returned indicated that the information being collected was previously unknown (cf. Rätsch 1996b* and 1996c*).

Question: *For which ailments or diseases do you use cannabis products as medicine?*

The following ailments, diseases, and indications were named:

absentmindedness
agitation/restlessness
allergies (wheat flour and cow milk)
asthma
back pain
bad moods
bad thoughts
bladder pressure (too high)
bronchitis
burned-out syndrome
cancer
chronic inflammation of the intestine
   (colitis ulcerosa)
colds
confusion
cough
cystitis
delusion
dementia
depression
depressive moods
digestive problems
disc (intervertebral) problems
exhaustion
glaucoma
headache
hay fever
high blood pressure
impotence
insufficient self-contact
jealousy
lack of appetite
loneliness
a feeling of meaninglessness of existence
menstrual problems
mental emptiness
migraine headache

multiple sclerosis (MS)
nervous stress conditions
nervousness
overburdening
pain
paraplegia
perplexity
phantom pain
illness prevention
problems falling asleep
psychic crises
psychosomatic complaints
quarrelsomeness
rheumatism
sciatica
shyness
sleeplessness
sorrow
spastic disorders
spastic disorders due to tetraporesis
   (paraplegia)
stomachache
stress
symptoms of exhaustion of perception
tenseness
tension (physical)
toothache
weight gain

Also:

to increase desire
for sexual stimulation, as an aphrodisiac
for a gentle birth, to overcome pains
   during birth
for prophylaxis against diseases
to relax the whole body
to calm

The consumption of marijuana and hashish is more representative of a characteristic of a subculture than of a medical or legal problem.
NICOLAUS NEUMANN
HASCH UND ANDERE TRIPS
(1970:105*)

Hemp as Medicine Questionnaire

Please fill out this questionnaire only if you yourself use hemp as a medicine. Multiple answers to the questions are allowed.

Do you use hemp products only as medicine?   Yes ___   No ___

Do you use also hemp products as agents of pleasure?   Yes ___   No ___
primarily ___   occasionally ___   seldom ___   never ___

Which hemp products do you use as medicine?
hashish ___   leaves and flowers ___   seeds ___   hemp oil ___
THC-containing medicaments ___   homeopathic products ___
other _____

In what form do you use hemp products as medicines?
smoked: yes ___   no ___
pure: yes ___   no ___
mixed with tobacco: yes ___   no ___
with other herbs: yes ___   no ___
if yes, with which _____

_____

eaten: yes ___   no ___

if yes, in what form _____

as tincture or alcohol extract _____

other _____

In what dosages do you use which hemp products as medicine? _____
_____

Where do you get your hemp products?

grow my own ___   from friends ___   from the black market ___
from the pharmacy ___   from my physician ___
other _____

Where did you learn that hemp can be used as a medicine?
from friends ___   from my parents/grandparents ___
from my physician ___   in school/university ___
from books ___   if yes, from which   _____

_____

from newspapers/magazines ___   if yes, from which

_____

discovered it myself ___   other sources _____

For which ailments or diseases do you use hemp products as medicine?

In doing so, which experiences were especially important for you?

Why do you think hemp is effective as a medicine?

Does your physician know about your medical use of hemp?
yes ___   no ___

Do you recommend the use of hemp products as medicine to others?
yes ___   no ___

Other comments on the topic of hemp as medicine
(if necessary, use an extra sheet)

Information about you:

age ___   sex : female ___   male ___

education _____

occupation _____

THC and Analogs

HEMP IN SCIENTIFIC MEDICINE

"Doctor, I need headache tablets, nose drops, and a pack of THC!" For AIDS and cancer patients, this sentence may soon be reality. The fact that cannabis has medicinal effects which cannot be ignored has now even made its way to the Federal Ministry of Health

SEBASTIAN SCHMIDT
DIE THC-PILLE AUF REZEPT
(1996:30)

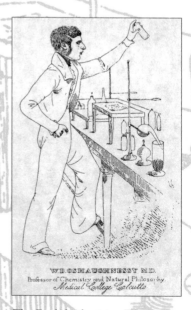

The English physician W. B. O'Shaughnessy (1809–90), who was stationed in India, is regarded as the founder of modern medical cannabis research. (contemporary illustration)

Western medicine has its roots in the late Middle Ages of Europe, back to the Italian schools of surgery that were established in Salerno and Bologna in the early thirteenth century. These schools in turn were based upon ancient traditions, Arabic-Islamic knowledge, and were especially indebted to Galen and Avicenna. In addition, much experimentation and empirical research was conducted in Salerno. Since anesthesia is especially important when performing surgery, a number of methods of anesthesiology were discovered in Salerno and Bologna:

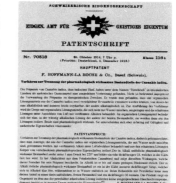

A separation method for producing medicinally usable hemp preparations was registered at the Swiss patent office in 1914.

> In the history of anesthesiology, it is of particular interest that the books of Theoderich [thirteenth century] are the first to clearly mention producing a narcosis by means of inhalation. The method involved the so-called sleep-spending sponge, which is reminiscent of ether narcosis. Sponges were impregnated with plant juices with narcotic effects, such as mandragora oil (which was also mentioned by Nicolaus of Salerno), and juice of henbane, opium, or Indian hemp. After soaking in the plant juices, the sponges were dried and stored, and would be placed in water an hour before use. After they were saturated, they would be held to the nose of the patient, who was then instructed to breathe deeply. The operation began when the subject was asleep, or rather dazed. . . . The Bolognese school, in any case, made a significant contribution towards reviving Occidental surgery. (Forgue and Bouchet 1990:948)

The positivistic natural sciences have a mechanistic view of the world, a worldview that is also at the heart of modern medicine: "Organisms that inhabit the earth are completely and without exception mechanical things, and as such machine constructions. As things, they are held together mechanically and perform all of their life functions through the workings of a mechanical construction. All life functions ultimately consist of the production of mechanical work" (Gutmann 1989:33).

In scientific medicine, with its natural scientific orientation, a human is regarded as a machine with specific functions. According to this view, when these functions are disturbed, a person becomes ill. Physicians then attempt to restore the functions to the machine. In the same way, a medicament is also defined by its function. The upshot of all this is that scientific medicine does not treat a person as someone who is ill, but as a symptom that can be influenced by medicaments. A remedy should have as specific an effect as possible, that is, it should perform a function that can be controlled. Since hemp does not necessarily function specifically, but rather holistically, its position in scientific medicine is a difficult one.

The bases of modern medicine and its materia medica were developed in the nineteenth century. Around 1827, hemp was used in German medicine: "The oily/slimy hemp seed is officinal and belongs to the soothing and emollient agents" (Chamisso 1987:70).

The British physician William O'Shaughnessy, who was stationed in India, learned there about the versatile ritual, hedonistic, and medicinal uses of hemp products made from *Cannabis indica*. He made a tincture from ganja that he tested on various ailments. O'Shaughnessy achieved sensational healing successes with rheumatism, hydrophobia (fear of water), cholera, tetanus, and cramps. He provided the first experimental confirmation of the indigenous uses. As a result of the publication of his results, Indian hemp came to Europe, where as a tincture it became a renowned remedy (O'Shaughnessy 1839*). Shortly after O'Shaughnessy's experiments, the first pharmacological and chemical investigations of the medicinal use of cannabis began in Germany (Martius 1855*). Toward the end of the nineteenth century, the physician G. Frank Lydston published a curious book in which he described his literary outpourings (which were inspired by a great deal of smoking pleasure) as well as a number of smoking devices, especially the Indian hookah (Lydston 1896). An essay on the general and medicinal use of hemp appeared in 1910, penned by the American physician Dr. Victor Robinson. In that essay, he stated unequivocally: "The medicinal hemp—the hemp with the potent narcotic principles—is *Cannabis indica*" (Robinson 1930:22*).

During the second half of the nineteenth century, the *Pharmacopoea germanica* listed as officinal both hemp seeds and "the herbage of the Indian, preferably female plants, known as hashish: *Herba Cannabis indicae*" (Pabst 1887:30). Extracts of hemp herbage (*Extractum Cannabis indicae*) as well as hemp tinctures (*Tinctura Cannabis indicae*) were used medicinally:

> The Indian hemp and its preparations primarily influence the activity of the brain and the nervous system. Small doses have stimulating effects upon the nerves, the sensory organs, and the imaginative faculty; they produce a cheerful mood. Following larger doses, a diminution of the sensory functions occurs, and numbness, relaxation, delirium, and finally sleep ensue. Indian hemp does not find frequent use as a medicament; because of its soporific effects, it is given in place of morphine and is sometimes used with advantage in cases in which morphine is ineffective or cannot be used. The seed was once frequently used in the production of emulsions, now it is less common. (Pabst 1887:30)

Toward the end of the nineteenth century, hemp preparations were chiefly used as sedatives and to treat weak and ailing nerves:

> Cannabis (Cannabinon). Indian hemp, hashishin.
> Its effects are different from those of opium and lactucarium[1] insofar as the soporific effect is generally preceded by great excitation associated with an alienation of the imaginative faculties and peculiar hallucinations. Habitual hashish inebriation very often leads to psychopathies. High doses are able to provoke manic outbursts and delirium with sensuous dreams. Because of its sedative effects, Cannabin. tannic. Merk is a superb agent for persons suffering from melancholy moods. Small doses of 0.02–0.04 usually produce a significant state of excitement; it is best combined with Pulvr. Coffeae tostae [roasted coffee beans] or cacao. It is prescribed in all cases where morphine and chloral are not effective. (Michaelis 1905:55f.)

All kinds of hemp preparations were available without prescription in European

---

1. Lactucarium is the pharmaceutical name for the thickened latex of wild lettuce (*Lactuca virosa* L., *Lactuca scariola* L. = *L. serriola* TORR.), which was formerly used in medicine as an opium substitute. Compared with opium, however, lactucarium has only mild analgesic and psychoactive effects (Rätsch 1998:311ff.*; Zubke 1998).

and American pharmacies into the twentieth century (Edes 1893*). In 1915, California began requiring a prescription for cannabis. In 1941, some thirty hemp preparations were removed from the pharmacopoeia. Since that time, hemp has been viewed as obsolete in Western medicine.

It was not until the hippie movement of the 1960s and the concomitant popularization of hashish and marijuana that hemp would again attract public and medical interest as a medicine. Bob Randell noted that his secret use of marijuana lowered his pathologically high intraocular pressure and thus helped him avoid blindness. After consulting with his physician, he underwent protracted clinical testing, which confirmed that his self-medication had been successful. His physicians were even able to arrange for Bob to be provided with marijuana grown on the government's own farms. Randell thus became the first legal "doper" (Stafford 1980:44f.*).

Since 1971, cannabis products have been investigated experimentally as treatments for alcoholism, heroin and amphetamine addiction, emotional disturbances, muscle spasms, and glaucoma (Furst 1988:35*; Hales 1991:357).

> Positive results using cannabis as an adjunct to psychotherapy have been obtained for depression, nervous tension disorders, and alcohol abuse, among others. (Haller 1996a:51*)

The German physician Dr. Gorm Grimm, who gained notoriety as a result of his scandalous "medicament-assisted therapy of drug addiction (MTD)," commented sarcastically, "Not only does hashish not function as a 'gateway drug,' but it also 'immunizes against later susceptibility to drugs' relatively well" (Grimm 1992:49*).

In 1990, Gerald Lancs, a microbiologist at the University of Southern Florida, discovered that marijuana can kill the herpes virus (afp report of May 16, 1990), thereby providing scientific confirmation of the ancient Roman recipe for treating herpes.

The traditional use of hemp preparations for asthma has now also received scientific support: "THC dilates the bronchial tubes. It can be inhaled as an aerosol like other medicines and works just as well" (Maurer 1989:48).

A Swiss team of researchers headed by Dr. Maja Maurer and Prof. Dr. Adolf Dittrich has now demonstrated that THC has anticonvulsive effects upon spasticity caused by the central nervous system (muscle cramps, for example, from multiple sclerosis or spinal injury) (Maurer et al. 1990). The group of researchers determined that THC (in a dosage of 5 mg) acts much like codeine, but is more effective and also better tolerated. The results of the study were so convincing that a spastic patient was given government permission to obtain the soothing drug from the pharmacy (Büttner 1991). The ability of THC to alleviate spasms is currently under assiduous investigation and is being tested on patients in Basel (Hagenbach 1996). The analgesic effects of THC and hemp are a main focus of both physicians and pain researchers (Simm 1997).[2] Another study is currently investigating the

---

2. Some of the discussions about these effects are becoming rather ridiculous. For example, during a workshop at the Frankfurter Schmerztag [Pain Day] '98 conference on "Cannabinoids in Pain Therapy" (held on March 5, 1998, with Robert Gorter, Rudolf Brenneisen, Wolfram Keup, Andreas Ernst, and others), it was argued that animal experiments are needed to study THC as an analgesic and spasmolytic agent, thus completely ignoring ten thousand years of experience with one of humanity's most important medicinal plants.

Remedy for Herpes?
(*Hamburger Abendblatt*, May 16, 1990)
AFP, LOS ANGELES: According to the microbiologist Gerald Lancz, marijuana kills the herpes virus. The scientist from the University of Southern Florida discovered the substance during experimentation.

therapeutic usefulness of cannabinoids for multiple sclerosis (Pertwee 1997).

The medicinal effectiveness of using hemp products, and especially THC and its analogs *(Nabinol, Dronabinol, Levonantradol/Cesa-Met)*, for treating glaucoma is now an established fact (Iversen 1993*; Santler 1995*). Studies have demonstrated that there is no other drug that is so easily tolerated and as effective as hemp (Roffman 1982*).

In the United States, a prescription drug that contains THC has been available for several years under the names Marinol and Canasol. It is prescribed by physicians for glaucoma. In 1991, this drug was even prescribed for President Bush. Nevertheless, Bush's war on drugs continued.

In 1992, American physicians were stripped of their authority to prescribe marijuana cigarettes or other medications that contain THC. Until that time, cancer patients who were suffering from the horrible side effects of chemotherapy—chronic nausea and vomiting—could be prescribed joints (Maurer 1989:48; Roffman 1979). The drug authorities at the Food and Drug Administration (FDA) had granted permission for only a few "hardship cases" to smoke marijuana under a doctor's supervision. That is no longer the case. The program is due to expire for the last fifteen patients, and new permits will not be issued. The reason given for the new policy is the recent increase in the number of applications for permits (Deutsche Presse Agentur report of April 7, 1992)!

Western physicians who have worked closely with cannabis and studied its effects are unequivocal:

> From the perspective of a physician, the evaluation of the relatively weakly euphoric cannabis products can only be summed up as follows: conditionally recommendable with the limitations that have been mentioned. Consequently: cannabis prohibition is indefensible, cannabis must be decontrolled. Every person must be able to decide for himself, whether he—using the proper dosage, of course—will ingest an alcoholic beverage, a cigarette, or a joint. (Grimm 1992:50*)

In recent years, persons suffering from AIDS have been experimenting increasingly with and using hemp and THC to stimulate their low or even absent appetites. This practice has now been studied scientifically (Doblin 1994; Gorter et al. 1997; Randall 1991), and the findings have important consequences for the decriminalization of a forbidden medicine:

> Many of these [medical] institutions, however, have shown no interest in distributing cannabis, often for financial reasons. For some time, however, things have been changing, for physicians are now increasingly learning from their patients. An AIDS patient will tell his doctor that he is using marijuana as a way to combat his weight loss. And the doctor can see the proof of this on his scale. This makes an impression, of course, and this is how opinions change. (Grinspoon 1998:17*)

In Germany, France, England, the United States, and Switzerland, numerous drugs whose main ingredient was hemp were prescribed by trained physicians from about 1845 to about 1951 (Fankhauser 1996*). Among the indications listed were: weak labor contractions, rheumatism, sleep disorders, metrorrhagy (chronic uterine bleeding not associated with menstruation), colic, cramps, cholera, asthma, lung and larynx disorders, neuralgia, corns, warts, hysteria, delirium tremens, psychosis, depression, gastric neurosis, dyspepsia, migraine headache, coughs, bronchitis, excessive milk secretion, carcinoma, difficult labor, vomiting during pregnancy, urethra deficiencies, women's disorders, gonorrhea, neurasthenia, debility, headache, tuberculosis, lung diseases, dysmenorrhea, gout, uratic diathesis, gall-stones, hair loss, hemorrhoids, angina pectoris, stenocardia, coronary sclerosis, heartburn, stomachache, enteritis, flatulence, nausea, lack of appetite, constipa-tion, kidney and bladder disorders, inflammations, cystitis, eczema, whopping cough, anemia, overexertion, anxiety states, tiredness, night sweats, hardening of the arteries, dizziness, nervousness, rachitis; in short: *Scientific medicine utilized cannabis as a universal remedy!*

In the nineteenth century, a variety of hashish preparations could be obtained without a prescription.[3] Some examples of the many preparations that contained cannabis are given below.

---

3. The Merck Company, in Darmstadt, introduced a hashish extract known as Cannabinon to the market in 1884–85, and a hashish oil that was marketed as Cannabinum in 1889. One of Cannabinum's uses was as an aphrodisiac (Fankhauser 1996:159f.*). Even the Royal Bavarian Court Pharmacy sold a hashish extract named Migränin, for treating migraines, in Munich around 1890 (ibid:163*).

Tinctura Cannabis Indicae

(Officinal preparation, 1856)

An extract of *Cannabis indica* dissolved in spirits was ingested as a narcotic and when labor contractions were too weak.

Rheumatism Oil

(1856)

Extract of *Cannabis indica* in oil
Poppy oil (from *Papaver somniferum*)
Henbane oil (from *Hyoscyamus niger*)

This oil mixture was applied externally to areas of the body affected by rheuma-tism and massaged into the skin.

Chlorodyne

(Dr. Collis Brown, 1856)

Tinctura Cannabis ind. 3%
morphine hydrochloride 0.5%
chloroform 6%

This tincture was used internally as a sedative and analgesic in doses of 5–20 drops several times a day.

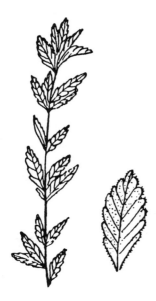

Mexican damiana (*Turnera diffusa*) is often used in place of tobacco to roll marijuana cigarettes, especially for medicinal use. (Mexican illustration)

Clavex
(Stern-Apotheke, St. Gallen, Switzerland, 1883)

A tincture was prepared from Indian hemp extract *(Cannabis indica)* and celandine juice *(Chelidonium majus)*

Asthma Fumigant "Pressant"
(1904)

40% Fol. Stramonii	*Datura stramonium*	thornapple
10% Herba Cannabis indic.	*Cannabis indica*	Indian hemp
2.5% Herba Hyoscyami	*Hyoscyamus nige*	henbane
30% kalium nitricum		potassium nitrate
2% anethol	*Anethum graveolens*	dill oil

The vapors of this fumigation mixture were inhaled to treat asthma and asthma attacks.

Neurosedat
(Josef Lang, Davos, Switzerland, 1910)

An elixir was prepared from the following ingredients (per teaspoon):
14.5 mg henbane extract (Hyoscyamus)
14.5 mg hemp extract
7.5 mg codeine
285 mg sodium bromide
285 mg potassium bromide

This potent psychoactive mixture was prescribed for use as a nerve sedative. The dose was 1 teaspoon two to three times a day.

Around the same time, in Indianapolis, a *Syrup Cannabis Compound* was recommended for asthma. It consisted of *Cannabis indica,* heroin hydrochloride, chloroform, *Lobelia* [*inflata,* Indian tobacco], antimony, and potassium tartrate (Fankhauser 1996:170*).

Neurotina
(1920)

Pills were made from the following ingredients:
8 mg *Cannabis indica* extract
4 mg extract of nux vomica (poison nut, *Strychnos nux-vomica*)
31 mg extract of saw palmetto *(Serenoa repens)*
31 mg iron phosphate
81 mg damiana extract *(Turnera diffusa)*
0.8 mg strychnine nitrate
Hyoscyamine
Scopolamine
Piperidine

These potent psychoactive pills were taken four times a day for neurasthenia and debilitation.

Asthma Fumigation Powder "Hadra"
(ca. 1920)

This powder was formerly available in Central European pharmacies. It was burned during asthma attacks and the smoke was inhaled. It may have possibly been used for "other purposes" as well (Fankhauser 1996*). Unfortunately, the list of ingredients is known, but not the amounts of each that were used:

Herb. Cannabis ind.	*Cannabis indica*	hemp herbage
Fol. Stramonii	*Datura stramonium*	thornapple leaves
Herb. Hyoscyami	*Hyoscyamus niger*	henbane
Herb. Lobelia	*Lobelia inflata*	lobelia herbage
Fol. Eucalypti	*Eucalyptus sp.*	eucalyptus leaves
Kal. nitric.		potassium nitrate
Menthol essential oil		

There were a large number of similar recipes, all of which have now been taken off the market.

Neo-Kawasol "Nyco"
(Nyegaard and Co., Oslo, 1933)

One pill contained the following ingredients:
0.02 g Res. Kava-Kava *(Piper methysticum)*
0.04 g Extr. Pichi-Pichi *(Fabiana imbricata)*
0.01 g Extr. *Cannabis indic.*
0.004 garbutin
0.1 g Phenyl. salicyl.

One to 2 tablets were swallowed three times daily to treat gonorrhea.

Neuragins
(A. Schmidt, Berlin, 1933)

A preparation of ginseng roots *(Panax ginseng)*, *Cannabis*, Spanish fly *(Cantharides)*, calcium phosphate, and lactose was administered for sexual neurasthenia (unfortunately, the dosages are unknown).

Psicotonico Sanat
(Pisa, 1933)

A tonic (probably in the form of an elixir) was made from:
Calcium glycerinophosphate
Sodium glycerinophosphate
Cola nut extract *(Cola acuminata, C. nitida)*
Muira puama *(Liriosma ovata or Ptychopetalum olacoides)*
Coca extract *(Erythroxylum coca)*
Guarana *(Paullinia cupana)*
Damiana *(Turnera diffusa)*
Indian hemp *(Cannabis indica)*

Unfortunately, the amounts that were used are unknown.

Two constituents of marijuana [THC and CBD] can help prevent the brain damage that often follows a stroke. The discovery by researchers at the National Institutes of Health (NIH) near Washington D.C. will add weight to the arguments of doctors who think the drug should be legal for medical use.

PHILIP COHEN
SMOKE FOR STROKES
(IN *NEW SCIENTIST*, JULY 11, 1998, P. 16)

REFERENCES

Büttner, Jean-Martin. 1991. Haschisch als Medikament, ein folgenreiches Experiment. *Tages-Anzeiger* Oct. 22, 1991:80.

von Chamisso, Adelbert. [1827] 1987. *Illustriertes Heil-, Gift- und Nutzpflanzenbuch*. Reprint, Berlin: Reimer.

Doblin, Rick. 1994. A Comprehensive Clinical Plan for the Investigation of Marijuana's Medical Use in the Treatment of the HIV-Related Wasting Syndrome. *Maps* 5(1):16–8.

Forgue, Emile, and Alain Bouchet. 1990. Die Chirurgie bis zum Ende des 18. Jahrhunderts. In *Illustrierte Geschichte der Medizin*, edited by R. Toellner. Vol. 2 Salzburg: Andreas und Andreas, pages 911–1001.

Gorter, Robert W., Martin Schnelle, Matthias Stoss, and Madelon van Wely. 1997. Cannabis in der Behandlung krebskranker und HIV-positiver Patienten. *Hanf!* 10/97:20–1.

Gutmann, Wolfgang F. 1989. *Die Evolution hydraulischer Konstruktionen*. Frankfurt am Main: Verlag Waldemar Kramer.

Hagenback, Ulrike. 1996. Spinale Spastik und Spasmolyse: Ist die Therapie mit THC eine unerwartete Bereicherung? *Jahrbuch des Europäischen Collegiums für Bewußtseinsstudien* 1995:199–207.

Hales, Dianne. 1991. *An Invitation To Health*. 5th ed. Redwood City, Calif.: Benjamin/Cummings Publishing Co.

Lydston, G. Frank. 1896. *Over the Hookah: The Tales of a Talkative Doctor*. Chicago: Fred. Klein.

Maurer, Maja. 1989. Therapeutische Aspekte von Cannabis in der westlichen Medizin. In *3. Symposion über psychoaktive Substanzen und veränderte Bewußtseinszustände in Forschung und Therapie*, edited by M. Schlichting and H. Leuner. Göttingen, Germany: ECBS, pages 46–9.

Maurer, M., V. Henn, A. Dittrich, and A. Hofmann. 1990. Delta-9-tetrahydrocannabinol Shows Antispastic and Analgesic Effects in a Single Case Double-blind Trial. *European Archives of Psychiatry and Clinical Neuroscience* 240:1–4.

Michaelis, Dr. Med. 1905. *Alte und neue Heilmittel für Schwache und kranke Nerven*. Berlin: Verlag J. Singer und Co.

Pabst, G, ed. 1887. *Köhler's Medizinal-Pflanzen*. Gera-Untermhaus: Fr. Eugen Köhler.

Pertwee, Roger G. 1997. The Therapeutic Potential of Cannabis and Cannabinoids for Multiple Sclerosis and Spinal Injury. *Journal of the International Hemp Association* 4(1):1, 4–8.

Randall, R.C., ed. 1991. *Marijuana and AIDS: Pot, Politics and PWAs in America*. Washington, D.C.: Galen Press.

Roffman, Roger A. 1979. *Using Marijuana in the Reduction of Nausea Associated with Chemotherapy*. Seattle: Murray Publishing Co.

Schmidt, Sebastian. 1996. Die THC-Pille auf Rezept. *Hanfblatt* 3(20):30–1.

Simm, Michael. 1997. Cannabis Beschäftigt die Schmerzforscher. *Deutsches Ärzteblatt* 94(48):B-2635.

Wassel, Gamila M. 1982. Plants Used in Mental Health. In *The History of Medicinal and Aromatic Plants*, edited by Abdallah Adly. Karachi, Pakistan: Hamdard Foundation Press, pages 171–7.

Zubke, Achim. 1998. Lactucarium. *HanfBlatt* 5(41):12–5.

The use of cannabis in the form of an alcohol tincture as an antispasmodic, analgesic, sedative, and narcotic agent was widespread in nineteenth century Europe and in the United States. In addition, cannabis was used to treat the symptoms of tetanus, neuralgia, uterine bleeding, rheumatism, and other complaints. It was considered a milder and much less dangerous analgesic than opium and regarded as an appetite stimulant. Between 1839 and 1900, more than one hundred articles appeared in Western scientific journals about the possibilities for utilizing marijuana.

LESTER GRINSPOON
CANNABIS ALS ARZNEI
(1996:43*)

PERSPECTIVES FOR HEMP AND WORLD HEALTH

The buffalo was the symbol of the Native Americans, the "other," the enemies of white civilization. With the bestial mass extermination of the American bison, Native Americans of the West were robbed of the foundation of their culture (Müller 1976).

Hemp became—barely one hundred years after the buffalo holocaust—a symbol of protesting youth, the enemies of the civilized establishment, the emergent counterculture. Since the 1960s, the American government has used flamethrowers and other machinery of war in their attempts to finish off the "weed" (Novak 1980*).

The U.S. government has declared war on "drugs," including hemp. The war against this harmless, peaceful plant is actually a war against people, people who not only have a right to inebriation, but also to cultural freedom. Little wisdom is needed to see that every war is senseless and harmful. No one benefits from wars against people, or from wars against plants. To the contrary, anyone who declares a war against nature risks cutting off the very branch upon which he sits. War is always synonymous with ecological catastrophe:

> It is not the drugs in a culture that are the problem, but rather how a culture deals with drugs, what kind of drug culture it is able to develop. (Kolte 1997:128)

This ethnomedical survey has demonstrated that there is no other plant that even comes close to having as wide a spectrum of medicinal uses as hemp. In addition, we have seen that modern medical and pharmacological research has confirmed the appropriateness of a great number of traditional uses. It has also become apparent that there may be no inebriant that is less harmful or better tolerated (cf. Rippchen 1992*). This knowledge alone, however, is of little use. The scientific evidence truly demonstrates that no other medicine is as easily tolerated and as effective in treating both glaucoma and the side effects of chemotherapy as THC. This notwithstanding, most hopelessly sick people are robbed of their last medicine because of absurd political decisions. If they decide to practice illegal self-medication, they risk being stamped as criminals, literally adding insult to their injuries. And so the misery grows.

These are the "real drug problems"; they are not created by the consumers, connoisseurs, and those in need of healing, but by the state, the politicians, and the drug laws:

> Today, the problems that are associated with the illegal status of cannabis certainly represent the greatest side effects of the medicinal use of the cannabinoids. There are many sedatives, sleeping pills, and painkillers that have a much higher addictive potential than cannabis, and these may be ordered on any standard prescription form. Thus, the classification of cannabis as a

The fame of Cannabis as a medicine spread with the plant.
RICHARD SCHULTES AND
ALBERT HOFMANN
PLANTS OF THE GODS
(1997*)

Marijuana, like all drugs of pleasure, is an active placebo that works with people that have learned to value it.
ANDREW WEIL
WAS UNS GESUND MACHT
(1991:357*)

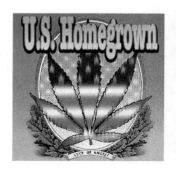

"controlled" narcotic is no longer medically tenable. A physician should be able to prescribe cannabis preparations of a specified quality just as he can prescribe other drugs. (Grotenhermen and Huppertz 1997:9f.*)

Among the basic rights possessed by humans is not just the right to alter our state of consciousness (Neskovic 1995), but also the right to health, and therewith the right to obtain and use suitable medicinal plants. When healing and health are concerned, every person has the right to access the medicines that will really help (cf. Szasz 1996). For this reason, every person has a right to use hemp products. If hemp preparations were freed from the morass of illegality, then they could make an enormous contribution to health around the globe—for no other plant has a similar worldwide distribution. People in all countries could be educated about the medicinally appropriate use of hemp, along the lines of the model proposed by the Swiss psychiatrist Dr. Peter Baumann, who has called for a "course in the proper use of inebriants" (1989:137*). Pipe dreams of the future? I don't think so.

Around the world, hemp is particularly valued as an antidepressant. From a medical perspective, this mood-enhancing ability may be hemp's most important effect. It is high time that our politicians, and especially our chronically misinformed drug counselors, themselves use the drug so that they might finally bid adieu to their depressive politics. One thing, however, must be kept in mind: There is no plant known that can counteract stupidity.

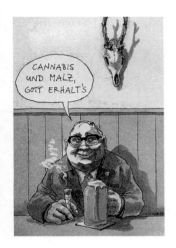

Postcard by Heribert Lenz and Achim Greser. The text reads: "Cannabis and malt, may God protect them." (Berlin, ca. 1997)

REFERENCES

Bertenghi, Paul, ed. 1996. *DroLeg: Die realistische Alternative*. Solothurn: Nachtschatten Verlag.

Kolte, Brigitta. 1997. Hanf—eine Pflanze mit Zukunft. In *DrogenVisionen: Zukunftswerkstatt für eine innovative Drogenpolitik und Drogenhilfe*, edited by AKZEPT e.V. Berlin: VWB (Studien zur qualitativen Drogenforschung und akzeptierenden Drogenarbeit, Vol. 12).

Müller, Werner. 1976. *Geliebte Erde: Naturfrömmigkeit und Naturhaß im indianischen und europäischen Nordamerika*. 2d ed. Bonn: Bouvier Verlag.

Neskovic, Wolfgang. 1995. Das Recht auf Rausch—Vom Elend der Drogenpolitik. In *Das Hanf-Tage-Buch*, edited by Ralph Cosack und Roberto Wenzel. Hamburg: Wendepunkt-Verlag, pages 141–64.

Szasz, Thomas. 1996. *Our Right To Drugs*. Syracuse, N.Y.: Syracuse University Press.

GLOSSARY

abortifacient   a substance that causes the expulsion of a fetus

aconite   plant drug from the rootstock of *Aconitum* sp.

alkaloid   nitrogen-containing, alkaline-reacting active substance in plants, animals, and humans

analgesic   a drug that alleviates pain

anesthetic   a drug that causes anesthesia; narcotic

animism   a religion that venerates nature, in which deities dwell in natural phenomena, stones, plants, animals (and humans); philosophical conception of an animated nature (filled with consciousness)

antidote   an agent that counteracts a poison

aphrodisiac   substance that in humans produces subjective sensations of an expansion or enrichment of the sensual, erotic, and sexual domains of experience

bhang   1. name of an Indian beverage made with hemp; 2. ancient Indo-European name for inebriant; 3. Indian name for marijuana leaves

binomial   taxonomy system for naming genera and species; introduced in the eighteenth century by Carolus Linnaeus

Bön   ancient Tibetan (pre-Buddhist) state religion with shamanic elements

catalepsy   sustained pathological fixity in a particular (usually uncomfortable) bodily position with increased muscular tension

charas   pure resin rubbed off female hemp flowers

composita   medicament made from a number of drugs

decoction   a plant extract; plant material is often soaked in cold water, then boiled

diuretic   a substance that increases the flow of urine and stimulates the activity of the kidneys

divination   telling the future or prophesizing via a divine medium

endemic   indigenous; limited to a precisely defined territory

ethnobotany   the study of culturally preserved domains of knowledge and activities that are related to plants

expectorant   a substance that promotes the secretion of mucus from the respiratory tract

flavonoids   natural substances that primarily occur as natural dyes in plants; in the human body, they counteract the oxidation of vitamin C and adrenaline

hierobotany   from the Greek: "study of sacred plants"; prophesize with or through plants (flower oracles, etc.)

induction   to influence or trigger a nerve event

laxative   1. an internally administered purgative agent; 2. having the effect of purging the bowels

lethal dose   the amount of a substance necessary to cause death

macerate   to make an extract in a cold liquid (water, alcohol)

materia medica   substances used for medicinal purposes

Morbus Basedow hyperthyroidism; a condition in which the thyroid is overactive, causing goiter and exophthalmia

moxibustion traditional Chinese healing method in which objects are burned on the body

necromancer magician who can establish contact with the world of the dead or the souls of the deceased and who can prophesize via this medium

Neolithic Late Stone Age; characterized by the beginnings of sedentary living and agriculture

officinal on the official list of medicaments

orchitis inflammation of the testicles with fever and painful swelling

panacea "cure-all"

pharmacology science of drugs

pharmacopoeia 1. (official) list of drug therapies; 2. the medicaments used by a culture or a medical system, during an epoch, or in a (cultural) geographical zone

pharmacy of filth the use of material discharged from human or animal bodies (primarily excrement)

phytotherapy use of plant drugs for medicinal purposes

psychedelic a drug that produces an expansion of consciousness

psychoactive moving the mind; stimulating mental activity

psychotropic affecting consciousness

purge cleanse internally, for example, with a laxative or enema

rhapsodist specialized or professional storytellers and singers who primarily recite legends and history texts

samadhi Sanskrit: "contemplation"; term used to characterized the highest state of consciousness (enlightenment)

Shintoism original religion of Japan, with a rich pantheon and rites for venerating nature

St. Anthony's fire disease caused by ergot poisoning (also known as *Ignis sacer*)

Taoism originally a Chinese philosophical doctrine of the Tao (Dao), the "unnamable"; later a polytheistic folk religion

tonic a general roborant (strengthener), with positive, preventive, and health-preserving effects on humans

toxicity the poisonous aspect of a substance; basically, every substance can be poisonous, depending upon the dose. Substances that are harmful in low doses are highly toxic; substances that are harmful in high or the highest doses (far above the dose required for other effects) have a low toxicity

traumatology doctrine about the cause, prevention, and treatment of damage to the body (from wounds, injuries)

trephination surgical opening of the skull

vapor bath use of warm vapors (from hot water or herbal teas) for healing purposes

LIST OF DISEASES AND MEDICAL SYSTEMS

The following diseases, symptoms, and indications are related to hemp thereapy in the various medical doctrines or systems that use the therapy. This list shows that there is no medicinal plant in the world that comes close to having as many different uses as hemp. However, it would be wrong to conclude that hemp is "the best medicine," a "wonder drug," or a panacea.

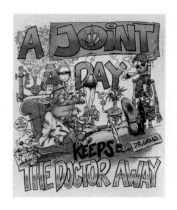

Indication	Medical System or chapter in which use appears
abdominal pains	Ancient Orient, Fathers of Botany
abscesses	Tibet
alcoholism	Ayurveda, Rastafarianism, Russia, Western medicine (psychotherapy)
altitude sickness	Shamanism, Tibet
amphetamine addiction	Western medicine
anemia	Ayurveda
animal bites	Curanderismo, Folk Medicine, Tibet
anthrax	Sub-Saharan Africa
antidote	Ancient Orient, Ayurveda, Islam, India
anxiety states	North Africa
aphrodisiac	Ayurveda, China, Curanderismo, Folk Medicine, Germanic, Islamic, North Africa, Rastafarianism, Russia, Self-Medication, Southeast Asia, Sub-Saharan Africa, Tibet
appetite (lack of)	Ayurveda, Homeopathy, Islamic, Western medicine, Self-Medication, Shamanism, Southeast Asia
arthritis	Curanderismo, Tibet
asthma	American Indian, Ayurveda, China, Curanderismo, Homeopathy, Islamic, Rastafarianism, Western medicine, Self-Medication, Southeast Asia, Sub-Saharan Africa
beriberi	China
black water fever	Sub-Saharan African
bladder disorders	Ancient Orient, Western medicine
bleeding	Curanderismo
blood poisoning	Southeast Asia, Sub-Saharan Africa
bronchitis	American Indian, Ancient Orient, Self-Medication
burns	Alchemy, Pre-Christian Europe, China
caesarean sections	Medieval Europe
cancer	Rastafariansim, Western medicine, Self-Medication, Southeast Asia, Sub-Saharan Africa
cholera	Ayurveda, Western medicine, Southeast Asia, Tibet
colds	Self-Medication, Sub-Saharan Africa
colic	Alchemy, Brazil, Curanderismo, Homeopathy
concentration (difficulties with)	Ayurveda
constipation	China, Islam, Japan

coughs	Alchemy, Native American, Ayurveda, Fathers of Botany, Folk Medicine, Homeopathy, Japan, Southeast Asia, Sub-Saharan Africa, Tibet
cramp (in the calf of the leg)	Folk Medicine
cramps	Ayurveda, Curanderismo, Folk Medicine, Western medicine, Southeast Asia, Tibet
dandruff	Ayurveda, Islam
delirium tremens	Ayurveda, Curanderismo, Western medicine
delivery (of a baby)	Ancient Orient, China, Southeast Asia, Sub-Saharan Africa, Tibet
delivery (to ease)	Africa, Ancient Orient, Folk Medicine, Self-Medication, Southeast Asia, Tibet
depressions	Ancient Orient, Folk Medicine, North Africa, Western medicine (psychotherapy), Scythia, Self-Medication, Shamanism
diarrhea	Pre-Christian Europe, Ayurveda, Brazil, Curanderismo, Sub-Saharan African, Tibet
digestion (weak)	Ayurveda, India, Southeast Asia, Tibet
discharge	China
dizziness	Southeast Asia, Tibet
ear ailments	Alchemy, Native American, Pre-Christian Europe, Ayurveda, China, Islamic, Tibet
ecstasy (to induce an ecstatic state)	Pre-Christian Europe, Scythia, Shamanism, Sub-Saharan Africa, Tibet
eczema on the head	China
epilepsy	Islam, Self-Medication
erysipelas	Fathers of Botany
exhaustion	Brazil, Homeopathy, Rastafarianism, Sub-Saharan Africa
exostosis	Folk Medicine
eye diseases	Ayurveda, Ancient Egypt, Self-Medication, Tibet
fever	Curanderismo, Fathers of Botany, Folk Medicine, Sub-Saharan Africa
flatulence	Ayurveda, China, Islam
flu	Rastafarianism
frenzy	Curanderismo
frostbite	Pre-Christian Europe
furuncle	Ayurveda
gallbladder disorders	Native American
glaucoma	Pharaohs, Rastafariansim, Western medicine, Self-Medication
gonorrhea	Ayurveda, Homeopathy, Islam
gout	Native American, Pre-Christian Europe, Ayurveda, China, Fathers of Botany, India, Russia, Tibet
gravel	China
hair loss	Folk Medicine
headaches	Alchemy, Ayurveda, Islam, Russia, Sub-Saharan Africa
hemorrhage	Ayurveda
hemorrhoids	Ayurveda, China, Southeast Asia, Tibet
hepatitis	Self-Medication
hernia (inguinal)	Ayurveda
heroin addiction	Western medicine
herpes	Pre-Christian Europe, Western medicine
hip pains	Native American, Fathers of Botany

hydrocele	Ayurveda
hydrophobia	Western medicine
hysteria	Homeopathy
impotence	Ancient Orient, Ayurveda, Homeopathy
inconstancy	Shamanism
inflammation of the middle ear	China
inflammations	Alchemy, Ayurveda, China, Ancient Egypt, Rastafarianism, Tibet
injuries	Native American, Japan
itching	Ayurveda, Tibet
jaundice	Alchemy, Ayurveda, Folk Medicine, Homeopathy, Self-Medication, Tibet
joint pains	Native American
kidney diseases	Japan, Tibet
lactation (absence of)	Cameroon, Southeast Asia, Tibet
laxative	China, Japan
leprosy	Curanderismo, Southeast Asia, Tibet
lice	Ayurveda
limb pains	Fathers of Botany, Germanic, Tibet
limbs (shaking)	Ancient Orient
liver diseases	Tibet
lower abdominal complaints	Ayurveda
malaria	Ayurveda, China, Southeast Asia, Sub-Saharan Africa
mania	Ayurveda
memory disturbances	Southeast Asia
menstrual problems	Ayurveda, Brazil, China, Southeast Asia
mental deficiency	Ayurveda
migraine headaches	Ayurveda, Self-Medication, Southeast Asia
multiple sclerosis	Western medicine, Self-Medication
muscle spasms	Curanderismo, Western medicine, Self-Medication
muscular atrophy	Native American
narcotic	Far East, China, Islam, Japan, Western medicine, Southeast Asia, Sub-Saharan Africa
nausea	Western medicine
nerve disorders	Ayurveda, China, Homeopathy, Western medicine, Tibet
nervous breakdown	Ayurveda, Sub-Saharan Africa
nervousness	China, Curanderismo, Sub-Saharan Africa
neuralgia	Southeast Asia
nightmares	Homeopathy
nipple pains	Pre-Christian Europe
nose (running)	Self-Medication, Tibet
nose bleed	Alchemy
orchitis	Ayurveda
otalgia	Ayurveda
pain	Native American, Ancient Orient, Ayurveda, Brazil, Curanderismo, Folk Medicine, Homeopathy, Japan, Rastafarianism, Russia, Western medicine, Southeast Asia, Sub-Saharan African, Tibet
panacea	Rastafarianism, Shamanism, Sub-Saharan Africa
paraplegia	Self-Medication

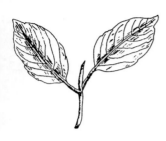

In Latin America, the dried leaves of *Nicotiana glauca* GRAH., known as *macuchi* or *palán-palán*, are smoked as a marijuana substitute.

pneumonia	Homeopathy
poisoning	Ayurveda, China, India
polyps	Southeast Asia
quadriplegia	Self-Medication
redness	China
rheumatism	Native American, Far East, Ayurveda, Brazil, China, Curanderismo, Russia, Western medicine, Southeast Asia, Sub-Saharan African, Tibet
scorpion stings	China, Curanderismo, Tibet
sedative	Brazil, China, Japan, Self-Medication, Southeast Asia
	Ancient Orient, Ayurveda, Curanderismo, India, Self-Medication
senility	China
shingles (herpes zoster)	Folk Medicine
skin eruptions	China
snakebite	Curanderismo, Sub-Saharan African
sorrow	Scythia, Self-Medication
spasmolysis	Western medicine
spleen (diseases of)	Japan
stiffness	Pre-Christian Europe, Southeast Asia
stimulant	Native American
stomachaches	Native American, India, Southeast Asia
stomach problems	Far East, Hildegard's Medicine, Japan, Tibet
swelling	Pre-Christian Europe
tension	Brazil, North Africa, Self-Medication, Southeast Asia
tetanus	Ayurveda, Curanderismo, India, Western medicine
tonic	Ayurveda, China, Curanderismo, Rastafarianism, Southeast Asia, Sub-Saharan Africa, Tibet
toothaches	Brazil, Russia, Sub-Saharan Africa
tuberculosis	Curanderismo, Rastafarianism, Sub-Saharan Africa
tumors	Ayurveda, China, Tibet
ulcers	China, Hildegard von Bingen, Southeast Asia
urine retention	China, Folk Medicine, Homeopathy, Tibet
uterine complaints	Fathers of Botany, Ancient Egypt
uterine contractions	Africa, Folk Medicine, Self-Medication, Southeast Asia
uterine cramps	Fathers of Botany
veterinary medicine	Native American, Fathers of Botany
vomiting	Ayurveda, China, Homeopathy, Western medicine, Self-Medication, Sub-Saharan Africa
wasting syndrome	Western medicine
weakness	China, Curanderismo, Japan, Rastafarianism
whooping cough	Ayurveda, Folk Medicine
women's disorders	Brazil, Fathers of Botany
worm infestations	Native American, India, Tibet
wounds	Pre-Christian Europe, Ayurveda, China, Rastafarianism, Russia

HEMP SUBSTITUTES

Just as a Western pharmacist can look in a list of medicines and determine which substitute she might be able to offer to a customer, other cultures and medical systems offer traditional substitutes for hemp preparations.

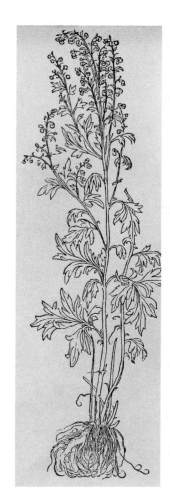

Substitute	Culture/system	Active Substance(s)	Reference
Anhalonium (peyote)			
Lophophora williamsii	Homeopathy	[mescaline]	Boericke 1992
Dagga (wild)			
Leonotis leonurus	South Africa	?	Du Toit 1975
Hedysarum			
Hedysarum ildefonsianum	Homeopathy	?	Boericke 1992
Kratom			
Mitragyna speciosa			
Grangea darerasparana	Thailand	alkaloids	Martin 1975
Linseed			
Linum usitatissimum	Chinese Medicine	organic acids, oil	Paulus and Ding 1987
Maconha brava			
Cestrum laevigatum	Brazil	saponine	Schultes & Hofmann 1995*
Macuchi			
Nicotiana glauca	Mexico	alkaloids, anabasine	Reko 1936:62
Patagallina (Kanef)			
Hibiscus cannabinus	Colombia	?	Rubin 1975:160*
Prickly Poppy (Chicalote)			
Argemone mexicana	Mexico	opiates	Rätsch 1991d*
Wormwood			
Artemisia mexicana			
Artemisia spp.			
Artemisia absinthium	Mexico	thujone, essential oil	Rätsch 1991d*
Zacatechichi	Mexico	bitter constituents,	Diaz 1979
Calea zacatechichi	(Chiapas)	essential oil	

The dried herbage of wormwood (*Artemisia absinthium*) is smoked as a marijuana substitute. Thujone, the main component of the essential oil (*Oleum absinthii*), has pharmacological effects similar to those of THC. (woodcut from Brunfels, *Kräuterbuch*, 1532)

REFERENCES

Boericke, William. 1992. *Handbuch der homöopathischen Materia medica*. Heidelberg: Haug. Translated from English and revised by D. J. Beha, R. Hickmann, and K. F. Scheible.

Diaz, José Luis. 1979. Ethnopharmacology and Taxonomy of Mexican Psychodysleptic Plants. *Journal of Psychedelic Drugs* 11(1-2):71–101.

Du Toit, Brian M. 1975. Dagga: The History and Ethnographic Setting of *Cannabis sativa* in Southern Africa. In *Cannabis and Culture*, edited by V. Rubin. The Hague: Mouton, pages 81–116.

Martin, Marie Alexandrine. 1975. Ethnobotanical Aspects of Cannabis in Southeast Asia. In *Cannabis and Culture*, edited by V. Rubin. The Hague: Mouton, pages 63–75.

Paulus, Ernst, and Ding Yu-he. 1987. *Handbuch der traditionellen chinesischen Heilpflanzen*. Heidelberg: Haug.

Reko, Victor. 1936. *Magische Gifte*. Stuttgart: Enke.

ORGANIZATIONS

National Organization for the Reform of Marijuana Laws (NORML)

NORML's mission is to move public opinion sufficiently to achieve the repeal of marijuana prohibition so that the responsible use of cannabis by adults is no longer subject to penalty.

Since its founding in 1970, NORML has been a voice for Americans who oppose marijuana prohibition. NORML is the oldest and largest national organization dedicated solely to reforming marijuana laws.

A nonprofit public-interest lobby based in Washington, D.C., NORML works closely with Congress, federal agencies, and the national media to reform current policy. NORML publishes a regular newsletter, issues special reports, and distributes a weekly press advisory to the media. Working with approximately sixty state and local affiliates, we also lobby state legislatures and support state-level voter initiatives. NORML also hosts a popular site on the Internet (www.norml.org) where visitors can inform themselves about the issue and send a free fax to Congress.

NORML's sister organization, the NORML Foundation, is a nonprofit educational, research, and legal foundation. The Foundation educates the public about the costs of and alternatives to marijuana prohibition, and provides legal support and assistance to victims of the current marijuana laws. Contributions to the foundation are tax deductible.

NORML
1001 Connecticut Ave. NW, Suite 710
Washington, D.C. 20036
Phone: (202) 483-5500
Fax: (202) 483-0057
www.norml.org

Multidisciplinary Association for Psychedelic Studies (MAPS)

MAPS is a membership-based, nonprofit research and educational organization. It assists scientists to design, obtain governmental approval, fund, conduct, and report on studies into the healing and spiritual potentials of psychedelic drugs. Since 1990, MAPS has disbursed more than a quarter of a million dollars to worthy research projects. Medical marijuana has been a part of MAPS's research efforts.

Founded in 1986, MAPS is an IRS approved 501 (c)(3) nonprofit corporation funded by tax-deductible donations from eighteen hundred members.

MAPS
2105 Robinson Avenue
Sarasota, FL 34232
Phone: 1-888-868 MAPS
Fax: (941) 924-6265
www.maps.org

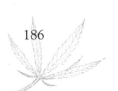

186

BIBLIOGRAPHY

Those articles specific to individual medical systems and traditional uses of hemp can be found at the end of each chapter. The literature references provided here are marked with an asterisk (*) in the text can be found among the resources listed here.

BIBLIOGRAPHIES

Gainage, J. R. and E. L. Zerkin. 1969. *A Comprehensive Guide to the English-Language Literature on Cannabis*. Madison, Wisc.: Stash Press.

Hefele, Bernhard. 1988. *Drogenbibliographie: Verzeichnis der deutschsprachigen Literatur über Rauschmittel und Drogen von 1800 bis 1984*. 2 vols. Munich: K G. Saur.

Società Italiana per lo Studio degli Stati di Coscienza (SISSC). 1994. *Bibliographia Italiana su Allucinogeni e Cannabis: Edizione commentata*. Bologna: Grafton 9 edizioni.

BOOKS AND ARTICLES

Abel, Ernest L. 1980. *Marihuana: The First Twelve Thousand Years*. New York: Plenum Press.

Aldrich, Michael R. 1977. Tantric Cannabis Use in India. *Journal of Psychedelic Drugs* 9(3):227–33.

———, ed. 1988. Marijuana—An Update. *Journal of Psychoactive Drugs* 20(1):1–138. Contains a number of interesting articles.

Amendt, Günter. 1974. *Haschisch und Sexualität*. Stuttgart: Enke.

ADH. 1997. Die Wende in Amerika? *Hanfblatt* 4(26):24–6.

Andrews, George, and Simon Vinkenoog, eds. 1968. *The Book Of Grass*. New York. Grove Press.

Arbeitsgruppe Hanf und Fuss, ed. 1994. *Unser gutes Kraut: Das Porträt der Hanfkultur*. Solothurn: Nachtschatten Verlag and Löhrbach: Werner Pieper's MedienXperimente.

Balabanova, S., F. Parsche, and W. Pirsig. 1992. First Identification of Drugs in Egyptian Mummies. *Naturwissenschaften* 79:358.

Baudelaire, Charles. 1972. *Die künstlichen Paradiese*. Cologne: Hegner.

Barber, Theodore X. 1970. *LSD, Marihuana, Yoga and Hypnosis*. Chicago: Aldine.

Baumann, Peter. 1989. Hanf heute—Wert und Unwert. *Schweizerische Ärztezeitung* 70(4):134–40.

———. 1989. Replik. *Schweizerische Ärztezeitung* 70(11):462–3.

Bayerle-Sick, Norbert. 1984. *Drogensubkultur*. Linden: Volksverlag.

Behr, Hans-Georg. 1982. *Von Hanf ist die Rede*. Basel: Sphinx.

———. 1995. *Von Hanf ist die Rede: Kultur und Politik einer Pflanze*. Frankfurt am Main: Zweitausendeins. This edition has been completely revised, updated, and expanded by about one-third over the version first published by Sphinx Verlag, Basel, in 1982.

Bello, Joan. 1996. *The Benefits of Marijuana: Physical, Psychological and Spiritual*. Cottonwood, Calif.: Sweetlight Books.

Benet, Sula. 1975. Early Diffusion and Folk Uses of Hemp. In *Cannabis and Culture*, edited by V. Rubin. The Hague: Mouton, pages 39–49.

Benjamin, Walter. 1972. *Über Haschisch*. Frankfurt am Main: Suhrkamp.

Bennett, Chris, Lynn Osburn, and Judy Osburn. 1995. *Green Gold—The Tree of Life: Marijuana in Magic and Religion*. Frazier Park, Calif.: Access Unlimited.

Berge, Fr., and W. A. Riecke. 1845. *Giftpflanzen-Buch oder allgemeine und besondere Naturgeschichte sämtlicher inländischer sowie der wichtigsten ausländischen phaneroganischen und cryptogamischen Giftgewächse*. Stuttgart: Hoffmann'sche Verlags-Buchhandlung.

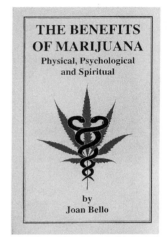

THE BENEFITS OF MARIJUANA
Physical, Psychological and Spiritual
by Joan Bello

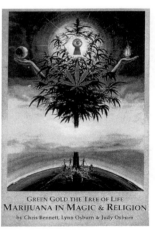

GREEN GOLD THE TREE OF LIFE
MARIJUANA IN MAGIC & RELIGION
by Chris Bennett, Lynn Osburn & Judy Osburn

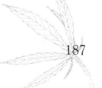

von Bibra, Ernst Freiherr. 1855. *Die narkotischen Genußmittel und der Mensch*. Nuremberg: W. Schmid.

Binder, Michael A. 1981. Haschisch und Marihuana. *Deutsches Ärzteblatt* 4(Jan. 22, 1981):117–26.

Blätter, Andrea. 1990. *Kulturelle Ausprägungen und die Funktionen des Drogengebrauchs*. Hamburg: Wayasbah.

———. 1992. Das Vergnügen, die Sucht und das Bewußtsein: Einstellungen zum Cannabiskonsum. *Jahrbuch für Ethnomedizin und Bewußtseinsforschung* 1:117–32, Berlin: VWB.

———. 1993. Der erlernte Rausch—Die Funktionen des Cannabiskonsums auf Jamaika und in Deutschland. *Jahrbuch für Ethnomedizin und Bewußtseinsforschung* 2:119–45, Berlin: VWB.

Bobcat Press, ed. 1997. *Das Joint Drehbuch: Tips, Tricks und Techniken*. Solothurn: Nachtschatten Verlag.

Böllinger, Lorenz, ed. 1997. *Cannabis Science—Cannabis Wissenschaft*. Frankfurt am Main: Peter Lang.

Boire, Richard Glen. 1992. *Marijuana Law*. Berkeley, Calif.: Ronin.

Bonnie, Richard J., and Charles H. Whitebread. 1974. *The Marihuana Conviction: A History of Marihuana Prohibition in the United States*. Charlottesville: University Press of Virginia.

Boyle, T. Coraghessan. 1990. *Grün ist die Hoffnung—Eine Pastorale*. Hamburg: Rogner und Berhard; Frankfurt am Main: Zweitausendeins.

Braude, M., and S. Szara, eds. 1976. *Pharmacology of Marihuana*. New York: Raven-Press.

Brenneisen, Rudolf. 1986. Hanf-Dampf in allen Gassen. *Uni-Press* Nr. 51:7–9.

———. 1996. Cannabis sativa—Aktuelle Pharmakologie und Klinik. *Jahrbuch des Europäischen Collegiums für Bewußtseinsstudien* 1995:191–8.

Brodmann, Thomas. 1997. Hanf—das verbotene Aphrodisiakum. *Highlife* 3(9):21–3.

Bührer, Tony. n.d. *Haschisch Studie: Zur Klassifizierung von Cannabis (Konsum, Anbau, Kleinhandel) als Bagatelldelikt*. Löhrbach: Werner Pieper's MedienXperimente (Der Grüne Zweig 125).

Burian, Wilhelm, and Irmgard Eisenbach-Stangl, eds. 1982. *Haschisch: Prohibition oder Legalisierung*. Weinheim and Basel: Beltz.

Calm, Sven E. 1995. Music Like Gunjah. *Hanfblatt* Nr. 7:25–6.

Carter, W. E., ed. 1980. *Cannabis Use in Costa Rica: A Study of Chronic Marijuana Use*. Philadelphia, Penn.: Institute for the Study of Human Issues.

Cherniak, Laurence. 1979. *The Great Books of Hashish*. 2 vol. Berkeley, Calif.: And/Or Press.

———. 1995. *Das Große Haschisch-Buch. Teil 1: Marokko, Libanon, Afghanistan und der Himalaya*. Markt Erlbach: Raymond Martin Verlag.

Chopra, G. S. 1969. Man and Marijuana. *International Journal of the Addiction* 4(2):215–47.

———. 1971. Marijuana and Adverse Psychotic Reactions. *Bulletin on Narcotics* 23:15–22.

Clarke, Robert C. 1977. *The Botany and Ecology of Cannabis*. Ben Lomond, Calif.: Pods Press.

———. 1981. *Marijuana Botany*. Berkeley, Calif.: Ronin Publ.

———. 1995. Hemp (*Cannabis sativa* L.) Cultivation in the Tai'an District of Shandong Province, Peoples Republic of China. *Journal of the International Hemp Association* 2(2):57, 60–5.

———. 1997. *Hanf: Botanik, Anbau, Vermehrung und Züchtung*. Aarau, Switzerland: AT Verlag.

Clarke, Robert C., and David W. Pate. 1994. Medical Marijuana. *Journal of the International Hemp Association* 1(1):9–12.

Coffman, C. B., and W. A. Gentner. 1979. Greenhouse Propagation of *Cannabis sativa* L. by Vegetative Cuttings. *Economic Botany* 33(2):124–7.

Cohen, Sidney. 1966. *The Beyond Within*. New York: Atheneum.

———. 1982a. Cannabis and Sex: Multifaceted Paradoxes. *Journal of Psychoactive Drugs* 14(1–2):55–8.

———. 1982b. Cannabis Effects on Adolescent Motivation. *Marijuana and Youth: Clinical Observations on Motivation and Learning*. Rockville, Maryland: NIDA.

Conrad, Chris. 1993. *Hemp: Lifeline to the Future*. Los Angeles: Creative Xpressions Publications.

———. 1997. *Hemp for Health: The Medicinal and Nutritional Uses of* Cannabis sativa. Rochester, Vt.: Healing Arts Press.

Cooke, Mordecai C. 1860. *The Seven Sisters of Sleep*. London: James Blackwood.

———. 1989. *The Seven Sisters of Sleep*. Lincoln, Mass.: Quarterman Publ. (facsimile of 1860).

———. 1997. *The Seven Sisters Of Sleep*. Rochester, Vermont: Park Street Press. With foreword by Rowan Robinson.

Corral, Valerie. 1994. A Patient's Story: Medical Marijuana. *Maps* 4(4):26–9.

Cosack, Ralph, and Roberto Wenzel, eds.

———. 1995. *Das Hanf-Tage-Buch: Neue Beiträge zur Diskussion über Hanf, Cannabis, Marihuana*. Hamburg: Wendepunkt-Verlag.

Cutrufello, Rosario. 1980. *Hashish: Testa d'Ariete dell'eroina*. Milan: Editrice Modelgrafica.

Dayanandan, P., and J. P. B. Kaufman. 1975. *Trichomes of* Cannabis sativa. Ann Arbor: University Of Michigan Press.

De Leeuw, Hendrik. 1939. *Flower of Joy*. New York: Lee Furman.

De Pasquale, Anna. 1982. Notices historiques sur la Chanvre Indien. In *The History of Medicinal and Aromatic Plants*, edited by Abdallah Adly. Karachi, Pakistan: Hamdard Foundation Press, pages 110–44.

De Ropp, Robert. 1961. *Drugs and the Mind*. New York: Grove Press.

Dittrich, Adolf. 1996. *Ätiologie-unabhängige Strukturen veränderter Wachbewußtseinszustände*. 2nd revised ed. Berlin: VWB.

Dobkin de Rios, Marlene. 1990. *Hallucinogens: Cross-Cultural Perspectives*. Bridport, Dorset: Prism Press.

Dornbush, R. L., A. Freedman, and M. Fink, eds. 1976. *Chronic Cannabis Use*. New York: New York Academy Of Sciences.

Drake, William Daniel. 1971. *The Connoisseur's Handbook of Marijuana*. San Francisco: Straight Arrow.

Edes, R. T. 1893. Cannabis Indica. *Boston Medical and Surgical Journal* 129(11):273.

Eliade, Mircea. 1964. *Shamanism: Archaic Techniques of Ecstasy*. Princeton, N.J.: Princeton/Bollingen.

———. 1975. *Schamanismus und archaische Ekstasetechnik*. Frankfurt am Main: Suhrkamp.

Emboden, William A. 1972a. *Narcotic Plants*. London: Studio Vista.

———. 1972b. Ritual Uses of *Cannabis Sativa* L.: A Historical-Ethnographic Survey. In *Flesh of the Gods*, edited by Peter Furst. New York: Praeger, pages 214–36.

———. 1974a. Cannabis—A Polytypic Genus. *Economic Botany* 28:304–10.

———. 1974b. Species Concepts and Plant Nomenclature. *California Attorneys for Criminal Justice Forum* 5(Aug/Sep 74):2–4.

———. 1979. *Narcotic Plants*. Revised and enlarged edition. New York: Macmillan.

———. 1981a. The Genus *Cannabis* and the Correct Use of Taxonomic Categories. *Journal of Psychoactive Drugs* 13(1):15–21.

———. 1981b. Cannabis in Ostasien—Ursprung, Wanderung und Gebrauch. In *Rausch und Realität*, edited by G. Vögler. Vol. 1. Cologne: Rautenstrauch-Joest-Museum für Völkerkunde, pages 324–9.

———. 1990. Ritual Use of *Cannabis sativa* L.: A Historical-Ethnographic Survey. In *Flesh of the Gods*, edited by P. Furst. Prospect Heights, Ill.: Waveland Press, pages 214–36.

———. 1996. Cannabis: The Generation and Proliferation of Mythologies Placed Before U.S. Courts. *Jahrbuch für Ethnomedizin und Bewußtseinsforschung* 4(1995):143–52.

Escohotado, Antonio. 1990. *Historia de las drogas*. 3 vols. Madrid: Alianza Editorial.

Evans, Fred J. 1991. Cannabinoids: The Separation of Central from Peripheral Effects on a Structural Basis. *Planta Medica* 57, Suppl. 1:S60–S67.

Fachner, Jörg, E. David, and M. Pfotenhauer. 1995. EEG-Brainmapping in veränderten

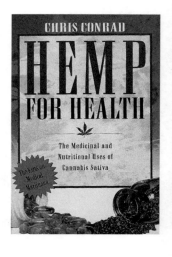

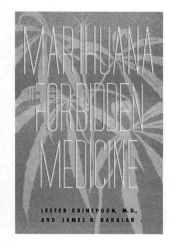

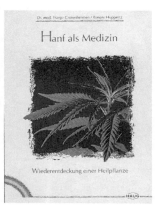

Bewußtseinszuständen unter Cannabiseinwirkung bei Hören ausgewählter Musikstücke—Ein Fallbeispiel. *curare* 18(2):331–358.

Fässler, Benjamin. 1997. *Drogen zwischen Herrschaft und Herrlichkeit*. Solothurn: Nachtschatten Verlag.

Fankhauser, Manfred. 1996. *Haschisch als Medikament: Zur Bedeutung von Cannabis sativa in der westlichen Medizin*. Bern: unpublished Inaugural-Dissertation.

Feuerlein, Wilhelm, ed. 1980. *Cannabis heute: Bestandsaufnahme zum Haschischproblem*. Wiesbaden, Germany: Akademische Verlagsanstalt.

Fisher, James. 1975. Cannabis in Nepal: An Overview. In *Cannabis and Culture*, edited by V. Rubin. The Hague: Mouton, pages 247–55.

Fromberg, Erik. 1996. Die Pharmakologie von Cannabis. In *Cannabis*, edited by Jürgen Neumeyer. Munich: Packeispresse Verlag Hans Schickert, pages 36–42.

Furst, Peter T. 1976. *Hallucinogens and Culture*. San Francisco: Chandler and Sharp.

———. 1988. *Hallucinogens and Culture*. 5th ed. Novato, Calif.: Chandler and Sharp.

———, ed. 1990. *Flesh of the Gods: The Ritual Use of Hallucinogens*. 2nd ed., with a new introduction. Prospect Heights, Ill.: Waveland Press.

Galland, Jean-Pierre, ed. 1993. *Première Journée Internationale du Cannabis*. Paris: Editions du Lézard.

———. 1994. *Fumée clandestine il était une fois le cannabis*. Paris: Editions du Lézard.

Gandjour, Joubin. 1997. Cannabis als Heilmittel. In *Berauschend gut backen mit Hanf*, edited by K. Gebhardt. Aarau, Switzerland: AT Verlag, pages 68–74.

Gelpke, Rudolf. 1967. Der Geheimbund von Alamut—Legende und Wirklichkeit. *Antaios* 8:269–93.

———. 1995. *Vom Rausch im Orient und Okzident*. Stuttgart: Klett-Cotta.

Geschwinde, Thomas. 1990. *Rauschdrogen: Marktformen und Wirkungsweisen*. 2nd ed. Berlin: Springer-Verlag.

Giger, Andreas. 1995a. Hanf—ein Nischenprodukt aus der Schweiz? *NZZ* Jan. 1, 1995.

———. 1995b. Bewußtseins-Design mit Cannabis: Das Portrait der Hanfkultur. *curare* 18(2):325–9.

Goode, Erich. 1970. *The Marijuana Smokers*. New York: Basic Books.

Grimm, Gorm. 1992. *Drogen gegen Drogen: Eine Bilanz*. Kiel: Veris Verlag.

Grinspoon, Lester. 1969. Marihuana. *Scientific American* 221(6).

———. 1971. *Marihuana Reconsidered*. Cambridge, Mass.: Harvard University Press.

———. 1992. A Brief Account of My Participation as a Witness in the Trial of Kerry Wiley. *Jahrbuch für Ethnomedizin und Bewußtseinsforschung* 1:199–202, Berlin: VWB.

———. 1996. Cannabis als Arznei. In *Cannabis*, edited by Jürgen Neumeyer. Munich: Packeispresse Verlag Hans Schickert, pages 43–55.

———. 1998. Interview: Marihuana, ein medizinisches Wunder. *HanfBlatt* 5(43):15–7.

Grinspoon, Lester, and James B. Bakalar. 1993. *Marihuana, the Forbidden Medicine*. New Haven, Conn.: Yale University Press.

———. 1994. *Marihuana, die verbotene Medizin*. Frankfurt am Main: Zweitausendeins.

Grotenhermen, Franjo. 1996. Schokolade, Haschisch und Anandamide. *Hanf!* Nr. 12/96:14–5.

———. 1997. Cannabis bei Schmerzen. *Hanf!* 10/97:16–8.

Grotenhermen, Franjo, and Renate Huppertz. 1997. *Hanf als Medizin: Wiederentdeckung einer Heilpflanze*. Heidelberg: Haug Verlag.

Grotenhermen, Franjo, and Michael Karus. 1995. *Cannabis als Heilmittel: Eine Patientenbroschüre*. Cologne: nova-Institut. Second slightly revised edition published Dec. 1995.

———. 1998. *Cannabis als Heilmittel: Ein medizinischer Ratgeber*. Edited by Nova-Institut. Göttingen: Verlag Die Werkstatt.

Grüne Hilfe, ed. [1996]. *Die Grüne Hilfe Fibel*. Löhrbach, Germany: Werner Pieper's MedienXperimente (Edition Rauschkunde).

Grupp, Stanley E., ed. 1971. *Marihuana*. Columbus, Ohio: Merrill Merrill Sociology Series.

Haag, Stefan. 1991. *Markt und Marketing des illegalen Drogenhandels*. Pforzheim: Diplomarbeit.

———. [1995]. *Hanfkultur weltweit: Über die Hanfsituation in fast 100 Ländern rund um den Äquator*. Revised ed. Löhrbach/Solothurn: Edition Rauschkunde.

Hager, Steven, ed. 1994. *High Times—Greatest Hits: Twenty Years of Smoke in Your Face*. New York: St. Martin's Press.

Hai, Hainer. 1981. *Das definitive Deutsche Hanf Handbuch*. Löhrbach: Die Grüne Kraft (Der Grüne Zweig 73).

Haining, Peter, ed. 1975. *The Hashish Club: An Anthology of Drug Literature*. 2 vols. London: Peter Owen.

Halikas, James, Ronald Weller, and Carolyn Morse. 1982. Effects of Regular Marijuana Use on Sexual Performance. *Journal of Psychoactive Drugs* 14(1–2):59–70.

Haller, Andi. 1996a. *Die kleine Hanffibel*. Markt Erlbach: Raymond Martin Verlag.

———. 1996b. *Hausgemachtes Haschisch und andere Methoden zur Cannabis-Verarbeitung*. Markt Erlbach: Raymond Martin Verlag.

Harner, Michael. 1994. *Der Weg des Schamanen*. Genf: Ariston.

Hartwich, Carl. 1911. *Die menschlichen Genußmittel*. Leipzig: Tauchnitz.

———. [1911] 1997. *Haschisch Anno 1911*. Reprint, Löhrbach: Werner Pieper's MedienXperimente (Edition Rauschkunde). Reprint of a chapter from *Die menschlichen Genußmittel*.

Hellmann, Arthur D. 1975. *Laws Against Marijuana: The Price We Pay*. Urbana: University Of Illinois Press.

Herer, Jack. 1990. *The Emperor Wears No Clothes: The Authoritative Historical Record of the Cannabis Plant, Hemp Prohibition, and How Marijuana Can Still Save the World*. Van Nuys, Calif.: HEMP Publishing.

Herer, Jack, and Mathias Bröckers. 1993. *Die Wiederentdeckung der Nutzpflanze Hanf Cannabis Marihuana*. Frankfurt am Main: Zweitausendeins.

———. 1996. *Die Wiederentdeckung der Nutzpflanze Hanf Cannabis Marihuana*, abridged and revised. Munich: Heyne.

Hesch, R., A. Meyer, F. Beckmann, and K. Hesch 1996. *Hanf: Perspektiven für eine ökologische Zukunft: Eine realistiche Betrachtung*. Lemgo: Taoasis Verlag.

Hess, Peter. 1973. *Experimentelle Untersuchungen akuter Haschischeinwirkung auf den Menschen*. Mannheim: Diss. MS. 1996.

———. 1996. Medizinische und psychiatrische Aspekte von Cannabis. *Jahrbuch des Europäischen Collegiums für Bewußtseinstudien* 1995:157–77.

Hofmann, Albert. 1996. Rudolf Gelpke und der Hanfrausch. *Jahrbuch des Europäischen Collegiums für Bewußtseinstudien* 1995:103–12.

Hollister, Leo E. 1986. Health Aspects of Cannabis. *Pharmacological Review* 38(1):1–20.

Holstrom, John. 1991. Marijuana and Sex. *High Times* No. 187 (March 1991):34, 52.

Homann, Ulf. 1972. *Das Haschischverbot: Gesellschaftliche Funktion und Wirkung*. Frankfurt am Main: Fischer.

Hoye, David. 1974. *Hasheesh: The Herb Dangerous*. San Francisco: Level Press.

Illmaier, Thomas. 1996. Cannabis und Kultur: Wissenschaft und Politik trafen sich in Hamburg. *Jahrbuch für Ethnomedizin und Bewußtseinsforschung* 4(1995):245–7.

Iversen, Leslie L. 1993. Medical Uses Of Marijuana? *Nature* 365:12–3.

Jansen, A. C. M. 1991. *Cannabis in Amsterdam: A Geography of Hashish and Marihuana*. Muiderberg: Dick Coutinho.

Jünger, Ernst 1980. *Annäherungen—Drogen und Rausch*. Frankfurt am Main: Ullstein.

Julien, Robert M. 1997. *Drogen und Psychopharmaka*. Heidelberg: Spektrum Akademischer Verlag.

Kabelic, J. et al. 1960. Cannabis as a Medicament. *Bulletin on Narcotics*. 12(3):5–23.

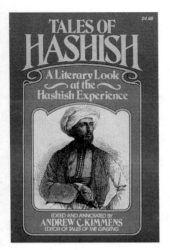

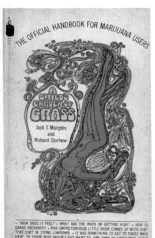

Kaplan, John. 1971. *Marijuana: The New Prohibition*. New York: Pocket Books.

Katalyse Institut für angewandte Umweltforschung. 1998. *Leitfaden Nachwachsende Rohstoffe*. Heidelberg: C. F. Müller Verlag.

Kessler, Thomas, ed. 1984. *Hanf in der Schweiz*. Grenchen: Nachtschatten Verlag.

———. 1985. *Cannabis helvetica*. Zurich: Nachtschatten Verlag.

Kettenes-van den Bosch, J. J., and C. A. Salemink. 1980. Biological Activity of the Tetrahydrocannabinols. *Journal of Ethnopharmacology* 2:197–231 (contains a very good bibliography).

Kimmens, Andrew C., ed. 1977. *Tales of Hashish: A Literary Look at the Hashish Experience*. New York: William Morrow.

Kotschenreuther, Helmut. 1978. *Das Reich der Drogen und Gifte*. Frankfurt am Maina: Ullstein.

Krüger, Thomas. 1998. Krampf ums Hanf. *Rolling Stone* No. 5, May 1998:38–43.

La Valle, Suomi. 1984. *Hashish*. London: Quartet Book.

Laatsch, Hartmut. 1989. Haschisch, Marihuana, THC. In *3. Symposium über psychoaktive Substanzen und veränderte Bewußtseinszustände in Forschung und Therapie*, edited by M. Schlichting and H. Leuner. Göttingen: ECBS, pages 41–3.

Lanz, Herbert. 1994. Hanf-Dampf in allen Gassen. *CoopZeitung*, No.17/28(April 1994):9–17.

Leipe, Peter. 1997. *Gegenwelt Rauschgift: Kulturen und ihre Drogen*. Cologne: VGS.

Lemberger, L. 1980. Potential Therapeutic Usefulness of Marijuana. *Annual Review of Pharmacology and Toxicology* 20:151–72.

Lenson, David. 1995. *On Drugs*. Minneapolis: University of Minnesota Press.

Leonhardt, Rudolf Walter. 1970. *Haschisch-Report: Dokumente und Fakten zur Beurteilung eines sogenannten Rauschgiftes*. Munich: Piper.

Leu, Daniel. 1984. *Drogen—Sucht oder Genuss*. 3d revised ed. Basel: Lenos.

Leuenberger, Hans. 1970. *Im Rausch der Drogen*. Munich: Humboldt.

Leuner, Hanscarl. 1981. *Halluzinogene*. Bern: Huber.

Lewin, Louis. 1980. *Phantastica*. Linden: Volksverlag.

Lewington , Anna. 1990. *Plants for the People*. London: Natural History Museum Publications.

Lewis, Barbara 1970. *The Sexual Power of Marijuana*. New York: Wyden.

Liggenstorfer, Roger. ed. 1991. *Neue Wege in der Drogenpolitik: Geschichte des Hanfs und der Drogenprohibition*. Solothurn: Nachtschatten Verlag.

———. 1996. Hanf in der Schweiz. *Jahrbuch des Europäischen Collegiums für Bewußtseinsstudien* 1995:147–56.

Liggenstorfer, Roger, and Christian Rätsch, eds. 1998. *Die berauschte Schweiz*. Solothurn: Nachtschatten Verlag.

Ludlow, Fitz Hugh. 1981. *Der Haschisch Esser*. Basel: Sphinx.

Lussi, Kurt. 1996. Verbotene Lust: Nächtliche Tänze und blühende Hanffelder im Luzerner Hexenwesen. *Jahrbuch für Ethnomedizin und Bewußtseinsforschung* 4(1995):115–42.

McKenna, Terence. 1990. *Plan—Plant—Planet*. Löhrbach: Der Grüne Zweig 135.

———. 1996. *Die Speisen der Götter: Die Suche nach dem Baum der Erkenntnis*. Löhrbach: Werner Pieper's MedienXperimente (Edition Rauschkunde).

Mann, Peggy. 1987. *Pot Safari: A Visit to the Top Marijuana Researchers in the U.S.* New York: Woodmere Press.

Margolis, Jack S., and Richard Clorfene. 1979. *Der Grassgarten*. Linden: Volksverlag.

Martius, Georg. [1855] 1996. *Pharmakologisch-medicinische Studien über den Hanf*. Reprint, Berlin: VWB.

Mattison, J. B. 1891. Cannabis Indica as an Anodyne and Hypnotic. *The St. Louis Medical and Surgical Journal*, 56(Nov.):265–71.

Mechoulam, Raphael. 1970. Marijuana Chemistry. *Science* 168(3936):1159–66.

———, ed. 1973. *Marijuana: Chemistry, Pharmacology, Metabolism and Clinical Effects*. New York: Academic Press.

———. 1986. *Cannabinoids as Therapeutic Agents*. Boca Raton, Florida: CRC Press.

Meister, George. [1677] n.d. *Der Orientalisch-Indianische Kunst- und Lust-Gärtner*. Reprint, Weimar: Kiepenheuer.

Merlin, Mark D. 1972. *Man and Marijuana: Some Aspects of Their Ancient Relationship*. Rutherford, N.J.: Fairleigh Dickinson University Press.

Mestel, Rosie 1993. Cannabis: the Brain's Other Supplier. *New Scientist* 7/93: 21–3.

Metzner, Wolfgang, and Berndt Georg Thamm. 1989. *Drogen*. Hamburg: Gruner und Jahr (Stern-Buch).

Meyrink, Gustav. 1984. Haschisch und Hellsehen. In *Das Haus zur letzten Latern*, 2:28–35. Moewig.

Mezzrow, Mezz. 1995. *Die Tüte und die Tröte—Kiffen & Jazz: Really the Blues*. Löhrbach: Werner Pieper's MedienXperimente (Edition Rauschkunde).

Michka and Hugo Verlomme. 1993. *Le Cannabis est-il une drogue?* Geneva: Georg Éditeur.

Mikuriya, Tod H., ed. 1973. *Marijuana: Medical Papers 1839-1972*. Oakland, Calif.: Medi-Comp Press. This book contains all of the important medical and pharmaceutical articles, from the pioneers to modern works.

———. 1982. Die Bedeutung des Cannabis in der Geschichte der Medizin. In *Haschisch: Prohibition oder Legalisierung*, edited by W. Burian and I. Eisenbach-Stangl. Weinheim, Germany: Beltz, pages, 87–102.

Moebius. 1983. *Reisen der Erinnerung*. Cologne: Taschen.

Moreau de Tours, Joseph J. 1973. *Hashish and Mental Illness*. New York: Raven Press.

———. [1845] 1974. *Du Hachisch et de l'Aliénation mentale*. Reprint, Yverdon, Switzerland: Kesselring, Editeur.

Morningstar, Patricia J. 1985. *Thandai* and *Chilam:* Traditional Hindu Beliefs About the Proper Uses of *Cannabis*. *Journal of Psychoactive Drugs* 17(3):141–65.

Mountain Girl. 1995. *Sinsemilla: Königin des Cannabis*. Markt Erlbach: Raymond Martin Verlag.

Müller-Ebeling, Claudia. 1992a. Visionäre und psychedelische Malerei. In *Das Tor zu inneren Räumen*, edited by C. Rätsch. Südergellersen: Verlag Bruno Martin, pages 183–96.

———. 1992b. Dic frühe französische Haschisch- und Opiumforschung und ihr Einfluß auf die Kunst des 19. Jahrhunderts. *Jahrbuch des ECBS* 1992:9–19, Berlin: VWB.

———. 1994. Kunst im Rausch. *Esotera* 4/94:90–5.

Müller-Ebeling, Claudia, and Christian Rätsch. 1986. *Isoldens Liebestrank: Aphrodisiaka in Geschichte und Gegenwart*. Munich: Kindler.

———. 1987. Kreisrituale. *Sphinx* 6/86:42–7.

Müller-Ebeling, Claudia, Christian Rätsch, and Wolf-Dieter Storl. 1998. *Hexenmedizin: Die Wiederentdeckung einer verbotenen Heilkunst—schamanische Traditionen in Europa*. Aarau, Switzerland: AT Verlag.

Mur. 1997. *Earthfreaks: Tales from the Pure Hashish Years of the Hippie Trip in the Orient from 1967 to 1973*. Berkeley, Calif.: Regent Press.

Nahas, Gabriel G., ed. 1976. *Marihuana: Chemistry, Biochemistry and Cellular Effects*. New York: Springer.

———. 1979. *Keep Off the Grass: A Scientific Enquiry Into the Biological Effects of Marijuana*. Revised ed. Oxford: Pergamon. Foreword by Jacques Cousteau, a bitter opponent of hemp use.

———. 1982a. *Marijuana and Health*. Washington, D.C.: National Academy Press.

———. 1982b. Hashish in Islam 9th to 18th Century. *Bulletin of the New York Academy of Medicine* 58(9):814–31.

National Academy of Sciences Institute of Medicine. 1982. *Marijuana and Health*. Washington, D.C.: National Academy Press.

Neumann, Nicolaus, ed. 1970. *Hasch und andere Trips*. Hamburg: Konkret Verlag.

Neumeyer, Jürgen, ed. 1996. *Cannabis*. Munich: Packeispresse Verlag Hans Schickert.

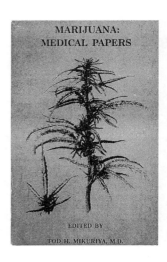

Novak, William. 1980. *High Culture: Marijuana in the Lives of Americans*. New York: Alfred A. Knopf.

O'Shaughnessy, W. B. 1839. On the Preparation of the Indian Hemp or Gunja. In *Marijuana: Medical Papers 1839-1972*, edited by T. Mikuriya. Oakland, Calif: Medi-Comp Press, pages 3–30.

Ohsawa, George, Herman Aihara, and Fred Pulver. 1985. *Rauchen, Marihuana und Drogen*. Holthausen, Münster: Verlag Mahajiva.

Ott, Jonathan. 1985. *Chocolate Addict*. Vashon, Wash.: Natural Products Co.

———. 1993. *Pharmacotheon*. Kennewick, Wash.: Natural Products Co.

———. 1995. *The Age of Entheogens and The Angels' Dictionary*. Kennewick, Wash.: Natural Products Co.

———. 1997. *Pharmacophilia or The Natural Paradises*. Kennewick, Wash.: Natural Products Co.

Ovadia, H., A. Wohlman, R. Mechoulam, and J. Weidenfeld. 1995. Characterization of the Hypothermic Effect of the Synthetic Cannabinoid HU-210 in the Rat. Relation to the Adrenergic System and Endogenous Pyrogens. *Neuropharmacology* 34(2):175–80.

Pelt, Jean-Marie. 1983a. *Pflanzenmedizin*, Düsseldorf: Econ.

———. 1983b. *Drogues et plantes magiques*. Paris: Fayard.

Petersen, R. C., ed. 1976. *Marijuana Research Findings: 1976*. Rockville, Maryland: NIDA Research Monograph 14.

Pieper, Werner, ed. 1997. *Die Grüne Hilfe Fibel*. 2nd ed. Löhrbach: Werner Pieper's Medienexperimente (Edition Rauschkunde).

Pliess, Rainer. 1993. Hanf als neues Heilmittel. *Integration* 4:67–9.

Pollak, Kurt. 1978. *Die Heilkunst der frühen Hochkulturen*. Wiesbaden; Löwit.

Rätsch, Christian. 1990a. *Pflanzen der Liebe*. Bern: Hallwag (after 1995 Aarau: AT Verlag).

———. 1990b. *"Die Orientalischen Fröhlichkeitspillen" und verwandte psychoaktive Aphrodisiaka*. Berlin: VWB.

———. 1991a. Ethnomedizinische Aspekte von Cannabis. In *Neue Wege in der Drogenpolitik*, edited by R. Liggenstorfer. Solothurn: Nachtschatten Verlag, pages 144–51.

———. 1991b. *Von den Wurzeln der Kultur: Die Pflanzen der Propheten*. Basel: Sphinx.

———. 1991c. De Hola Herb—Vom Hanf in der Bibel. In *Das Böse Bibel Buch*, edited by R. Ranke-Rippchen. Löhrbach: *Der Grüne Zweig* 145, pages 101–4.

———. 1991d. *Indianische Heilkräuter*. 2d revised ed. Munich: Diederichs.

———. 1992. *Hanf als Heilmittel: Eine ethnomedizinische Bestandsaufnahme*. Löhrbach: Werner Pieper's MedienXperimente and Solothurn: Nachtschatten Verlag (Joint Venture) (4th edition, 1995).

———. 1994. Der Nektar der Heilung. *Dao* 4/94:44–6.

———. 1995a. Get High Beyond Style! Hanf, Musik und Kultur. In *Hanfkultur weltweit: Über die Hanfsituation in fast 100 Ländern rund um den Äquator*, by Stefan Haag. Revised ed. Löhrbach/Solothurn: Edition Rauschkunde, pages 179–89.

———. 1995b. BIOROHSTOFF HANF 1995: Internationales Technisch-wissenschaftliches Symposium und Produkt- und Technologieschau 2.-5. März—Frankfurt a.M./Messe. *curare* 18(1):231–3.

———. 1996a. Die Hanfkultur—Eine kulturanthropologische Betrachtung. *Jahrbuch des Europäischen Collegiums für Bewußtseinsstudien* 1995:113–46.

———. 1996b. Die Pflanze der Götter. *Esotera* 6/96:52–7.

———. 1996c. Hanf als Heilmittel: Ethnomedizinische Befunde. In *Cannabis*, edited by Jürgen Neumeyer. Munich: Packeispresse Verlag Hans Schickert, pages 72–87.

———. 1996d. *Urbock: Bier Jenseits von Hopfen und Malz*. Aarau: AT Verlag.

———. 1996e. *Raucherstoffe—Der Atem des Drachen*. Aarau: AT Verlag.

———. 1997. *Steine der Schamanen: Kristalle, Fossilien und die Landschaften des Bewußtseins*. Munich: Diederichs Verlag (Gelbe Reihe Magnum).

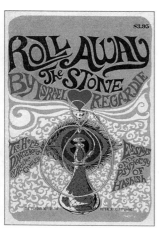

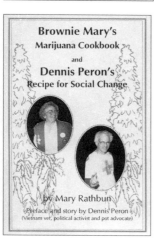

—————. 1998. *Enzyklopädie der psychoaktiven Pflanzen*. Aarau: AT Verlag.

Rathbun, Mary, and Dennis Peron. 1993. *Brownie Mary's Marijuana Cookbook and Dennis Peron's Recipe for Social Change*. San Francisco: Trail of Smoke Publishing Co.

Regardie, Israel. 1968. *Roll Away The Stone*. Saint Paul, Minn.: Llewellyn. Contains the entire text of *The Herb Dangerous* by Aleister Crowley; cf. Hoye 1974.

Reininger, W. 1941. Haschisch. *Ciba Zeitschrift* 7(80):2765–95.

—————. 1968. Remnants from Prehistoric Times. In *The Book of Grass*, edited by G. Andrews and S. Vinkenoog. New York: Grove Press, pages 14–5.

Reuband, Karl-Heinz, et al. 1976. *Rauschmittelkonsum*. Wiesbaden: Akademische Verlagsgesellschaft.

Rippchen, Ronald, ed. 1992. *Das Recht auf Rausch: Materialien zur Haschischdiskussion*. Löhrbach: Werner Pieper's Medienexperimente (Der Grüne Zweig 147). Contains the text of the Lübeck court decision.

—————. 1994. *Das Haschisch-Urteil*. Löhrbach: Werner Pieper's Medienexperimente (Edition Rauschkunde).

—————. 1996. *Mein Urin gehört mir*. Löhrbach: Edition Rauschkunde.

Robinson, Rowan. 1996. *Hanf: Droge, Heilmittel, Mode, Faser*. Cologne: VGS.

Robinson, Victor. 1930. *An Essay on Hasheesh*. New York: Dingwall-Rock.

Römpp, Hermann. 1950. *Chemische Zaubertränke*. 5th revised ed. Stuttgart: Kosmos Franckh'sche Verlagsbuchhandlung.

Roffman, Roger A. 1982. *Marijuana as Medicine*. Seattle: Madrona.

Rosenthal, Ed. 1984. *Marijuana Beer*. Berkeley, Calif.: And/Or Press.

—————. 1990. *Marijuana Questions? Ask Ed: The Encyclopedia of Marijuana*. San Francisco: Quick American Publishing Company.

—————. 1991. *Closet Cultivator*. San Francisco: Last Gasp.

—————, ed. 1994. *Hemp Today*. Oakland, Calif.: Quick American Archives.

—————. 1996. *Marijuana Beer* (revised edition), Oakland: Quick American Archives.

Rosevear, John. 1967. *Pot: A Handbook of Marihuana*. New York: Lancer Books.

Roth, Lutz, Max Daunderer, and Kurt Kormann. 1994. *Giftpflanzen—Pflanzengifte*. 4th ed. Munich: ecomed.

Rubin, Vera, ed. 1975. *Cannabis and Culture*. The Hague: Mouton.

Sagunski, Horst, Eva-Susanne Lichtner, and Corinna Hembd. 1996. *Hanf: Das Praxisbuch*. Munich: Ludwig Verlag.

Samorini, Giorgio. 1998. *Halluzinogene im Mythos*. Solothurn: Nachtschatten Verlag.

Santler, Helmut. 1995. Hanf Als Medizin. *HanfBlatt* No. 9, July 1995:8–13.

Scherer, Sebastian, and Irmgard Vogt, eds. 1989. *Drogen und Drogenpolitik*. Frankfurt am Main: Campus.

Scheuch, Erwin K. 1970. *Haschisch und LSD als Modedrogen*. Osnabrück, Germany: Verlag A. Fromm.

Schmidt, Stephan. 1992. Cannabis. In *Hagers Handbuch der pharmazeutischen Praxis*. 5th ed. Vol. 4. Berlin: Springer, pages, 640–55.

Schneider, Wolfgang. 1984. *Biographie und Lebenswelt von Langzeitcannabiskonsumenten: Eine ereignisbezogene Deutungssaktanalyse im Vergleich*. Berlin: EXpress.

—————. 1995. (together with Wolfgang Haves) *Risiko Cannabis? Bedingungen und Auswirkungen eines kontrollierten, sozial-integrierten Gebrauchs von Haschisch und Marihuana*. Berlin: VWB.

Schmidbauer, Wolfgang, and Jürgen vom Scheidt. 1997. *Handbuch der Rauschdrogen*. 8th expanded and revised ed. Munich: Nymphenburger.

Schultes, Richard Evans. 1973. Man and Marijuana. *Natural History* 82(7):58–64.

—————. 1976. *Hallucinogenic Plants*. Racine, Wisc.: Western Publishing.

Schultes, Richard E., and Albert Hofmann. 1980. *The Botany and Chemistry of Hallucinogens*. Revised and enlarged ed. Springfield, Ill.: Charles C. Thomas.

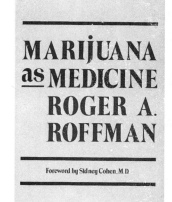

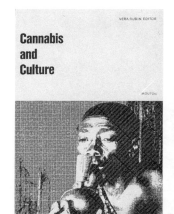

———. 1992. *Plants of the Gods: Their Sacred, Healing and Hallucinogenic Powers*. Rochester, Vt.: Healing Arts Press.

———. 1995. *Pflanzen der Götter*. Aarau, Switzerland: AT Verlag.

———. 1998. *Pflanzen der Götter. Die magischen Kräfte der bewußtseinserweiternden Gewächse.* Revised by Christian Rätsch. Aarau: AT Verlag.

Schultes, Richard E., William M. Klein, Timothy Plowman, and Tom E. Lockwood. 1975. Cannabis: An Example of Taxonomic Neglect. In *Cannabis and Culture*, edited by V. Rubin. The Hague: Mouton, pages 21–38.

Segelman, Alvin, R. Duane Sofia, and Florence H. Segelman. 1975. Cannabis sativa L. (Marihuana): VI. Variations in Marihuana Preparations and Usage—Chemical and Pharmacological Consequences. In *Cannabis and Culture*, edited by V. Rubin. The Hague: Mouton, pages 269–91.

Seyfried, Gerhard, and Matthias Bröckers. 1996. *Hanf im Glück: Das Hohe Lied vom hehren Hanf.* Frankfurt am Main: Zweitausendeins.

Sharma, G. K. 1977a. Cannabis Folklore in the Himalayas. *Botanical Museum Leaflets*, Harvard University. vol. 25(7):203–15.

———. 1977b. Ethnobotany and Its Significance for Cannabis Studies in the Himalayas. *Journal of Psychedelic Drugs* 9(4):337–9.

Shik, J. Fred E., David E. Smith, and Frederick H. Meyers. 1968. Use of Marijuana in the Haight-Ashbury Subculture. *Journal of Psychedelic Drugs* 1(2):49–66.

Siegel, Ronald K. 1989. *Intoxication: Life in Pursuit of Artificial Paradise.* New York: E. P. Dutton.

———. 1995. *Rauschdrogen: Sehnsucht nach dem Künstlichen Paradies*, Frankfurt am Main: Eichborn.

Silver, Gary, ed., and Michael Aldrich (text) 1979. *The Dope Chronicles 1850-1950.* New York: Harper and Row.

Simmons, J. L. 1967. *Marihuana: Myths and Realities.* North Hollywood, Calif.: Brandon House.

Smith, David E. 1968. Acute and Chronic Toxicity of Marijuana. *Journal of Psychedelic Drugs* 2(1):37–47.

———, ed. 1970. *The New Social Drug: Cultural, Medical, and Legal Perspectives on Marijuana.* Englewood Cliffs, N.J.: Prentice-Hall.

Solomon, David, ed. 1966. *The Marihuana Papers.* Indianapolis: Bobbs-Merrill.

Spinger, Alfred. 1980. Zur Kulturgeschichte des Cannabis in Europa. *Kriminalsoziologische Bibliographie* 26–7.

———. 1982. Zur Kultur und Zeitgeschichte des Cannabis. In *Haschisch: Prohibition oder Legalisierung*, edited by W. Burian and I. Eisenbach-Stangl. Weinheim, Basel: Beltz, pages 34–43.

Stafford, Peter. 1980. *Cannabis: Haschisch und Marijuana.* Markt Erlbach: Raymond Martin Verlag.

———. 1983. *Psychedelics Encyclopedia.* Revised ed. Los Angeles: Tarcher.

Starks, Michael. 1981. *Marihuana Potenz.* Linden: Volksverlag.

Stone Mountain. 1970. *Pot Art: Marijuana Reading Matter.* Tucson, AZ: Apocryph Press.

Tart, Charles. 1971. *On Being Stoned: A Psychological Study of Marijuana Intoxication.* Palo Alto, Calif.: Science and Behavior Books.

Täschner, Karl-Ludwig. 1979. *Das Cannabis-Problem: Die Kontroverse um Haschisch und Marihuana aus medizinisch-soziologischer Sicht.* Wiesbaden: Akademische Verlagsanstalt.

———. 1981a. Das Haschischproblem aus klinischer Sicht. *Deutsches Ärzteblatt* 4 (Jan. 22, 1981):126–9.

———. 1981b. *Haschisch: Traum und Wirklichkeit.* Wiesbaden: Akademische Verlagsanstalt. An abridged version of Täschner, 1979.

Tossmann, H. P. 1987. *Haschischabhängigkeit? Lebensgeschichten von Drogenkonsumenten*. Frankfurt am Main: Fischer TB.

Touw, Mia. 1981. The Religious and Medicinal Uses of Cannabis in China, India and Tibet. *Journal of Psychoactive Drugs* 13(1):23–34.

Trebach, Arnold S., and James K. Inciardi. 1993. *Legalize It? Debating American Drug Policy*. Washington, D.C.: The American University Press.

Turner, D. M. 1997. *Der psychedelische Reiseführer*. Solothurn: Nachtschatten Verlag. Translated by Claudia Müller-Ebeling.

Wagner, Hildebert. 1970. *Rauschgift-Drogen*. 2d ed. Berlin: Springer (Verständliche Wissenschaft, Vol. 99).

———. 1985. *Pharmazeutische Biologie: Drogen und ihre Inhaltsstoffe*. 3d ed. Stuttgart: G. Fischer.

Waskow, Frank. 1995. *Hanf und Co.— Die Renaissance der heimischen Faserpflanzen*. Göttingen: Verlag Die Werkstatt/AOL-Verlag. Edited by the Katalyse-Institut.

Weil, Andrew. 1972. *The Natural Mind*. Boston: Houghton Mifflin.

———. 1976. *The Natural Mind*. Boston; Houghton Mifflin. (German: *Das erweiterte Bewußtsein*, Stuttgart: dva.)

———. 1980. *The Marriage of the Sun and Moon*. Boston: Houghton Mifflin.

———. 1986. *The Natural Mind*. Revised ed. Boston: Houghton Mifflin.

———. 1988. *Health and Healing*. Boston: Houghton Mifflin.

———. 1991. *Was uns gesund macht*. Weinheim, Germany: Beltz (Psychologie Heute Taschenbuch).

Weil, Andrew, and Winifred Rosen. 1993. *Chocolate to Morphine: Understanding Mind-Active Drugs*. Revised and updated. Boston: Houghton Mifflin.

Weil, A. T., N. E. Zinberg, and J. M. Nelson. 1968. Clinical and Psychological Effects of Marijuana in Man. *Science* 162:1234.

Wheelwright, Edith Grey. 1974. *Medicinal Plants and Their History*. New York: Dover.

Woggon, B. 1974. *Haschisch—Konsum und Wirkung*. Berlin: Springer.

Wolke, William, ed. 1995. *Cannabis Handbuch*. Revised ed. Markt Erlbach: Raymond Martin Verlag.

Wolstenholme, Gordon, and Julie Knight, eds. 1965. *Hashish: Its Chemistry and Pharmacology*. London: Churchill (CIBA Foundation Study Group No. 21).

Zinberg, Norman E. 1984. *Drug, Set, and Setting*. New Haven: Yale University Press.

Zinberg, N. E. and A. T. Weil. 1976. A Comparison of Marijuana Users and Non-Users. *Nature* 266:119–23.

HEMP PERIODICALS

The magazine *High Times* has appeared in the United States since 1974. Its primary subject area is hemp, but it also covers other aspects of psychedelic culture. *HanfBlatt* is a monthly magazine published in northern Germany since 1994. The scientific *Journal of the International Hemp Association* has been published in Amsterdam since 1994 (two issues per year). The magazine *Hanf! Das zeitkritische Journal*, which was first published in April/May 1995, appears every two months. The magazine *Grow! Marihuana Magazin* is a quarterly that has appeared since the summer of 1995. The first issue of *CannaNet—Das Magazin der Hanfkultur* (Switzerland) was published in the fall of 1995. The magazine *Hemplife Magazine*, which first appeared in December 1995, is published every two months in German. Produced in Holland, it has recently been marketed under the name *Highlife*. Other

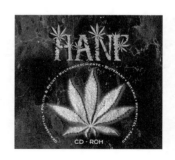

magazines have appeared on the market and quickly disappeared: *Hemp Nation Magazine, Hanf-Bulletin, BTM-Kurier, Hanfblatt* (Switzerland), *A-Bulletin, Hanfforum, Österreichisches Hanfmagazin.*

MULTIMEDIA

CD-ROM *Marihuana für DOS—Was Sie schon immer über Hanf fragen wollten, aber nie zu wissen wagten!* (Marihuana for DOS—Everything You Ever Wanted to Ask About Hemp, But Never Dared to Know!), Mannheim: TopWare PD-Service GmbH (TopWare 539), 1994.

Hanfnet presents: *Hanf CD-ROM,* Gelsenkirchen: Media Factory 1996 (ISBN/Switzerland 3-907080-20-3; ISBN/Germany 3-9805466-0-8).

INTERNET ADDRESSES

Cannabis Culture (online magazine): www.hempBC.com
Council on Spiritual Practices: www.csp.org
European College for the Study of Consciousness: www.magnet.ch/ecbs
Heffter Research Institute: www.heffter.org
High Times Magazine: www.hightimes.com
Island Web: www.island.org
Lycaeum—Entheogenic Database: www.lycaeum.org
MAPS: www.maps.org
Medical Marihuana site: www.rxmarihuana.com
Multidisciplinary Association for Psychedelic Studies: www.maps.org
Netherlands Coffee Shops: www.coffeeshop-nl.com
Netherlands Smart Shops: www.consciousdreams.nl
NORML: www.norml.org
Rave Culture: www.hyperreal.com
Society for Ethnomedicine (Germany): www.med.uni-muenchen.de/medpsy/ethno
The Vaults of Erowid: www.erowid.com
Working Groups Cannabis as Medicine (Germany): www.hanfnet.de/acm

INDEX